Functional Surgery of
Cerebellopontine Angle
by Minimally Invasive Retrosigmoid Approach

Functional Surgery of
Cerebellopontine Angle
by Minimally Invasive Retrosigmoid Approach

Jacques Magnan MD
Professor Emeritus
University Aix-Marseille (F)
Head of ORL & Head and Neck Surgery
Hopital Nord, Marseilles (1989-2011)
Past President–EAONO
Past President–Politzer Society, President–MSOA
Chairman 2nd EAORL-HNS, Nice 2013
Causse/Champeau Clinics, Beziers, France

Bhavin Parikh MS (ENT) Fellowship in Otology
Bharti ENT Care Center
Vadodara, Gujarat, India

Hidemi Miyazaki MD (ORL)
Department of Otorhinolaryngology
Jikei University School of Medicine
Tokyo Kyosai Hospital
Tokyo, Japan

Foreword
Prof. Georges Albert Bremond

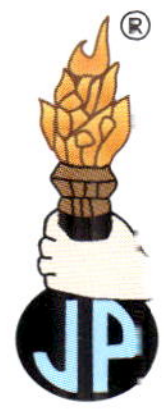

JAYPEE BROTHERS MEDICAL PUBLISHERS (P) LTD

New Delhi • London • Philadelphia • Panama

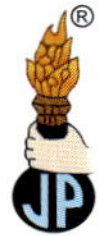

Jaypee Brothers Medical Publishers (P) Ltd

Headquarters

Jaypee Brothers Medical Publishers (P) Ltd
4838/24, Ansari Road, Daryaganj
New Delhi 110 002, India
Phone: +91-11-43574357
Fax: +91-11-43574314
Email: jaypee@jaypeebrothers.com

Overseas Offices

J.P. Medical Ltd
83, Victoria Street, London
SW1H 0HW (UK)
Phone: +44-2031708910
Fax: +02-03-0086180
Email: info@jpmedpub.com

Jaypee-Highlights Medical Publishers Inc.
City of Knowledge, Bld. 237, Clayton
Panama City, Panama
Phone: +507-301-0496
Fax: +507-301-0499
Email: cservice@jphmedical.com

Jaypee Medical Inc.
The Bourse
111 South Independence Mall East
Suite 835, Philadelphia, PA 19106, USA
Phone: + 267-519-9789
Email: joe.rusko@jaypeebrothers.com

Jaypee Brothers
Medical Publishers (P) Ltd
17/1-B Babar Road, Block-B
Shaymali, Mohammadpur
Dhaka-1207, Bangladesh
Mobile: +08801912003485
Email: jaypeedhaka@gmail.com

Jaypee Brothers
Medical Publishers (P) Ltd
Shorakhute, Kathmandu
Nepal
Phone: +00977-9841528578
Email: jaypee.nepal@gmail.com

Website: www.jaypeebrothers.com
Website: www.jaypeedigital.com

Inquiries for bulk sales may be solicited at: jaypee@jaypeebrothers.com

Functional Surgery of Cerebellopontine Angle by Minimally Invasive Retrosigmoid Approach

First Edition: **2013**

ISBN 978-93-5090-525-8

Printed at: Ajanta Offset & Packagings Ltd., New Delhi

Dedicated to

Our late ENT colleagues: Jean-Pierre Pradoura and Richard De Gasquet.
The nurses and personnel of ORL operation theater at Hopital Nord, Marseilles for their selfless support in all our endeavors.

Foreword

De longue date les complications de l'otite chronique nous avait fait franchir la dure-mère, mais cela était la main forcée car à cette époque, nous sommes dans les années 60-70, la dure-mère était considérée comme une frontière que seuls les neurochirurgiens savaient et pouvaient franchir.

En fait, c'est par la pathologie du nerf facial avec ses paralysies que le froid n'expliquait pas plus que la décompression ne les guérissait, puis surtout par les vertiges invalidants qui bénéficiaient de la neurotomie vestibulaire, qu'il nous est apparu qu'en prenant les précautions nécessaires il n'y avait pour l'otologiste aucun interdit à franchir la dure-mère. Déçu par la voie sus-pétreuse, je pris alors la décision avec mon élève Jacques Magnan d'explorer la face postérieure du rocher. Or pour cela il fallait pénétrer dans l'espace ponto-cérébelleux baigné de LCR, encombré de tout un complexe de nerfs et de vaisseaux d'une extrême importance. Nous avons franchi la dure-mère retro-sigmoïde et ce fut une véritable révélation.

Par la suite des avancées techniques ont facilité nos actions aussi bien diagnostiques comme le scanner ou l'IRM qu'opératoire avec l'endoscopie et le monitoring. Maintenant, à l'heure actuelle, je mesure les progrès accomplis, l'angle ponto-cérébelleux n'est plus « le coin sombre » de notre spécialité tel que je l'avais appris et même enseigné.

Prof. Georges Albert Bremond

Foreword

(As translated from original Foreword in French)

In the past, complications of chronic otitis made us go beyond the dura mater. We were forced to do so, because in the 1960s–1970s, the dura mater was otherwise considered an implacable border that only neurosurgeons knew how to and were allowed to cross. Later in facial nerve pathology with accompanying paralysis of idiopathic cause and where mastoid segment decompression did not heal, and then in patients with incapacitating vertigo that required vestibular neurotomy made us realize that if we took the necessary precautions there was no reason why an otologist could not go beyond the dura mater. Disappointed by the middle fossa approach, I decided with my pupil Jacques Magnan to explore the posterior side of the petrous bone in early 1970s. To do this we had to penetrate into the cerebellopontine space immerged in cerebrospinal fluid, filled by complex nerves and blood vessels of the utmost importance. We crossed the retrosigmoid dura mater and what a revelation it was.

Subsequently technical progress has facilitated our work, be it for diagnosis with the CT scan and MRI, or for surgery, with endoscopy and monitoring. Today, I take full measure of the progress and accomplishments made. The cerebello-pontine angle is no longer "the dark corner" of our specialty as I had once learned and even taught.

Prof. Georges Albert Bremond

Preface

As an ENT resident, I had the privilege to witness the first retrosigmoid approach performed by Professor Michel Garcin in 1970 at Hopital Nord in Marseilles, France. It was Professor Georges Bremond through his stature and charisma that espoused and developed it. I can thus say that I began my career with the retrosigmoid approach and that I am terminating it by writing this book. The retrosigmoid approach is undoubtedly the most simple and direct access to the cerebellopontine angle. Curiously, this approach is also the least well known amongst otologists.

The purpose of this book is to discover, popularize and practice the retrosigmoid approach as it was originally conceived "by otologists for otologists", but of course it can be used by all surgical specialties involved with pathologies of the cerebellopontine angle. To understand why this approach has become indispensable for us, i.e. the otologists, we have to go back in time. During the 1970s, the operating microscope was widely used in all ENT centers, while its utility was just appearing in neurosurgery. The original concept of the "a minima" (French word for minimally invasive) retrosigmoid approach was to adapt the techniques of microsurgery of ear to surgery of the acousticofacial nerve bundle. Another purpose of developing the retrosigmoid approach was to reduce morbidity so as to distinguish it from the legendary seriousness of the suboccipital approach.

Though the retrosigmoid approach by its topography and its objective was the daughter of the suboccipital approach, it is contrary to it in many aspects. The patient's position, the type of operating microscope, the instruments, the size of the craniotomy and its guiding landmarks, the absence of mechanical retraction, the postoperative consequences and no age limit. To try to do a minimally invasive retrosigmoid approach with neurosurgical "armamentarium" is quite difficult. Obviously the intrusion of ENT specialists in this deep and delicate space, the surgical elite's reserve, was subject to criticism not only by neurosurgeons but also by ENT specialists themselves. Thus to criticize the "exiguous nature" of the retrosigmoid approach, and to differentiate it from the large opening of the classical suboccipital approach, it was given the nickname of "keyhole" approach. Though originally used as pejorative, the term Keyhole approach has gradually become an incredible promotion underlining the minimally invasive character of the surgery. In fact nowadays the distinction between retrosigmoid approach and suboccipital approach tends to merge into the common denomination of posterior retrosigmoid approach, confirming the value of this approach even if it is practiced in different ways.

The retrosigmoid approach benefitted from the formidable challenge initiated by William House and perfected by Ugo Fisch. We were all beginners, residents and heads of department alike. But we were lucky; we could go to the morgue and practice anatomical dissections to master the translabyrinthine approach, the middle fossa approach, the retrolabyrinthine approach progressively. The initial operations for cerebellopontine angle pathologies were long and laborious resulting in a narrow and deep operating field in which it was difficult to identify the elements of the acoustico-facial nerve bundle, even with the help and collaboration of a neurosurgeon. The only practical access as practiced on cadavers that seemed simple and with least danger for the cochlea and facial nerve was the retrosigmoid approach.

My revered teachers—Professors Bremond and Garcin, inaugurated the retrosigmoid approach on elderly and fragile patients suffering from trigeminal nerve neuralgia referred by neurosurgeons to otologists for treatment using less invasive approaches. After partial retrogasserian rhizotomy, indications for the retrosigmoid approach were extended to vestibular neurotomy, and then to small acoustic neuroma in the 'otological stage' (when the patients do not have any neurological complaints). We had to wait until the 1990s when intraoperative endoscopic procedure was added to our armamentarium to be convinced of the reality of neurovascular conflicts as the main cause of trigeminal neuralgia and hemifacial spasm. Thus, the minimally invasive retrosigmoid approach became the endoscope-assisted retrosigmoid approach.

During these 40 years, technical progress has been considerable and has been taken into consideration by all specialties involved in this surgery, above all anesthesiology. Deep anesthesia and assisted ventilation make the cerebellum retract spontaneously and eliminate the need for peroperative lumbar puncture or Mannitol hypertonic solutions. This spontaneous retraction of the cerebellum is an essential step of this cerebellopontine angle surgery to have access to and open the posterior fossa cistern. It is difficult to believe in the spontaneous retraction of the cerebellum during surgery particularly when looking at a preoperative MRI showing the cerebellum in contact with the petrous bone or when the cerebellum obstructs the access to the cerebellopontine angle during anatomical dissection.

The retrosigmoid approach has been more than just a technical adventure, it had been a fantastic human journey with its moments of nobleness and baseness. We will only remember the former when adversity has been changed into opportunity. During these years, I had been graceful to develop:

- Enduring friendship with Professor Carlo Zini's team in Parma and his brilliant student turned master Professor Mario Sanna and his "Gruppo Otologico".
- The European Academy of Otology and NeuroOtology (EAONO) with the support of 90 European experts and the authority of Professors Mirko Tos and Ugo Fisch.
- Broadcasting of teaching by video-conferencing with the help of the Live International Otolaryngology Network (LION) and the Tempus TransmedEast project.

The originality of the retrosigmoid approach attracted many visitors to my department at the Hopital Nord in Marseilles. Drs Bhavin Parikh and Hidemi Miyazaki made themselves particularly available and were very eager to see this book appear. They followed me to the Causse-Champeaux Clinics in Beziers when I retired from the Hopital Nord. Dr Bhavin has been the driving force in editing this work. Over and above his epistolary talent, he was responsible for collecting the data and the clinical cases included. Dr Hidemi has brought the most recent developments of the retrosigmoid approach with intraoperative monitoring of cranial nerves, especially cochlear nerve. Thank you so much to both of you and my best wishes for a brilliant career.

Finally, I would like to thank more than 2000 patients who were operated using this surgical procedure for their trust and their gratitude.

Jacques Magnan

Preface

Newer horizons have opened due to conjunction of the use of endoscope and microscope in the surgery of cerebellopontine angle (CPA) in the last two decades. Endoscope provides brilliant illumination and excellent preview of anatomy of CPA unforeseen before its advent. Endoscope-assisted retrosigmoid approach gives an opportunity to perform surgery for functional disorders (non life-threatening benign conditions that cause significant worsening of quality of life) of CPA in minimally-invasive manner with small external incision, accurate precision and significantly reduced morbidity and is increasingly practiced even in elderly population.

My maiden voyage in the field of lateral skull base surgery initiated when I first met Professor Jacques Magnan at a live surgery workshop in New Delhi in the December of 2008. He was operating a case of hemifacial spasm using endoscope-assisted retrosigmoid approach. This approach allowed clear and concise view of anatomy of the contents of cerebellopontine angle and was performed from a completely different perspective. With the intent of getting opportunity to work with Professor Magnan to enhance my knowledge and skills regarding skull base surgeries, I contacted him and after 8 months I was pleased to receive an invitation to work in his department of ENT at Hopital Nord, Marseilles, France. During my visit to Marseilles at his department and later at Beziers, I experienced his generosity as a host, his kind-heartedness and charisma as a leader. He will always inspire me with his didactic character and adorable surgical skills.

Professor Magnan sensed the necessity to convey this core knowledge of endoscope-assisted retrosigmoid approach to future generation of neuro-otologists and neurosurgeons. Professor Magnan being a pioneer in this novel approach and with such tremendous experience would be the ultimate source for imparting this invaluable information, that too in a “how I do it” format and in a “step-by-step” manner. The completion of this work was made possible because of my close academic association with Professor Magnan. I am indebted to him for being a wonderful teacher and mentor, and for generously sharing his profound knowledge and wisdom with me. His presence was a constant source of inspiration, and his untiring interest, healthy criticism and invaluable guidance provided the impetus to shape this work to the desired level of accuracy and completeness. My colleague and friend Hidemi, has been pioneer in developing and implementing a newer design of electrodes useful in continuous cochlear and facial nerve monitoring that I am sure is going to significantly alter the rate of functional preservation of hearing and facial nerve function in various functional surgeries of CPA by retrosigmoid approach. His collaboration in preparing this book on functional surgery of CPA was irreplaceable and I would like to express my sincere appreciation to him for sharing and imparting us with detailed knowledge on the same.

I would like to thank my wife and father for enduring long periods of my absence at home and for their love and support. Lastly, blessings of the Almighty and my late mother’s influence has been a source of continuous inspiration and has been the driving force in all my efforts.

Bhavin Parikh

Preface

It was in the autumn of 2004 that I first had the opportunity to knock the door of Professor Jacques Magnan's department. I was astonished to see the world of Jacques where cerebellopontine angle (CPA) surgeries by retrosigmoid approach (RSA) were performed almost daily and for a moment I felt like I had come to a wrong department. But repeatedly devoting my mind in drawing the sketches of the surgical field, I became fascinated with the elegant surgical field and the talented operating hands. The five months of my stay just flew passed. Following this stay till the end of 2005, I was fortunate to have introductory lessons on various other otologic approaches to skull base under the masters of skull base surgery worldwide. In the same period, I happened to meet a skull base surgeon named Dr Hirofumi Nakatomi. A year and a half after I returned to Japan, we met again by chance, and from spring 2007 we jointly embarked on the development of continuous electrophysiological monitoring system which measures the dorsal cochlear nucleus action potential (DNAP). The person who appreciated our concept the most and gave us the chance to demonstrate our system was Jacques. In February 2008, through the case which became clear during the operation to be facial schwannoma, we were able to show not only the continuous electrophysiological monitoring by DNAP but also the effectiveness of continuous electrophysiological monitoring on facial nerve we were developing at the same time. On this technique, I presented the results in the Politzer Society Meeting in autumn of 2009 and at that time Jacques commented "When I heard about the technique from him, to be honest, I did not believe it. But, when I saw their technique with my eyes in Tokyo and had it performed in Marseilles, I was convinced that it was real. His words were real."

I rejoined Jacques's surgical team from spring 2012. Coauthoring this book with Bhavin and writing the preface are all things unimaginable for me nine years ago. In return for the kindness Jacques gave me up to now, I have written in this book the concept of continuous electrophysiological monitoring centered on the experience I had so far.

I would like to devote this book to all otologists and otoneurosurgeons who handle operations in this field. Combining the allies of continuous electrophysiological monitoring, a new cochlear nerve mapping technique together with minimally invasive retrosigmoid approach systematized by Professor Magnan, I wish that the quality of life can be significantly improved for all our patients undergoing surgical procedures for the cerebellopontine angle pathologies by preserving the neural function and conducting the targeted surgery in minimally invasive way. I wish that more and more surgeons conduct function-preservation cerebellopontine angle surgery confidently resulting in excellence and wish this book to provide the basis for achieving this goal.

Lastly, I would like to thank my family who supported me in all my endeavors, especially adjusting to the difficulties arising due to my dual duties in Europe and Japan.

Hidemi Miyazaki

Acknowledgments

With the collaboration of:

Francois Caces (Beziers/Villefranche-Rouergue, France), Andre Chays (Marseilles/Reims, France), Arnaud Deveze (Marseilles, France), John Economides (Athens, Greece), Amr Hegab (Cairo, Egypt), Renaud Meller (Marseilles, France), Hirofumi Nakatomi (Tokyo, Japan), Agadurappa Mahadevaiah (Bengaluru, India), Honnurappa Vijayendra (Bengaluru, India) and Gruppo Otologico (Piacenza/Rome, Italy).

With the contributions by:

Miguel Aristegui, Gregorio Babighian, Jean-Pierre Bebear, Gerard Bonnaud, Per Cayer-Thomassen, Carlos Cenjor, Cor Cremers, Christian Dubreuil, Emilio Garcia-Ibanez, Thomas Lenarz, Masahiro Miura, Shreeram Murthy, Masaaki Nakajima, Kazimierz Niemczyk, Gerard O'Donoghue, Erwin Offeciers, Munehito Okada, Nuri Ozgirgin, Ranjan Aiyer, Archana Desai, KK Ramalingam, Philippe Romanet, Hitoshi Sano, Witold Szyfter, Jens Thomsen, Mirko Tos, Patrice Tran Ba Huy, Alain Uziel, Francois Vaneecloo and Hans Peter Zenner.

For their work:

Alfredo Vega Alarcon, Nacim Ait Mesbah, Hacene Ait Mimoune, Fayed Ashraf, Yakoot Ashraf, Sinnathuray Ar, Andrea Bacciu, Omar Bacha, Fathi Baki, Marco Barbieri, Jean-Francois Belus, Makhlouf Benzamit, Lukadz Borucki, Brahim Boutassetta, Laurent Broder, Michel Bruzzo, Mercedes Alvarez Buylla, Valeriu Buza, Francesco Canani, Rameh Charbel, Marina Cihanek, Olivier Coulet, Claire Lise Curto, Pavel Dimov, Jacob Economides, Christine Fatou-Balansard, Cristina Ferrario, Hani El Garem, Bhat Gautham, Davide Giordano, Melvin Guardado, Nicolas Guevara, Hella Hajri, Dirk Kunst, Benoit Lafont, Daniel Latil d'Alberta, Bob Lerut, Ali Mardassi, Mounir Marrakchi, Stavros Mavroidakos, Cyrille Menelli, Jean-Rene Millet, Badr El Din Mostafa, Mohamed Moussa, Sofiane Ouhah, Nazim Rous, Elaini Sherif, Laurent Tardivet, Franco Trabalzini and Pradeep Vundavalli.

For their support:

Denise Alpe, Roger Authie, Michel Autric, Jean Luc Breitenstein, Gerard Barki, Michel Lucciano, Jean Christophe Girardot, Frederic Giraud, Michel Salvati, Andreas Tedde, Christian Vuolo and Michel Lacour.

For their teaching:

Georges Bremond, Michel Garcin, Kimitaka Kaga, Nobumasa Kuwana, Agadurappa Mahadevaiah, Jean Marquet, Hiroshi Moriyama, Michel Portman, Jacob Sade, Jean-Marc Sterkers, Mirko Tos, Michel Wayoff, Ugo Fisch and Carlo Zini.

Contents

Surgical Anatomy of Cerebellopontine Angle

1

The cerebellopontine angle (CPA) is the angular space located between the superior and inferior limbs of the cerebellopontine fissure formed by the petrosal cerebellar surface folding around the pons and middle cerebellar peduncle. The cerebellopontine fissure is open medially and has superior and inferior limbs that meet at a lateral apex. Broadly, however, the CPA is constituted by the brainstem, cerebellar peduncles, fissures between the cerebellum and brainstem, cerebellar surfaces, and is traversed by various cranial nerves (CN IV to XII) and the cerebellar arteries (Fig. 1.1). It is essential to comprehend the relationships of various structures that inhabit the CPA and their individual variations. It is not the purpose of this book to present the detailed review of the surgical anatomy of the CPA but we present a brief introduction required for surgical procedures and suggest excellent literature by various stalwarts for further reading (prominent among them being wonderfully illustrated articles from Rhoton et al.).[1-8]

NEUROVASCULAR ANATOMY OF POSTERIOR CRANIAL FOSSA: SUPERIOR, MIDDLE AND INFERIOR ZONES

To better understand the intricacies of the posterior cranial fossa, it is divided into three zones (Figs 1.2 and 1.3) based on the relationship of the three cerebellar arteries to its adjacent structures: superior zone includes the superior cerebellar artery (SCA) and its relations, middle zone includes the anteroinferior cerebellar artery (AICA) and its relations, and inferior zone includes the posteroinferior cerebellar artery (PICA) and its relations. Each of the three zones has its anatomical landmarks in the form of an artery (one of SCA, AICA or PICA), part of the brainstem (either midbrain, pons or medulla), the cerebellar surface (either tentorial, petrosal or suboccipital), the fissures between the brainstem and the

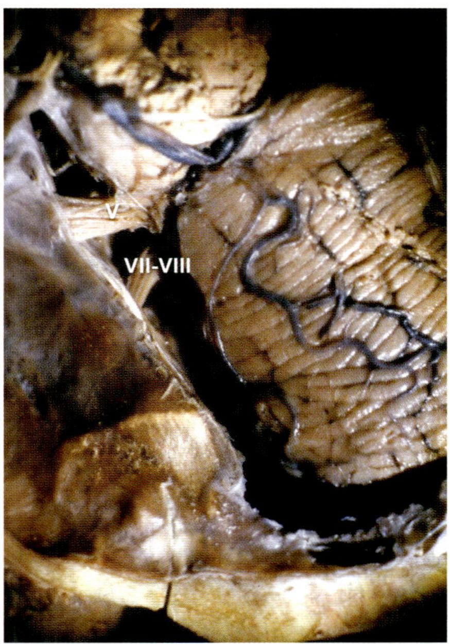

Fig. 1.1: Superior view of the left cerebellopontine angle (CPA) showing the trigeminal nerve (V) in the Meckel's cave area and the vestibulocochlear nerve along with facial nerve (VII–VIII) entering into internal auditory meatus (IAM). Note that the CPA is a very narrow space traversed by various cranial nerves and the cerebellar arteries, thus making it one of the most difficult areas to assess surgically for any pathology without adding any morbidity

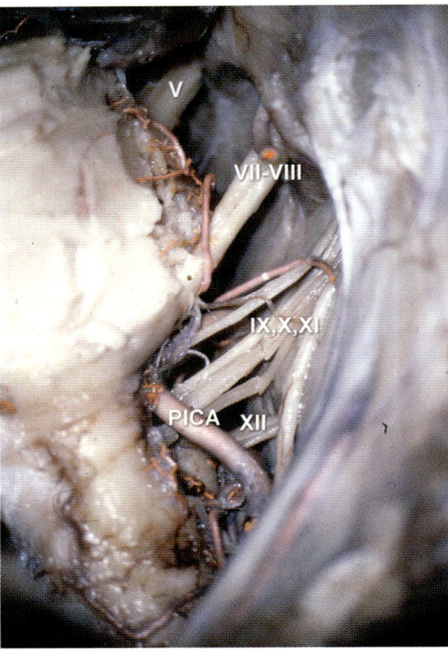

Fig. 1.2: Posterior view of the right cerebellopontine angle (CPA) after removal of cerebellum: Anterosuperiorly trigeminal nerve (V) joins the lateral surface of mid pons and runs obliquely up to petrous apex to enter into the tentorial dural fold called Meckel's cave to reach middle cranial fossa. Also seen is the Dandy's vein draining into the superior petrosal sinus. The vestibulocochlear nerve along with facial nerve (VII–VIII) originates from the lateral pontomedullary junction and traverses laterally to enter into internal auditory meatus (IAM) maintaining constant relation with each other throughout the CPA and the IAM. The vestibulocochlear and facial nerves are in a constant relationship with the anteroinferior cerebellar artery (AICA), which arises usually from basilar artery in the midline to traverse laterally to supply petrosal surface of cerebellum and lateral part of pons. The AICA also gives branch to the inner ear called labyrinthine artery. The posteroinferior part of CPA is occupied by the lower cranial nerves namely the glossopharyngeal, vagus, spinal accessory (IX, X, XI) and hypoglossal nerve (XII). The glossopharyngeal, vagus and spinal accessory nerves arise from the uppermost part of medulla lateral to the olive and enter the jugular foramen medial to the jugular bulb. The hypoglossal nerve arises from the upper medulla between the olive and the pyramid and enters neck through the hypoglossal canal which lies anteroinferior to the jugular foramen. The lower cranial nerves are closely related to the posteroinferior cerebellar artery, which usually arises from the vertebral artery and supplies the suboccipital surface of cerebellum and the lateral medulla

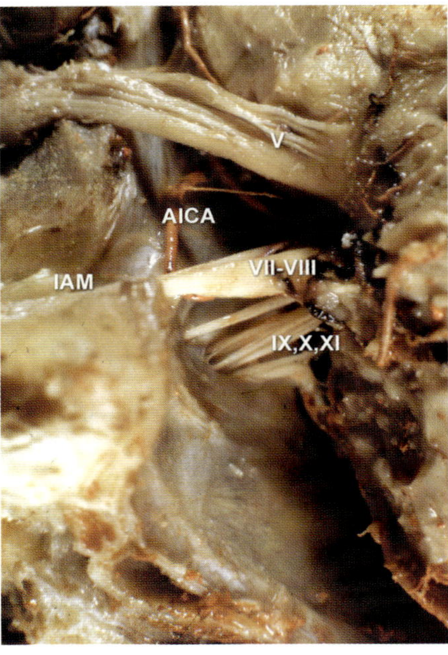

Fig. 1.3: Posterosuperior view of the left cerebellopontine angle (CPA) after removal of the tentorium showing the trigeminal nerve (V) in the Meckel's cave area, the vestibulocochlear nerve along with facial nerve (VII–VIII) entering into internal auditory meatus (IAM) and the lower cranial nerves (IX, X, XI) entering into jugular foramen. Note that the bone forming the roof of IAM has been removed. The branch of anteroinferior cerebellar artery can be seen between the facial and vestibulocochlear nerve

cerebellum (cerebellomesencephalic, cerebellopontine or cerebellomedullary), cerebellar peduncles that connect the brainstem to the cerebellum (superior, middle or inferior) and associated cranial nerves (IV to XII).

Superior Zone

The superior zone includes the SCA, midbrain, cerebellomesencephalic fissure, superior cerebellar peduncle, tentorial surface of the cerebellum, and the oculomotor, trochlear and trigeminal nerves. The SCA arises from the basilar artery in front of the midbrain, passes below the oculomotor and trochlear nerves and above the trigeminal nerve to reach the cerebellomesencephalic fissure, where it runs on the superior cerebellar peduncle and terminates by supplying the tentorial surface of the cerebellum. The SCA divides at a variable level of its path between the basilar artery and cerebellomesencephalic fissure into two branches, rostral and caudal. The trigeminal root joins the brainstem about halfway between the lower and upper borders of the pons. In its intradural course, the trigeminal nerve uniformly runs obliquely upwards from the lateral part of the pons toward the petrous apex. It exits the posterior fossa to enter the middle cranial fossa by passing forward beneath the tentorial attachment to enter the Meckel's cave. This nerve has two roots: the wide sensory root or "portio major" located laterally and the narrow motor root or "portio minor" located at the medial edge of the sensory root. The superior petrosal vein or Dandy's vein is formed by the anastomosis of various veins draining the cerebellum and brainstem. It drains into the superior petrosal sinus posterior to the trigeminal nerve as one or more venous pedicles. The superior petrosal vein is sometimes a barrier to accessing the trigeminal nerve during surgery for trigeminal neuralgia (Fig. 1.4).

Middle Zone

The middle zone includes the AICA, pons, middle cerebellar peduncle, cerebellopontine fissure, petrosal surface of the cerebellum, and the abducens, facial and vestibulocochlear nerves. The AICA arises at the pontine level, usually from the basilar artery, occasionally from the vertebral artery, courses in relation to the abducens, facial and vestibulocochlear nerves to reach the surface of the middle cerebellar peduncle, where it courses along the cerebellopontine fissure and terminates by supplying the petrosal surface of the cerebellum. In 40% of cases, the AICA forms a vascular loop running toward the porus acousticus. The AICA usually passes inferior to the VII–VIII complex, but it can also run superior to them or between the VII and VIII. The branches of the AICA near the VII–VIII complex are the labyrinthine artery, perforating arteries to the brainstem and "subarcuate" artery.

The acousticofacial nerve bundle arises from the brainstem near the lateral end of the pontomedullary sulcus, anterior and slightly superior to the end of the lateral recess of the fourth ventricle, inferomedial to the peduncle of the cerebellar flocculus, and above the rootlets of the glossopharyngeal nerve. The facial nerve arises in the pontomedullary sulcus 1–2 mm anterior to the point at which the vestibulocochlear nerve joins the brainstem at the lateral end of the sulcus. Just after leaving the CPA, the facial nerve remains in close contact with the pons over a few millimeters in length, the so-called subpial course of the facial nerve. The end of this subpial part corresponds to the point of contact between the nerve and the pons that usually is hidden by the cerebellar flocculus and choroid plexus. This segment of facial nerve including the subpial course and the first 2–3 mm of the origin from the pons is considered the root exit zone of the facial nerve, and has clinical importance as the point of vascular conflict in hemifacial spasm. The interval between the vestibulocochlear and facial nerves is greatest at the level of the pontomedullary sulcus and decreases as these nerves approach the meatus.

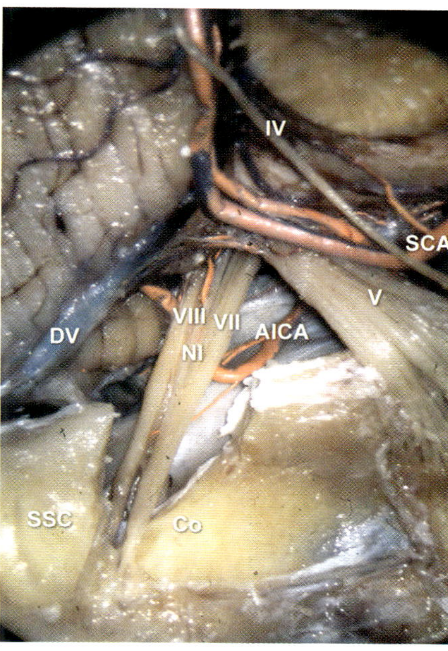

Fig. 1.4: Superior view of the right cerebellopontine angle (CPA) after removal of the tentorium showing the trigeminal nerve (V) being in close contact with the superior cerebellar artery (SCA) (divided into rostral and caudal branches). The SCA arises from basilar artery in front of the midbrain, passes above the trigeminal nerve to reach the cerebellomesencephalic fissure and terminates by supplying the tentorial surface of the cerebellum. The vestibulocochlear nerve along with facial nerve (VII–VIII) enters into internal auditory meatus (IAM) (the bone forming the roof of IAM has been removed). The anteroinferior cerebellar artery (AICA) arises usually from basilar artery in the midline to traverse laterally inferior to the VII–VIII complex to supply the petrosal surface of cerebellum and lateral part of pons. The AICA also gives branch to the inner ear called labyrinthine artery. The branch of AICA can be seen between the facial and vestibulocochlear nerve (DV: Dandy's vein; SSC: Superior semicircular canal; Co: Cochlea, NI: Nervus intermedius)

In the CPA, the facial and vestibulocochlear nerves run forward and lateral to reach the posterior surface of the petrous bone to enter the internal auditory canal (IAC). During their cisternal course, the facial is located anteromedially and the vestibulocochlear nerve is located posterolaterally. Among them the vestibular nerve is superior, while cochlear nerve is inferior. As they approach the porus of the internal auditory meatus (IAM), the vestibulocochlear nerve divides into the superior and inferior vestibular nerves and the cochlear nerve. The four nerves (facial and branches of the vestibulocochlear nerve) occupy the four quadrants of the IAM. The facial nerve is anterosuperior, the cochlear is anteroinferior, the superior vestibular is posterosuperior and the inferior vestibular

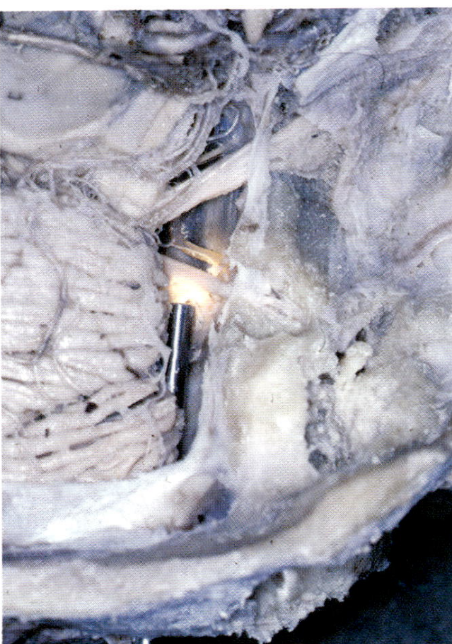

Fig. 1.5: Endoscopic anatomy from retrosigmoid approach: The cerebellopontine angle (CPA) is a narrow space traversed by various cranial nerves and the cerebellar arteries, thus making it one of the most complex neuroanatomical areas. The use of endoscope through retrosigmoid approach provides panoramic view of the contents of the left CPA from tentorium to the foramen magnum giving access to cranial nerves V to XI arising from lateral aspect of pons and medulla along with associated cerebellar arteries and veins

nerve is posteroinferior. The anteriorly placed facial nerve (VII) is hidden by the vestibulocochlear nerve in the posterior approaches to the CPA. The vestibulocochlear nerve is separated by a furrow, the cleavage plane between two components first described by Bremond. Between the facial nerve and the auditory nerve travels the nerve of Wrisberg (nervus intermedius). The three nerves are included in the same arachnoid cover. The cisternal route has a length of 8–12 mm. The flocculus is the lobe of the cerebellum that hides the zone of emergence of the acousticofacial nerve bundle during the posterior surgical approach.

Inferior Zone

The lower zone includes the PICA, medulla, inferior cerebellar peduncle, cerebellomedullary fissure, suboccipital surface of the cerebellum, and the glossopharyngeal, vagus, spinal accessory and hypoglossal nerves. The PICA arises from the vertebral artery at the medullary level, encircles the medulla, passing in relation to the glossopharyngeal, vagus, accessory and hypoglossal nerves to reach the surface of the inferior cerebellar peduncle, where it dips into the cerebellomedullary fissure

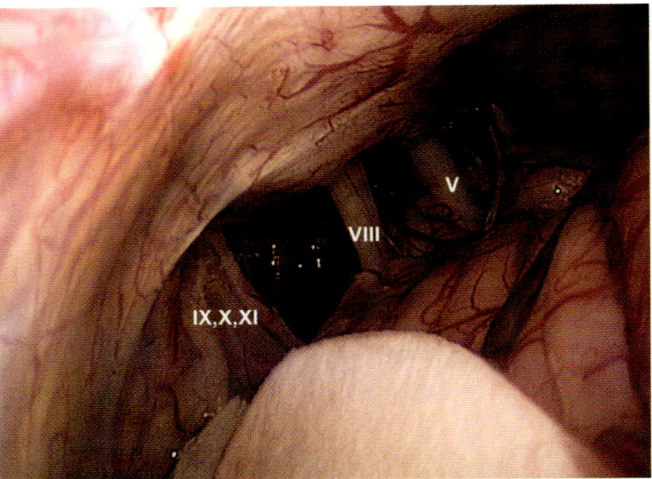

Fig. 1.6: Panoramic view of the contents of the left cerebellopontine angle (CPA). Root entry zones and cisternal courses of cranial nerves V to XI can be seen

and terminates by supplying the suboccipital surface of the cerebellum. The "glossopharyngeal nerve" arises as one or rarely two rootlets from the upper medulla, posterior to the upper one-third of the olive, just caudal to the origin of the facial nerve. It courses ventral to the choroid plexus protruding from the foramen of Luschka on its way to the jugular foramen. The "vagus nerve" arises inferior to the glossopharyngeal nerve as a line of tightly packed rootlets along a line 2–5.5 mm in length posterior to the superior one-third of the olive. The vagus is composed of multiple combinations of large and small rootlets that pass ventral to the choroid plexus protruding from the foramen Luschka on its way to the anteromedial part of the pars venosa. The "spinal accessory nerve" arises as a widely separated series of rootlets that originate from the medulla at the level of the lower two-thirds of olive and from the upper cervical cord. The cranial rootlets of the spinal accessory nerve arise as a line of rootlets just caudal to the vagal fibers. The spinal accessory fibers pass superolaterally from their origin to reach the jugular foramen.

OPERATIVE ENDOSCOPIC ANATOMY

The 30° angled endoscope is a valuable and indispensable optical device to visualize the CPA and it permits us to observe the blind spots in the CPA by "looking around the corner" giving a panoramic view of its contents (Figs 1.5 and 1.6). Through retrosigmoid approach using the endoscope, the acousticofacial nerve bundle is the reference level, crossing the middle of the CPA, giving distinct separate anatomical endoscopic surgically assisted areas (Figs 1.7 to 1.12). O'Donoghue and O'Flynn[7] divided the CPA area into four levels on the basis of neuroendoscopic inspection.

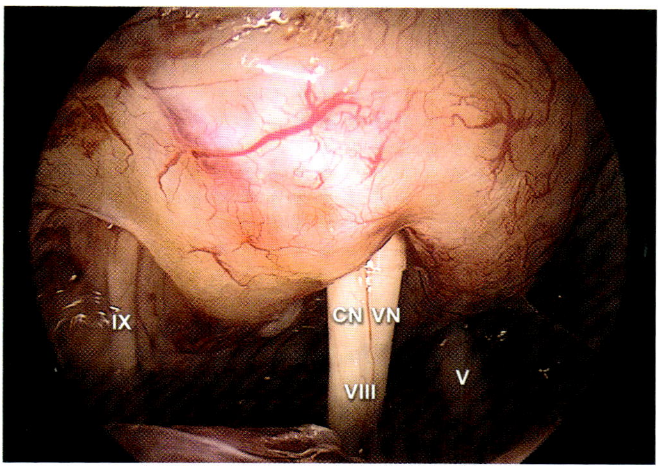

Fig. 1.7: Endoscopic view of the left cerebellopontine angle (CPA) centered at the vestibulocochlear nerve (VIII). The vestibulocochlear nerve is always demarcated into the superior vestibular division (VN) (toward trigeminal nerve) and inferior cochlear nerve (CN) (toward lower cranial nerves) by an arteriole along the cleavage. Also seen are the trigeminal (V) and glossopharyngeal (IX) nerve

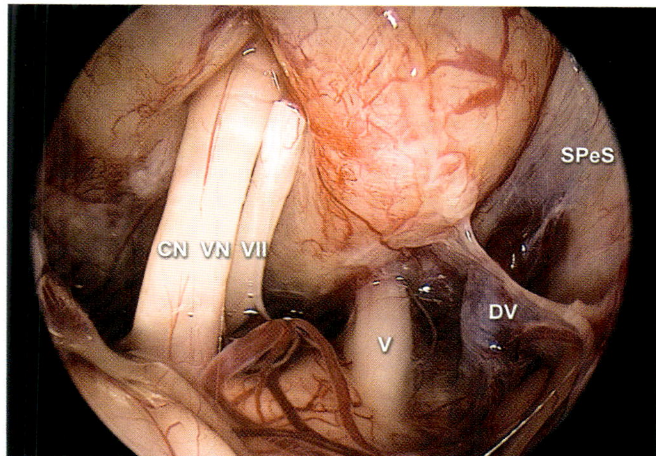

Fig. 1.8: Endoscopic view of the left cerebellopontine angle (CPA) superior to the vestibulocochlear nerve. The facial nerve arises anteroinferior to the vestibulocochlear nerve at the pontomedullary junction and crosses the latter from inferior to superior as it enters into internal auditory meatus (IAM) in anterosuperior quadrant at porus acousticus. Also visible are anteroinferior cerebellar artery (AICA) superior to VII–VIII complex, flocculus, trigeminal nerve and Dandy's vein (DV) entering into superior petrosal sinus (SPeS)

Level 1

Level 1 contains the trigeminal and abducens nerves, Meckel's cave, Dandy's vein and the SCA (Fig. 1.8).

Level 2

Level 2 contains the acousticofacial bundle traversing the CPA from the pontomedullary sulcus to the ICA, the length varying between 10 and 15 mm (average 13 mm) The facial nerve can be seen entering the anterosuperior compartment of the IAM as it passes laterally (Fig. 1.7). The facial nerve is separated laterally from the superior vestibular nerve in the fundus of the IAM and the AICA is entwined within the acousticofacial bundle. The AICA arises at the pontine level, usually from the basilar artery, occasionally from vertebral artery, courses in relation to the facial and vestibulocochlear nerves to reach the petrosal surface of the cerebellum (Fig. 1.10). In 40% of cases, the AICA forms a vascular loop running toward the porus acousticus. The AICA usually passes inferior to the VII–VIII complex, but it can also run superior to them or between the VII and VIII (Fig. 1.11).

Level 3

The dominant anatomic features at this level are the lower cranial nerves as they pass laterally from the medulla to the jugular foramen (Fig. 1.9). The lower cranial nerves along with root entry/exit zone of the facial and vestibulocochlear nerves are intimately related to the loop of the PICA (Fig. 1.12).

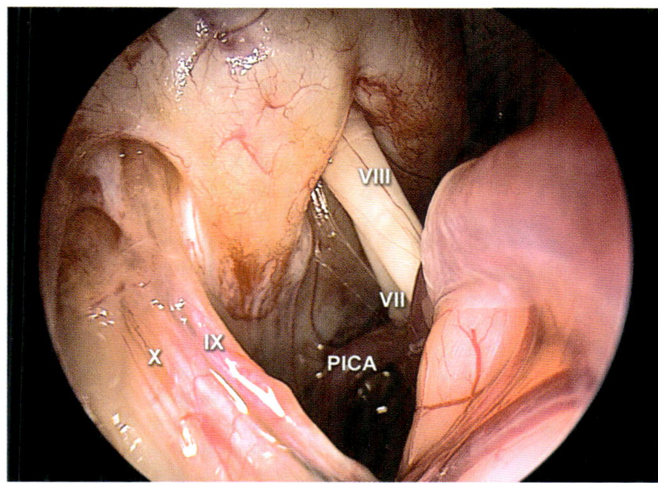

Fig. 1.9: Endoscopic view of the left cerebellopontine angle (CPA) inferior to the vestibulocochlear nerve. The facial nerve (VII) arises anteroinferior to the vestibulocochlear nerve (VIII) at the pontomedullary junction. The posteroinferior cerebellar artery (PICA) is seen inferior to the VII–VIII complex. The lower cranial nerves (glossopharyngeal, vagus and spinal accessory nerves) are seen entering into the jugular foramen

Level 4

An inferior extension of the CPA in which the lower medulla and spinal cord are readily apparent. The accessory nerve exits through the foramen magnum and the rootlets of the hypoglossal nerve run horizontally to gain entry to the

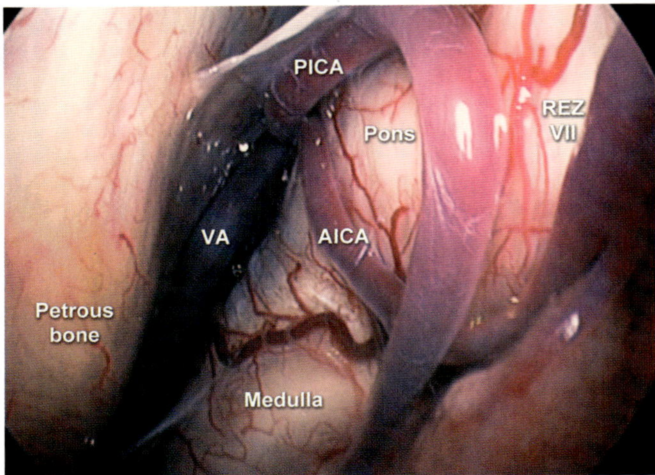

Fig. 1.10: Endoscopic view of the left cerebellopontine angle (CPA) inferior to the vestibulocochlear nerve showing vascular anatomy in inferior CPA. Posteroinferior cerebellar artery (PICA) usually arises from vertebral artery (VA) [occasionally from anteroinferior cerebellar artery (AICA) or basilar artery] and passes inferior to vestibulocochlear nerve and superior to lower cranial nerves to supply inferior surface of cerebellum. The AICA usually arises from the basilar artery (occasionally from vertebral artery or PICA) and courses in relation to the abducens, facial and vestibulocochlear nerves to reach the petrosal surface of the cerebellum. Here both the AICA and PICA cross the root entry zone (REZ) of VII

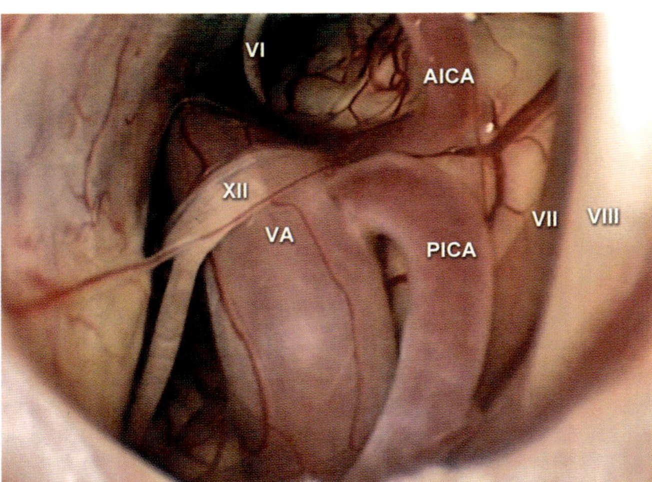

Fig. 1.12: Endoscopic view of the left cerebellopontine angle (CPA) showing posteroinferior cerebellar artery (PICA) arising from vertebral artery (VA) and anteroinferior cerebellar artery (AICA) arises from the basilar artery. Note the different cranial nerves and their relations to AICA and PICA. The hypoglossal (XII) nerve is seen turning around the vertebral artery to enter hypoglossal canal. Also seen are root entry/exit zone of facial (VII) and vestibulocochlear nerves (VIII). VI–Abducens nerve

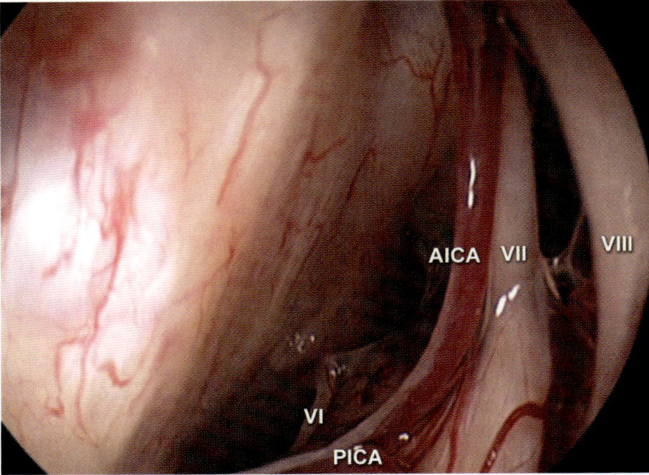

Fig. 1.11: Endoscopic view of the left cerebellopontine angle (CPA) showing anteroinferior cerebellar artery (AICA) following the cisternal course of facial nerve inferiorly. VI–Abducens nerve is seen in the background

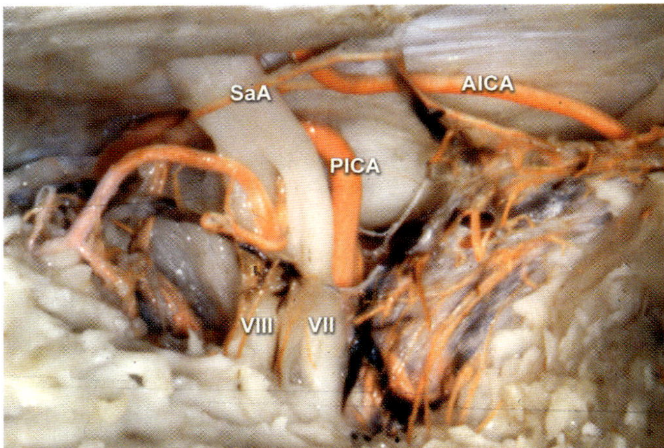

Fig. 1.13: Superior view into left cerebellopontine angle (CPA) showing VII–VIII nerve complex entering into the internal auditory meatus (IAM) at porus acousticus. Note its relation to the subarcuate artery (SaA), labyrinthine artery (LA) and anteroinferior cerebellar artery (AICA)

hypoglossal foramen. The PICA can be seen intimately related to the rootlets of the lower cranial nerves.

ANATOMY OF INTERNAL AUDITORY MEATUS

The internal auditory meatus (IAM) is a bony canal that forms a transition zone before the vestibulocochlear nerve enters the respective inner ear structures and transmits the facial nerve from CPA through the temporal bone to the face (Figs 1.13 to 1.17). It also carries the labyrinthine branch of AICA that acts as an end artery for cochlea and

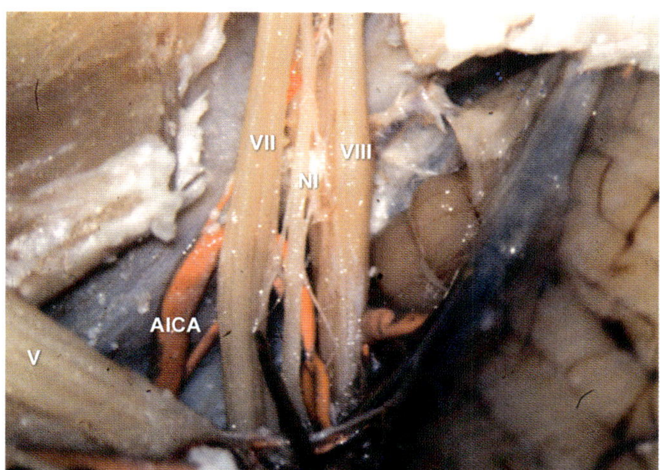

Fig. 1.14: Superior view into right internal auditory meatus (IAM) after drilling its superior roof showing the facial nerve (VII), nervus intermedius (NI), cochlear and vestibular nerves (VIII). The facial nerve is located in anterosuperior quadrant and is separated from superior vestibular nerve by Bill's bar. Facial nerve is joined by nervus intermedius in the internal auditory meatus (IAM). Note the extent of drilling and its probable relation to cochlea, superior semicircular canal and posterior semicircular canal. Also seen are the geniculate ganglions of the facial nerve, greater superficial petrosal nerve, trigeminal nerve, arcuate eminence with blue lining of the superior semicircular canal. The loop of anteroinferior cerebellar artery (AICA) can be seen between the VII–VIII nerves along with the labyrinthine branch to inner ear

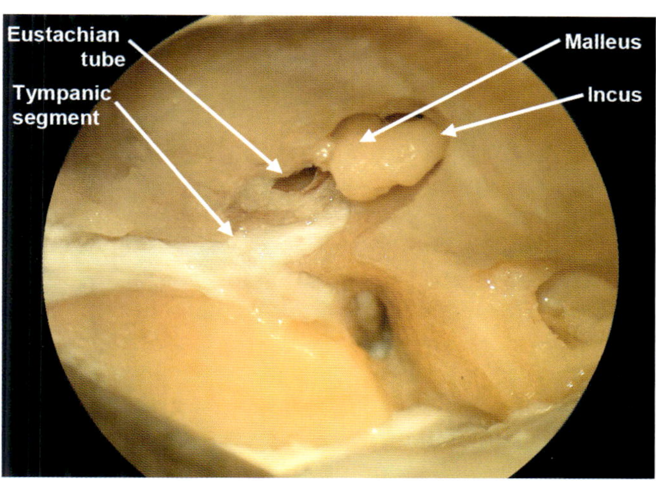

Fig. 1.15: Superior view of the internal auditory meatus (IAM) through middle fossa approach showing labyrinthine segment of facial nerve, geniculate ganglion and initial segment of tympanic portion of facial nerve. Greater superficial petrosal nerve arises from geniculate ganglion

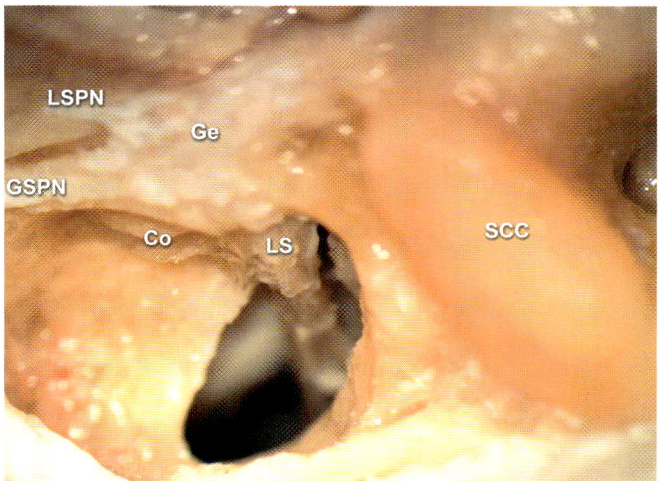

Fig. 1.16: Closer view of internal auditory meatus (IAM) through middle fossa approach showing labyrinthine segment of facial nerve (LS), geniculate ganglion (Ge) and initial segment of tympanic portion of facial nerve. (SSC: Superior semicircular canal; Co: Cochlea; GSPN: Greater superficial petrosal nerve; LSPN: Lesser superficial petrosal nerve)

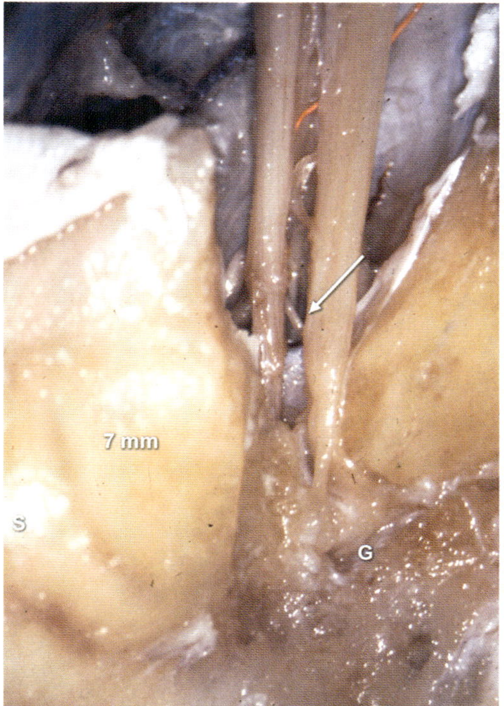

Fig. 1.17: Superior view into right cerebellopontine angle (CPA) showing internal auditory meatus (IAM) after drilling its superior roof. The length of IAM that can be drilled without causing injury to labyrinth is approximately 7–8 mm and the width of IAM is around 4 mm. Arrow points to Oort's bundle that carries efferent cochlear nerve fibers leaves the vestibular nerve to join the cochlear nerve in IAM

labyrinth. Its medial end toward the CPA is known as porus acousticus and is located on the posterior surface of the temporal bone. Its lateral end is known as fundus and it forms the medial end of bony labyrinth. The neurovascular contents of IAM are surrounded by the dura mater and arachnoid wrapping up to the fundus. The falciform (transverse) crest, a transverse ridge of bone, divides the lamina cribrosa into upper and lower compartments and provides an attachment site for the dura. The upper compartment is divided into anterior (containing the facial nerve) and posterior (containing the superior vestibular nerve) quadrants by the vertical crest (also known as Bill's bar). In the lower compartment, the cochlear nerve courses in the anterior quadrant, while the inferior vestibular nerve lies in the posterior quadrant. The average width of IAM is less than 4 mm (around 3.65 mm) and the average length of the IAM is around 8 mm with minor individual variations (Fig. 1.17). These dimensions are important when drilling the IAM blindly through the retrosigmoid approach as there are no landmarks to guide the drilling to avoid injury to bony labyrinth. The posterior semicircular canal and crus commune are intimately related to the IAM when drilling it through the retrosigmoid approach.

REFERENCES

1. Rhoton AL. The cerebellopontine angle and posterior fossa cranial nerves by the retrosigmoid approach. Neurosurgery. September 2000;47(3). Supplement.
2. Rhoton AL Jr. Microsurgery of the internal acoustic meatus. Surg Neurol. 1974;2:311–8.
3. Rhoton AL Jr. Microsurgical anatomy of the brainstem surface facing an acoustic neuroma. Surg Neurol. 1986;25:326–39.
4. Rhoton AL Jr. Microsurgical anatomy of decompression operations on the trigeminal nerve. In: Rovit RL, Murali R, Jannetta PJ (Eds). Trigeminal neuralgia. Baltimore: Williams & Wilkins; 1990, pp 165–200.
5. Rhoton AL Jr. Microsurgical anatomy of acoustic neuromas. In Jackler RK (Ed). Otolaryngologic clinics of North America. Philadelphia, W.B. Saunders Co.; 1992, pp 257–94.
6. Rhoton AL Jr. Microsurgical anatomy of posterior fossa cranial nerves. In Barrow DL (Ed). Surgery of the cranial nerves of the posterior fossa: neurosurgical topics. Park Ridge, AANS; 1993, pp 1–103.
7. O'Donoghue G, O'Flynn P. Endoscopic anatomy of the cerebellopontine angle. Am J Otol. 1993;14:122–5.
8. Magnan J, Sanna M. Endoscopy in neuro-otology. New York: Thieme Stuttgart; 1999.

Instruments 2

MICROSCOPIC SET-UP

The operating microscope is the prime and single-most important equipment for any surgery for cerebellopontine angle (CPA). As the operating period of surgery for cerebellopontine angle is usually long leading to physical discomfort and fatigue, operating surgeon should be comfortable both with image quality as well as freedom of movement. The microscope should provide excellent image quality along with adequate degree of maneuverability. Parfocal set-up of operating microscope, appropriate use of magnification and binocular three-dimensional microscopic vision for depth perception improves safety and accuracy of the surgery. The optical unit should be compact and not too bulky to allow adequate freedom of movement (Fig. 2.1).

VIDEO-ENDOSCOPIC EQUIPMENT AND SET-UP

Endoscopic-assisted procedure has helped to develop the concept of noninvasive surgery. Apart from endoscopes, the video-endoscopic set-up includes autoclavable optic fiber cable, cold light source (halogen or xenon light), endoscopic camera (preferably with high resolution) and the video monitor with video recording system. The endoscope (Fig. 2.2) and the optical fiber cable (Fig. 2.3) used are sterilized by autoclaving. By covering the camera cable and the camera adaptor with a sterilized polyethylene cover (Fig. 2.4), endoscopes can be exchanged easily under the clean handling condition. In order to maintain asepsis, the endoscopic examination is followed on a monitor rather than directly.

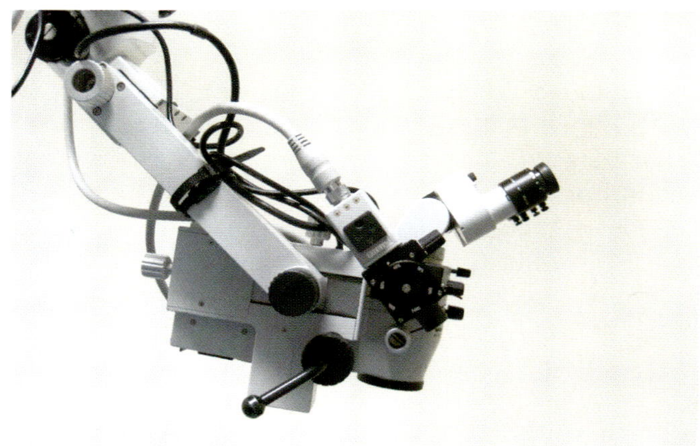

Fig. 2.1: Operating microscope

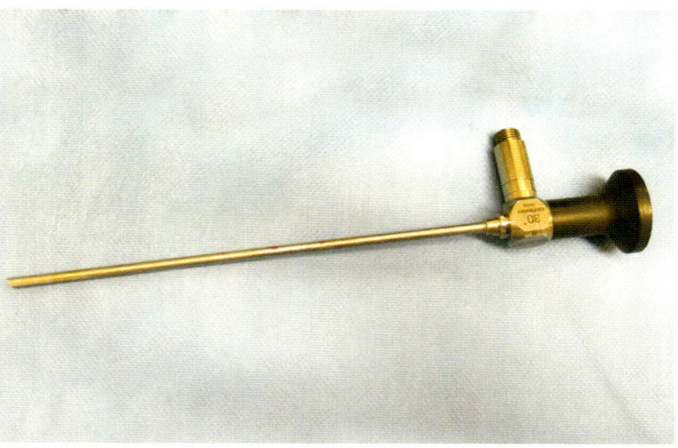

Fig. 2.2: Autoclavable 30° angled endoscope for endoscopy of cerebellopontine angle endoscopy

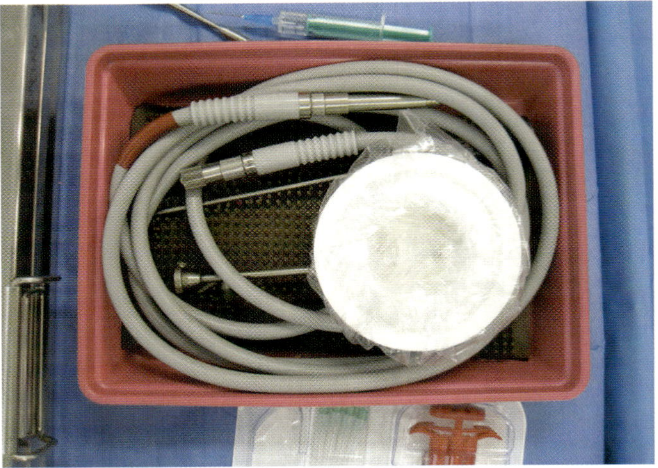

Fig. 2.3: Autoclavable optical fiber cable with sterile cover

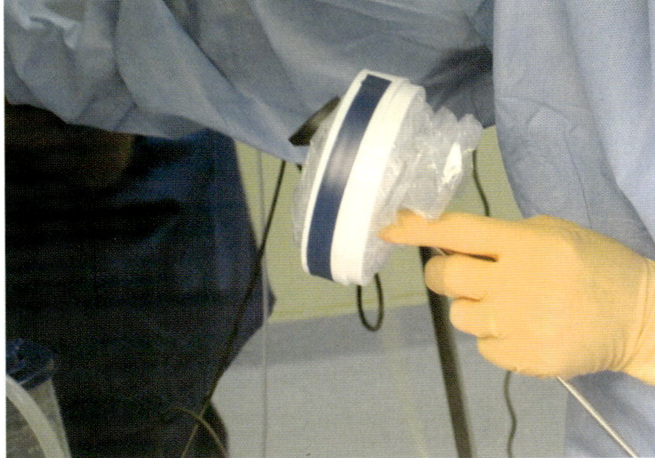

Fig. 2.4: Care is taken to maintain absolute asepsis by using autoclaved endoscope and optical fiber cable and by covering the camera cable and the camera adaptor with a presterilized polyethylene cover

Endoscopic Equipment

Rigid and autoclavable endoscopes are used. The most helpful is 30° endoscope, 4 or 2.7 mm in diameter and 11 or 18 cm in length. The endoscopes used are mainly the four described below.

1. 6 cm in length, 4 mm in diameter, 0°
2. 6 cm in length, 4 mm in diameter, 30°
3. 11cm in length, 2.7 mm in diameter, 30°
4. 18 cm in length, 4 mm in diameter, 30°.

We prefer 30° 18 cm endoscope, but when the operator is novice and not familiar with CPA endoscopic procedure, we recommend using 0° or 30° endoscope with shorter length (6 cm or 11 cm) as it is easier to manipulate and safer in preventing injury in CPA. Rotating the 30° endoscope around the longitudinal axis changes the field of vision, in contrast to the 0° endoscope and allows the surgeon to "look around the corner". The more angled endoscopes like 45° and 70° ones allow still more lateral view but we condemn them as they are dangerous in CPA as the surgeon could not appreciate the exact position of the tip and could cause injury to surrounding structures while introduction or during maneuvering the scope for side vision.

MONOPOLAR AND BIPOLAR CAUTERY (FIGS 2.5 AND 2.6)

In monopolar cautery, the electrical current passes through the patient to the ground electrode. There is a possibility of transmission through electrically and thermally sensitive adjoining neural tissues in CPA and so it is preferred only in the initial steps for subcutaneous tissue dissection and bleeding control. The bipolar system, first developed by Malis, uses a 1 MHz waveform for cutting and coagulation. A benefit of bipolar cautery is that it does not require a grounding pad as is required in monopolar cautery. The energy at the tips is separate, so the current passes only between the two tips of the instrument, eliminating the heat and current spreading to the surrounding area. If the actual tips of the bipolar forceps come into contact with each other without a vessel passing between the tips, coagulation does not occur. A bipolar cautery by high frequency passes electrical current through tissue from an active to passive electrode. In otoneurosurgery, bipolar cautery forceps perform delicate procedures concerning macroscopic blood vessels and tissues. Bipolar cautery uses electrical current through a medical device which is used to cut/coagulate tissue or vessels. The electricity and heat of the electrodes help to burn/coagulate tissues. In certain situations, the forceps generate a significant amount of heat while coagulation is being performed. This causes them to adhere to and even tear blood vessels and tissue with which it comes into contact during the procedure. Local heat is generated and causes tissue burns and clot formation which adhere to the tips of forceps. Thus, it is important to help irrigate the site where a neurosurgeon intends to coagulate, since this prevents the adherence of the tips of the forceps. A system known as the electroconvergent cautery system is now used as bipolar cautery. This cautery system uses a radiofrequency

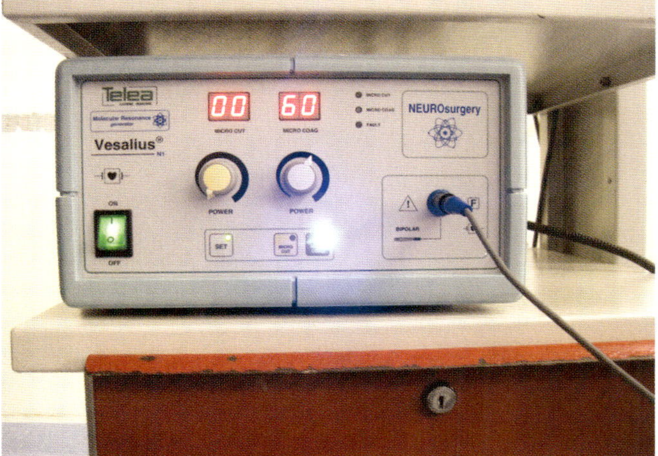

Fig. 2.5: Bipolar cautery unit

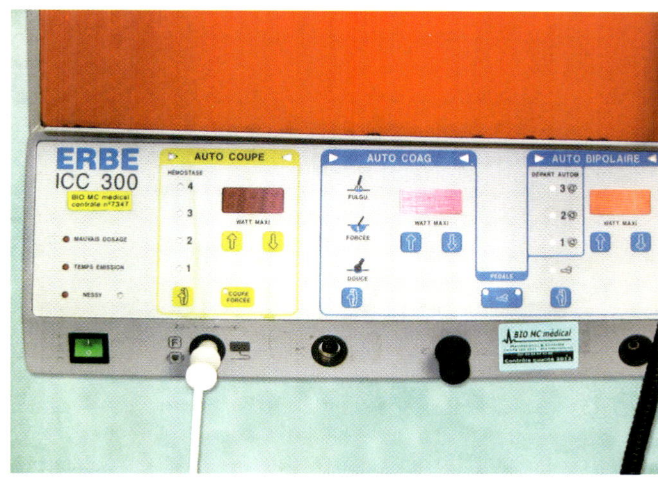

Fig. 2.6: Combined monopolar and bipolar units

current of 13.56 MHz. The current is passed through an amplifier, an impedance matching system, and a loading and tuning coil into a probe. After the probe tip is touched to the tissue, the mismatch of impedance between the probe tip and the generator is minimized to almost zero, resulting in high-current density at the probe tip, which causes pinpoint heating of the tissue at the point where it is touched by the probe without spread of heat to the surrounding tissue. This heat can cut and vaporize tissue and coagulate vessels. Because convergence of energy is used for tissue heating, a grounding pad is not needed. The system can also be used under cerebrospinal fluid or saline. Bipolar cautery is a significant invention in the field of CPA surgery. It responds to the key principle of gentle tissue management, less tissue dehydration and damage, it permits the control of hemorrhage and provides a clear and improved view of the operative site.

SURGICAL DRILL AND HANDPIECES

High-powered surgical drills along with cutting- and diamond burrs offer the versatility and precision needed for mastoidectomy, craniotomy, and other otoneurosurgical procedures like drilling of internal auditory meatus (IAM). The surgical drill should be relatively small, easy to handle and offer excellent balance and maneuverability, with adjustable speeds. We prefer pneumatic or electric high-speed surgical drills with facility for attachment of burrs with curved shaft for outstanding visibility and access in tight anatomic spaces like drilling of IAM through retrosigmoid approach.

FOOT CONTROLS

In CPA surgery, the surgeon has to control various devices with their foot controls. These include foot control for monopolar/bipolar cautery, high speed drill and suction control (Fig. 2.7). Different surgeons prefer different devices to be controlled by them while delegating some of them to scrub nurse. We prefer to control the drill and suction foot control and delegate the cautery foot switch to the scrub nurse. Foot control of suction unit is a very important (Fig. 2.8) and critical step to avoid injury to delicate structures like cranial nerves, especially in CPA surgery.

GENERAL INSTRUMENT SET

The general instruments (Fig. 2.9) used for retrosigmoid exposure include:

- Knife handles number 3, 4 and 7 with blades number 11 and 22
- Adson's tissue holding forceps with and without tooth—fine and regular
- De Bakey forceps
- Dissecting Allaine's scissors—short and long
- Large mastoid self-retaining retractors of Wulstein or Beckmann type
- Farabeuf's and Lempert's periosteal elevator
- Freyer's elevator/elevator for dura mater
- Suction adaptors and cannula of various sizes: Three Frazier's nasal suction cannula number 10, 12 and 15 and otoneurology suction cannula (long) of size : 1 × 2.0, 1 × 1.8 , 2 × 1.5 , 3 × 1.2
- Needle holder
- Different sizes of bowls.

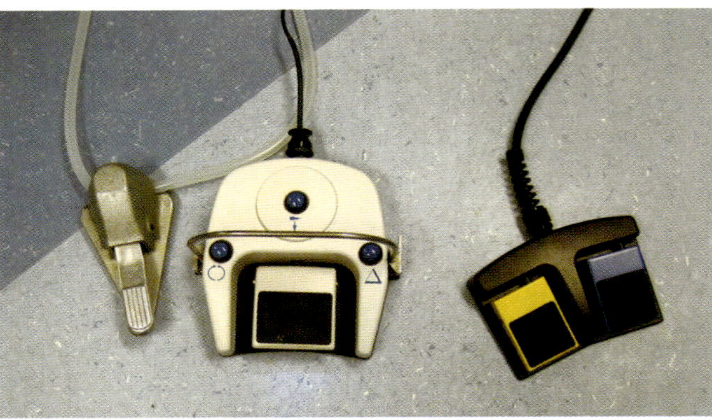

Fig. 2.7: Various foot controls for suction control, high speed drill and monopolar/bipolar cautery

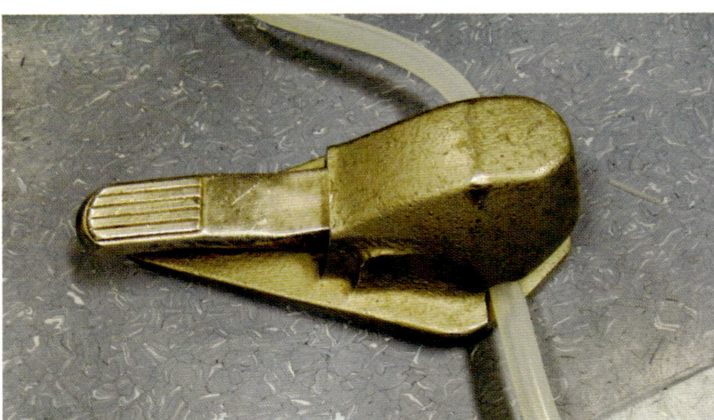

Fig. 2.8: Foot control of suction unit is a very important and critical step to avoid injury to delicate structures like cranial nerves, especially in cerebellopontine angle (CPA) surgery

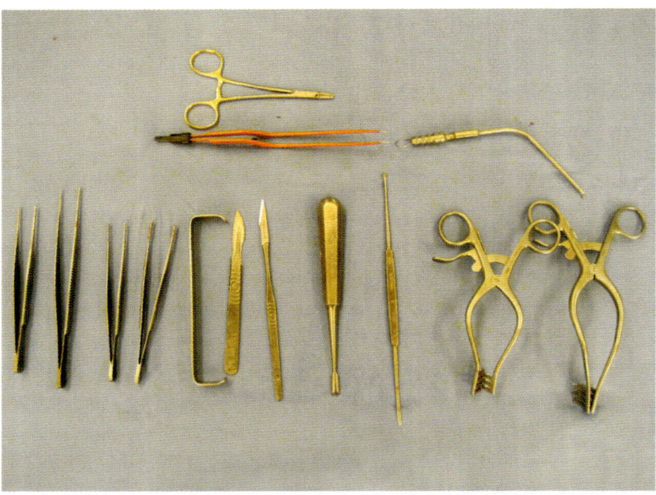

Fig. 2.9: General instruments set used for retrosigmoid exposure

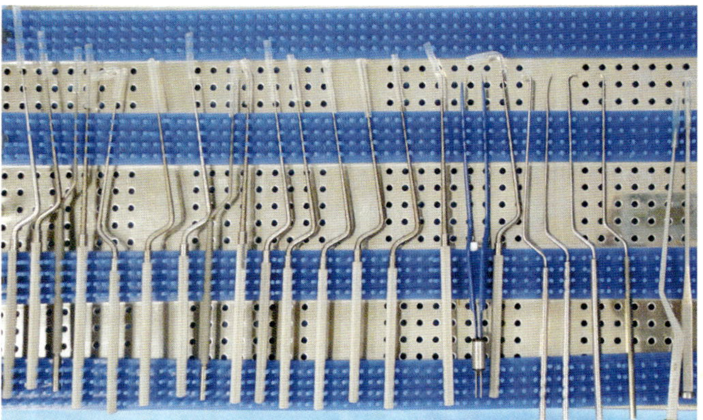

Fig. 2.11: Special bayonet-shaped instruments with the length of 19 cm and with working distance of 9.5 cm have been adapted to the keyhole retrosigmoid approach

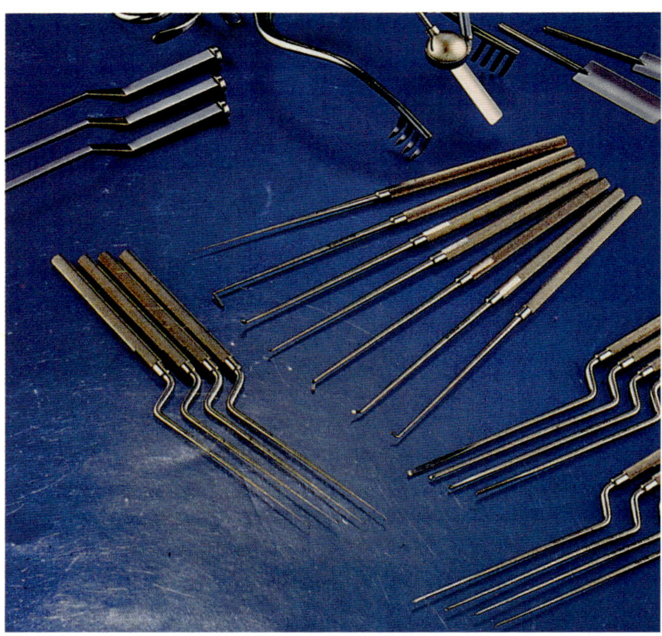

Fig. 2.10: Special instruments set used for retrosigmoid exposure

MICROSURGICAL INSTRUMENTS FOR RETROSIGMOID APPROACH

Specific suitable instruments are required because otologic microinstruments are too short, neurosurgical ones are too long and too cumbersome. Special bayonet-shaped instruments with the length of 19 cm have been adapted to the keyhole retrosigmoid approach (Figs 2.10 to 2.12). The bayonet shape facilitates visualization while working in the CPA by retrosigmoid approach and their distal end is pointing upwards,

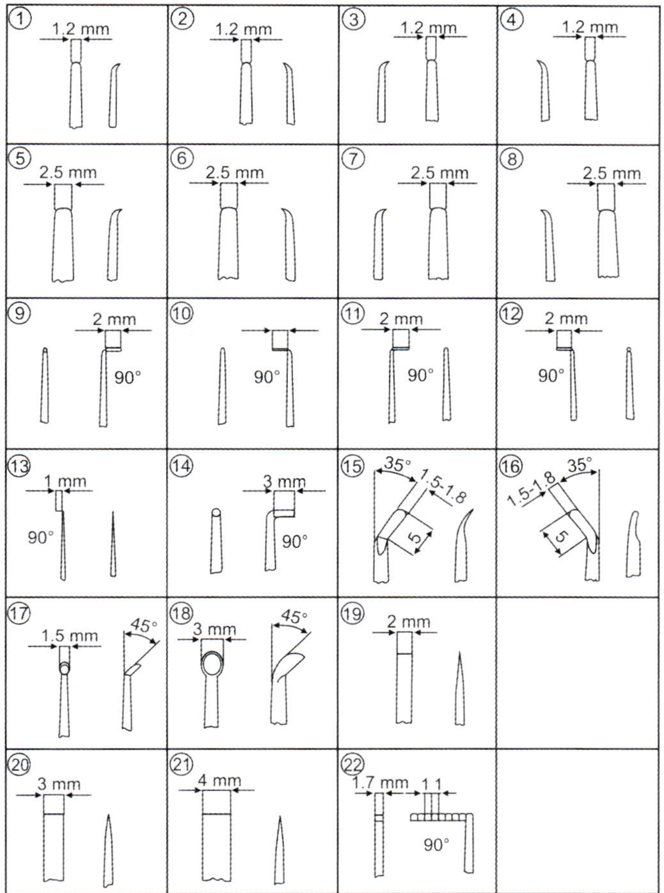

Fig. 2.12: Bayonet-shaped instruments include elevators of two sizes (1.2 mm and 2.5 mm breadth), blunt right-angled probes of different lengths, special curved dissector/elevators and bayonet chisels of various sizes

below, right or to the left to allow operating in the CPA with accuracy and delicacy.

The entire bayonet-shaped instruments have a length of 19 cm with working distance of 9.5 cm. The retrosigmoid instrumental armamentarium includes:

Straight Dissecting Instruments

- Straight right-angled probes with tip of 1 mm and 3 mm
- Right and left Marquet dissectors (Fig. 2.13).

Bayonet-shaped Instruments (Figs 2.14 and 2.15)

- A set of four bayonet-shaped elevators with a width of 1.2 mm with its end oriented right, left, up and down respectively
- A set of four bayonet-shaped elevators with a width of 2.5 mm with its end oriented right, left, up and down respectively

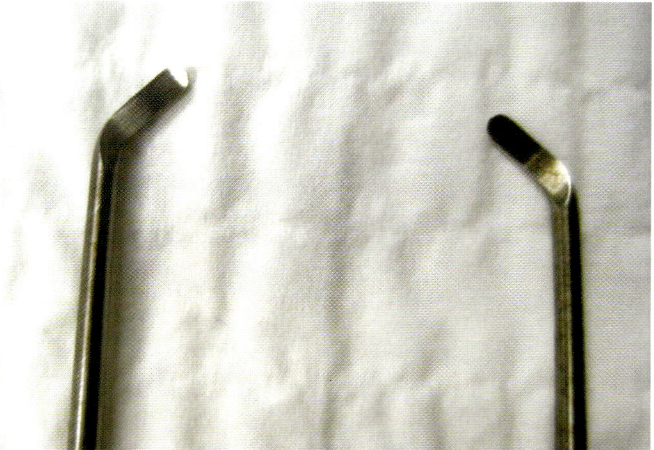

Fig. 2.13: Two special straight dissector elevator instruments with the length of 19 cm and with working distance of 9.5 cm and curved to right and left respectively

- Bayonet-shaped curved elevator
- A set of four bayonet-shaped right-angled hooks with blunt probes at the end with a length of 2 mm oriented right, left, up and down respectively
- Bayonet-shaped chisels of width 2 mm, 3 mm and 4 mm
- Bayonet-shaped special curved and straight dissector for dissection in internal auditory canal (IAC) for acoustic neuroma (Figs 2.16 and 2.17)
- Bayonet-shaped right-angled ring curette with length of shaft of ring curette of 10 mm with angulation at 8 mm and ring size of 2 mm (Figs 2.16 to 2.19)
- Bayonet-shaped blunt probe.

Dissecting Scissors

- Two bayonet-shaped Yasargil scissors with short and long straight blades (Figs 2.20 and 2.21)
- Straight long Sterker's alligator scissors (Fig. 2.21).

CONSUMABLE MATERIALS

Neuropatch (Braun®)

The synthetic dura substitute that is well tolerated and stable made from a highly purified polyester-urethane. The Neuro-Patch® cannot be degraded within the body either enzymatically or by direct cellular activity. We use Neuro-Patch® for protecting the cerebellum while assessing the CPA through retrosigmoid approach by cutting a 1.2 cm by 7.5 cm strip (Fig. 2.22). We occasionally use Neuro-Patch® for microvascular decompression of facial or cochlear nerve instead of Teflon felt, especially in cisternal course or in the IAM.

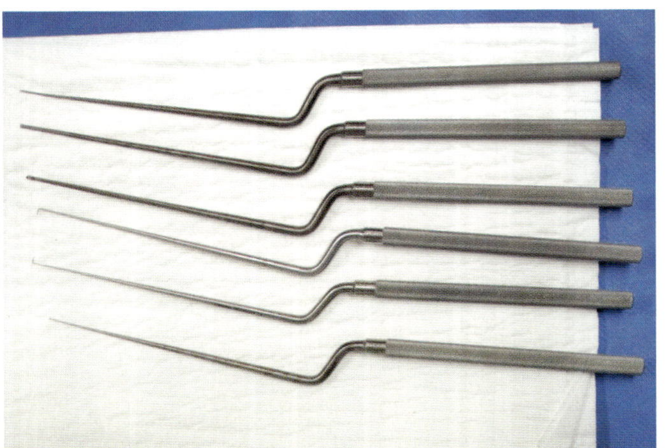

Fig. 2.14: Actual size of instruments with their tips

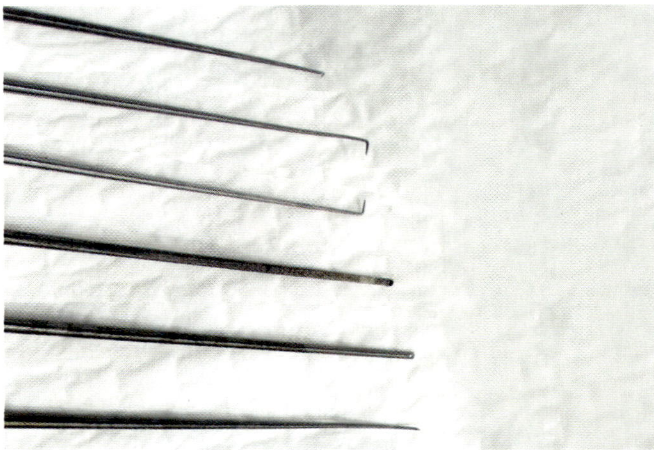

Fig. 2.15: Magnified view highlighting the tips of the special bayonet-shaped instruments

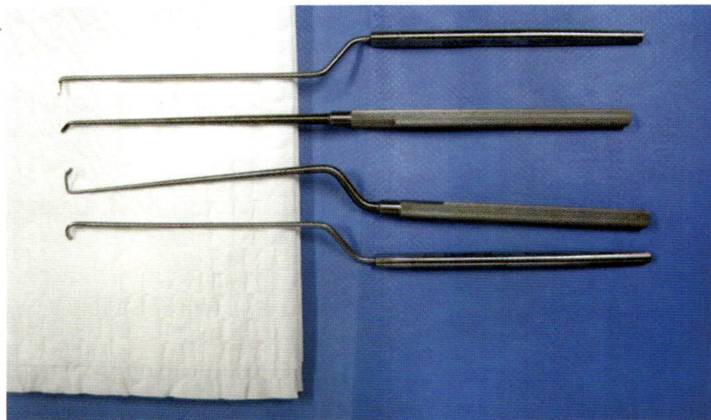

Fig. 2.16: Instruments used for endoscopic dissection of acoustic neuroma tumor remnant near fundus of internal auditory meatus

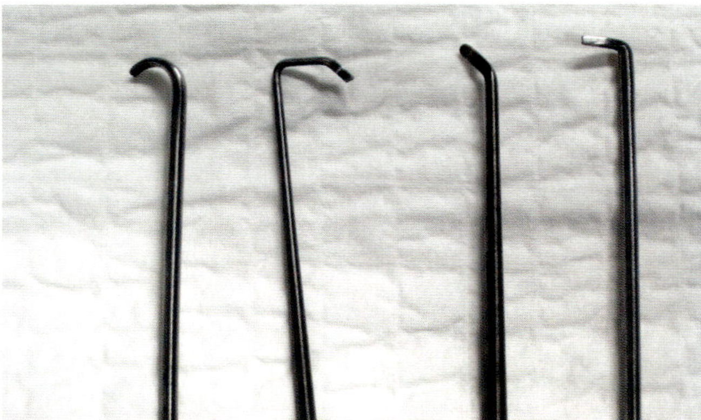

Fig. 2.17: Magnified view highlighting the tips of the special instruments used for endoscopic dissection of acoustic neuroma tumor remnant near fundus of internal auditory meatus. The instruments include bayonet-shaped right-angled curved dissector, bayonet-shaped right-angled ring curette, straight dissector and bayonet-shaped right-angled straight dissector

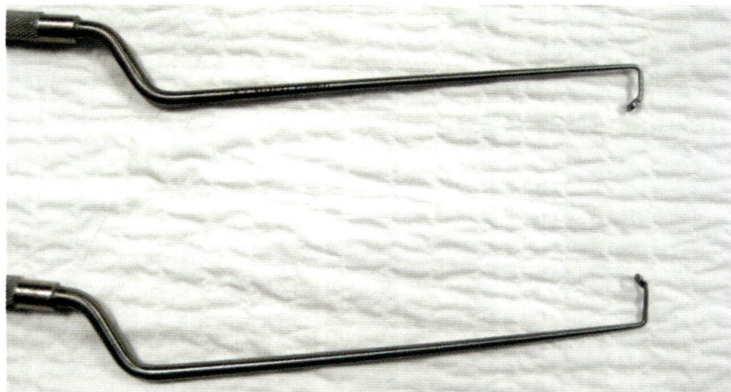

Fig. 2.18: Bayonet-shaped right-angled ring curette for right and left internal auditory meatus

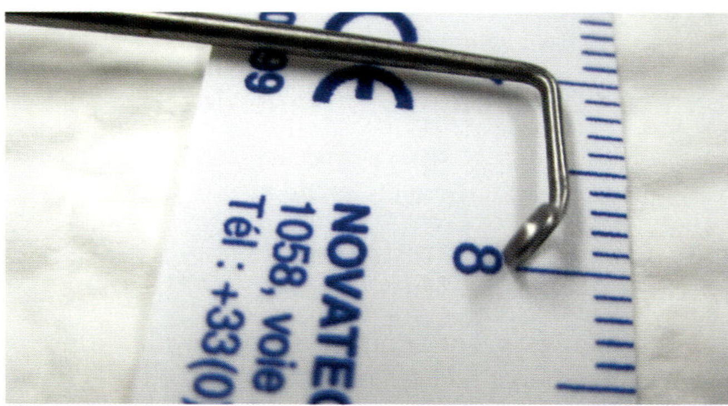

Fig. 2.19: Magnified view highlighting the tip of bayonet-shaped right-angled ring curette with length of shaft of ring curette of 10 mm with angulation at 8 mm and ring size of 2 mm

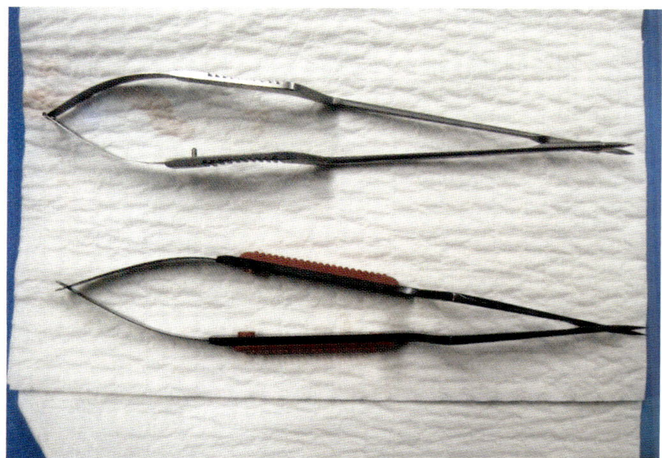

Fig. 2.20: Two bayonet-shaped Yasargil scissors with short and long straight blades

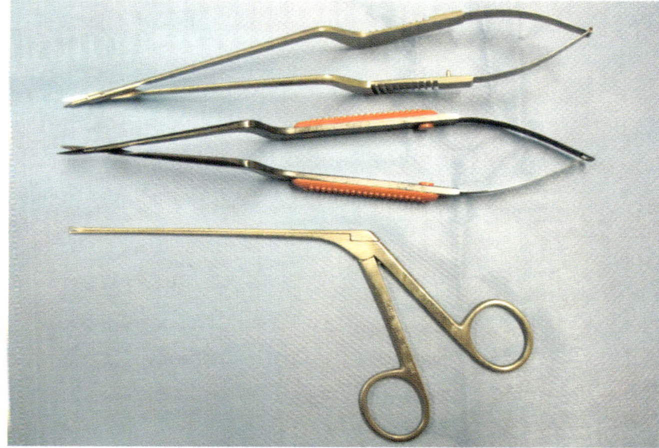

Fig. 2.21: Bayonet-shaped Yasargil scissors with short and long straight blades and straight long Sterker's alligator scissors

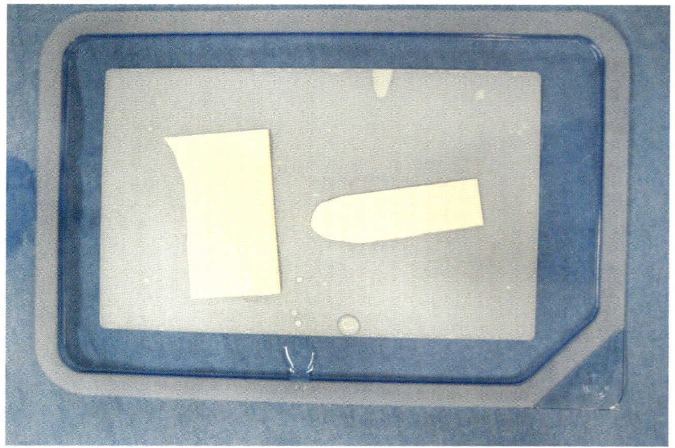

Fig. 2.22: Nonabsorbable synthetic dura substitute, Neuro-Patch (Braun®) is used for protecting the cerebellum while assessing the cerebellopontine angle through retrosigmoid approach by cutting a 1.2 cm by 7.5 cm strip

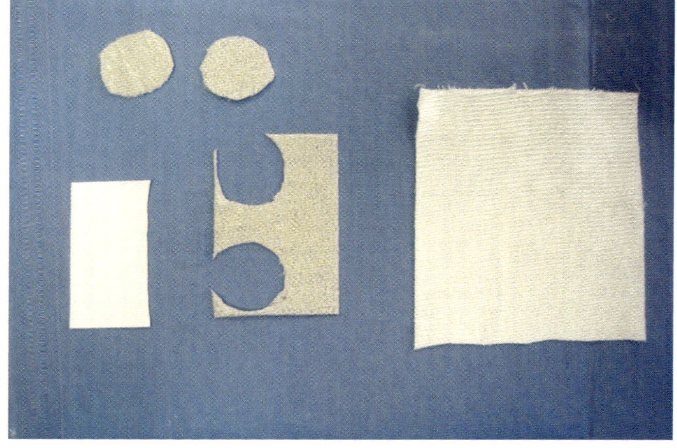

Fig. 2.23: A disc of absorbable synthetic dura substitute, Durapatch (Codman® Ethisorb™) is used to close the craniotomy defect, by suturing the circular disc cut slightly larger than the size of craniotomy defect with the dura to minimize the risk of CSF leak. Also seen is the Neuro-Patch® on left of cut sheet of Durapatch®

Durapatch (Codman® Ethisorb™)

It is a synthetic absorbable dural substitute for bridging the defects of dura mater and is a composite of a fleece of undyed vicryl (Polyglactin 910) and undyed PDS (Polydioxanon) along with a violet-dyed PDS foil. The porous vicryl fleece allows tissue on-growth while the PDS film coating minimizes leakage of cerebrospinal fluid (CSF). Absorption is complete approximately 90 days after implantation. The absorbable, fleece-like, porous structure allows for the progressive integration of the implant by the newly formed fibrous, connective tissue with minimal risk of inflammation; when fully absorbed, the implant leaves no foreign body in situ. The basic component materials of the implant (being commonly used as suturing materials, Coated Vicryl™ and PDS II™), have been extensively tested to prove their biocompatibility and nontoxicity. The implant may elicit a minimal initial tissue reaction, which is transient and is followed by the deposition of fibrous, connective layers of tissue. We utilize a disc of Durapatch to place it in the craniotomy defect (Fig. 2.23), which is sutured with the dura to minimize the risk of CSF leak.

Bard® PTFE Teflon Felt

Teflon felt is cut into pledgets of necessary size and compressed slightly (Figs 2.24 and 2.25) to be used as an insulating material for microvascular decompression of the cranial nerve from the conflicting artery.

Fine Neurosurgical Cottonoids (Codman®)

Cottonoids of different lengths are used as neurosurgical patties for giving local pressure/dissection (Fig. 2.26). A count is kept of the total number of patties of different sizes used (Fig. 2.27). Codman® surgical patties and strips provide the softness, gentleness, protection and absorbency to meet the demands of delicate CPA surgery. Codman® patties absorb more than five times their weight in less than a second. Codman® patties' precision cut provides smooth edges and helps prevent linting. Codman® Cottonoid® is a compressed rayon that provides the natural softness, absorbency and pliability of cotton. A special process interweaves individual rayon fibers to resist shedding, stretching or linting—whether wet or dry. Codman® Sutureweld®'s strong bond holds the indicator string to the pattie so the surface which lies next to the tissue is completely smooth and free of stitches. These

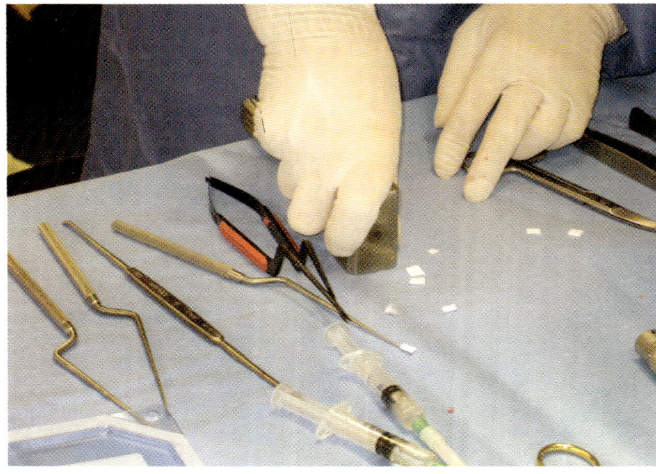

Fig. 2.24: Teflon felt is cut into pledgets of necessary size and compressed slightly to be used as an insulating material for microvascular decompression

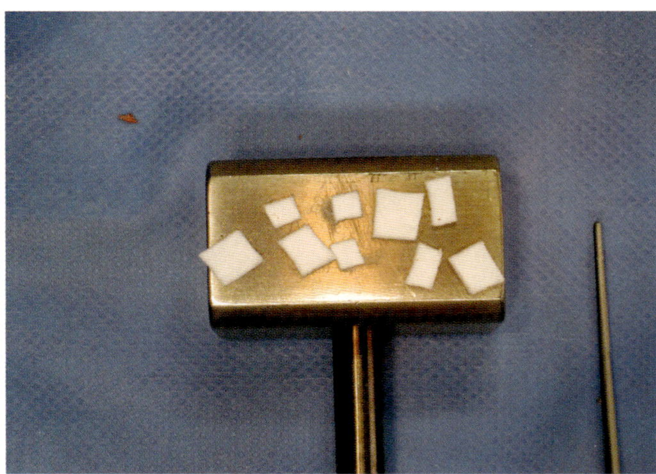

Fig. 2.25: Teflon felt is cut into pledgets of necessary size to be used as an insulating material for microvascular decompression

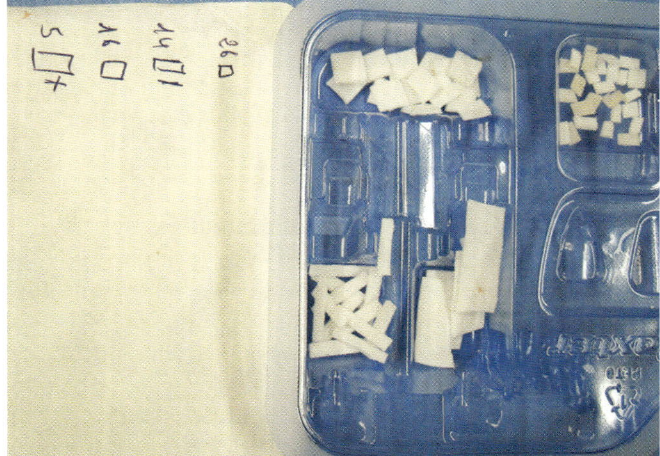

Fig. 2.26: Fine neurosurgical cottonoids (Codman®) of different length are used as neurosurgical patties for giving local pressure/dissection

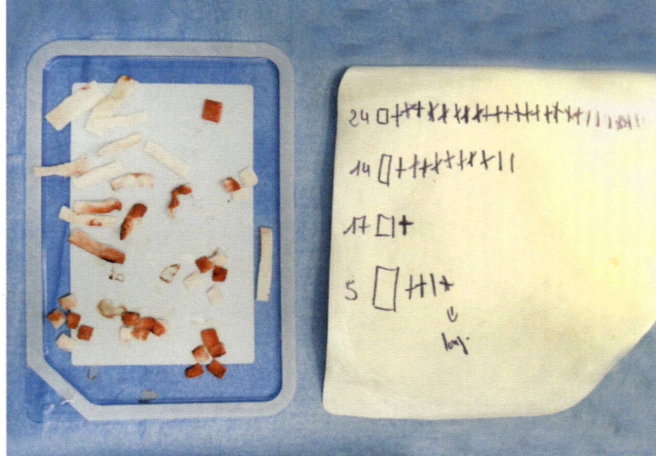

Fig. 2.27: A count is kept of the total number of cottonoids of different sizes used for keeping record

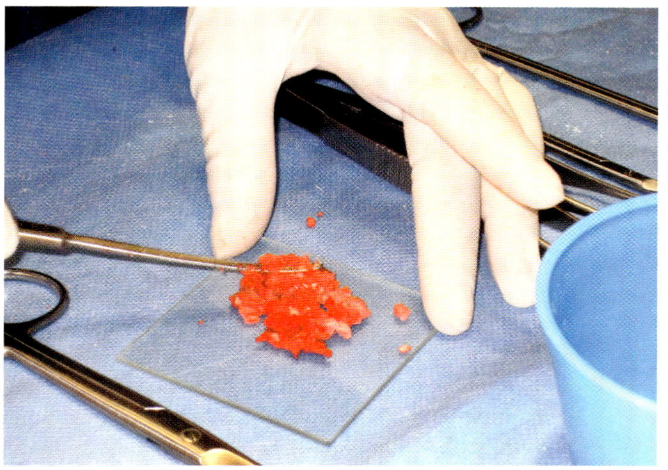

Fig. 2.28: Fibrin glue (Tissucol®) is used to form bone paste from collected bone dust

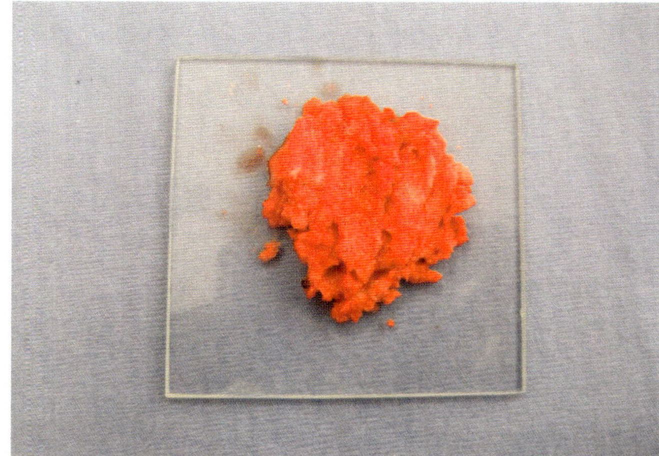

Fig. 2.29: Bone paste created by mixing fibrin glue and bone dust is used to cover the craniotomy defect

patties are porous and pliable and one can safely suction through them without aspirating the tissue or the pattie strip. They are radiologically detectable.

Fibrin Glue (Tissucol®)

It is composed of 1 mL solutions each (total 2 mL) of:

- Tisseel® powder consists of clottable protein (including fibrinogen, plasma fibronectin, factor XIII and plasminogen) to be reconstituted with aprotinin solution (bovine 3000 KIU/mL^2), 1 mL.
- Thrombin 4 IU/500 IU powder for thrombin solution to be reconstituted with calcium chloride solution, 1 mL.

Tisseel® kit is used to achieve hemostasis, to seal or glue tissue, and to support wound healing.

We prefer to use fibrin glue to:

- Form bone paste from collected bone dust (Figs 2.28 and 2.29)
- Fortify dural closure after retrosigmoid approach along with suturing of dura and use of Durapatch®
- Cause adhesions between transposed artery in microvascular decompression
- Prevent CSF leak from the IAC after drilling it open to remove acoustic neuroma by plugging it with free muscular tissue along with fibrin glue.

Bone Wax

Bone wax is a sterile mixture of beeswax and a wax-softening agent such as paraffin or vaseline, used to help control bleeding from bone surfaces. It is smeared across the bleeding edge of the bone, blocking the holes and causing immediate bone hemostasis through a tamponade effect. Bone wax is supplied in sterile sticks, and most often requires softening before it can be applied. It does not act biochemically and is minimally resorbable.

Surgicel (Ethicon®)

The absorbable hemostats made from oxidized regenerated cellulose achieve hemostasis by providing a matrix for platelet adhesion and aggregation for heavy bleeding. It has proven bactericidal against a broad range of gram-positive and gram-negative organisms. It is a plant-based product and is fully absorbable within 7–14 days. The newer Nu-knit (Ethicon®) Surgicel is more dense knit material and so provides high tensile strength in the presence of heavy bleeding. Its soft, pliable weave is designed to hold a suture and for placement on delicate tissue. It is three times denser than original Surgicel and takes 36% lesser time to hemostasis.

SUTURE MATERIALS (FIG. 2.30)

- Silk 5-0 on 3/8 circle taper round bodied 12-mm needle for suturing the dura
- Polyamide (Flexocrin) 2-0 on 3/8 circle taper cut 30-mm needle for suturing the periosteum and subcutaneous tissue
- Polyamide (Ethilon) 3-0 on 3/8 circle taper cut 24-mm needle for suturing the skin incision.

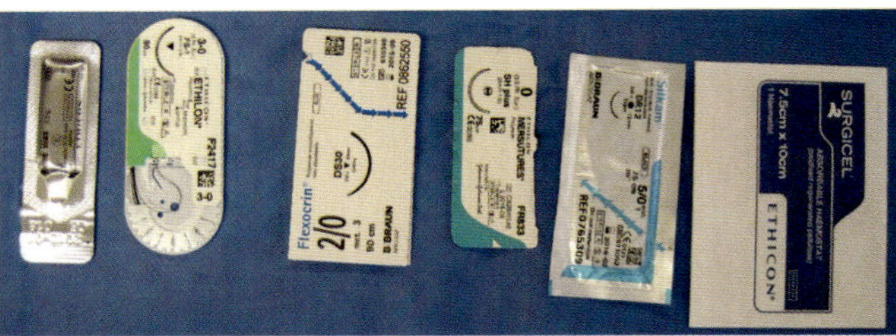

Fig. 2.30: Suture materials used for retrosigmoid craniotomy: Silk 5-0 on 3/8 circle taper round bodied 12-mm needle for suturing the dura, polyamide (Flexocrin) 2-0 on 3/8 circle taper cut 30-mm needle for suturing the periosteum and subcutaneous tissue and polyamide (Ethilon) 3-0 on 3/8 circle taper cut 24-mm needle for suturing the skin incision. Also seen in the picture are Surgicel (Ethicon®) and bone wax

OTHER MEDICAMENTS

- Xylocaine 1% with 1:100,000 adrenaline for local anesthesia
- Papaverin for vasodilatation of intracranial arteries
- MESNA mucolytic solution for acoustic neuroma dissection.

OTHER DISPOSABLE MATERIALS

- Disposable drape set for craniotomy
- Adhesive tapes
- Disposable covers for microscope and endoscope
- Pouch for putting instruments and probes.

3 Nerve Monitoring for Cerebellopontine Angle Surgery

INTRODUCTION

During the early part of acoustic neuroma surgery, the larger size of tumors and crude surgical techniques made saving the life of the patient a priority. Once there was a consistent improvement in mortality rates for this surgery, facial nerve function preservation was the next priority. The use of facial nerve-monitoring system has now got universal acceptance for acoustic neuroma surgery. Recent developments in the last decade in diagnosis and treatment have considerably reduced the average size of tumor detection and improved the facial nerve preservation significantly. So naturally the ever enthusiastic surgeons have now made hearing preservation as their next target. But the role of monitoring in achieving cochlear nerve function preservation had multiple technical and surgical hindrances leading to relatively poor acceptance among surgeons involved in acoustic neuroma surgery. The acceptance of cochlear nerve monitoring in the last few years is due to evolution of much more rapid and stable feedback systems for considering hearing preservation in acoustic neuroma surgery.

INTRAOPERATIVE CONTINUOUS COCHLEAR AND FACIAL NERVE MONITORING FOR SURGERY OF ACOUSTIC NEUROMA

Acoustic neuroma is a benign tumor that usually originates in the internal auditory canal and is essentially a vestibular schwannoma. The hearing function declines in vestibular schwannoma because the cochlear nerve is also an eighth cranial nerve similar to the vestibular nerve, and the cochlear nerve gets distorted at the internal auditory meatus (IAM) or cerebellopontine angle (CPA) by the vestibular schwannoma. The facial nerve abutting the vestibulocochlear nerve also gets distorted by the pressure caused by the tumor, but facial nerve paresis occurs far less compared to the declining of the hearing, which shows that the cochlear nerve function is highly sensitive and cochlear nerve gets damaged to even minimum of disturbance by tumor growth or tumor manipulation during surgery. So as long as the cochlear nerve is treated by the same method applied to the facial nerve, which is relatively resistant to damage, it is difficult to expect an improvement in the cochlear nerve function preservation ratio namely hearing preservation ratio.

Intraoperative Continuous Cochlear Nerve Monitoring by Measuring Dorsal Cochlear Nucleus Action Potentials (DNAP)

The ability to preserve the cochlear nerve function with certainty depends on the existence of a rapid and sensitive nerve-monitoring system that is obtained in a stable and persistent way to allow visualization of the status of the nerve function. The auditory brainstem response (ABR) is generally used as an intraoperative continuous cochlear monitoring, but it is often affected by electromagnetic waves generated from equipments in the operation room. It is not considered to be a good choice for intraoperative monitoring because if the preoperative hearing is bad, the ABR soon gets lost. Also the time needed to measure ABR is too long for rapid information about cochlear nerve status during acoustic neuroma surgery as it requires 500–1000 additional counts. To improve on these problems, an intraoperative monitoring using cochlear nerve action potential (CNAP) has been developed by putting an electrode on the cochlear nerve. If the electrode is set on the nerve, a good intraoperative monitoring could be conducted, but it is difficult to set a fine electrode stably on the cochlear nerve, which is only 1 mm wide. It becomes a huge obstacle when the electrode along with its connecting cord gets into the surgical field and interferes with the microsurgery. To obtain a stable intraoperative continuous cochlear monitoring by solving the problems that ABR and CNAP have, we developed a monitoring method that sets a recording electrode right on the dorsal cochlear nucleus (DCN) at the medial end of the cochlear nerve in the foramen of Luschka to measure Dorsal cochlear Nucleus Action Potentials (DNAP) (Fig. 3.1). The DNAP obtained from DCN has approximately 10–50 times larger amplitude compared to ABR, and is agile and only requires 100–200 addition counts, reducing the measurement time significantly to 6–12 s. There were reports[1,2] on active potentials being obtained from DCN but the methods never became prevalent. Probably it would have been difficult previously to set an electrode safely and reliably without damaging the normal cranial nerve tissues. So we embarked on the task of designing the electrode for that purpose and accomplished making the special electrode (Fig. 3.2), which has a platinum electrode in the center of a silicone plate with the size 3 mm × 5.5 mm and with excellent biocompatibility (Patents: JP4185562, EP2100555,US-2009-0234421-A1).

Intraoperative Continuous Facial Nerve Monitoring by Measuring Facial Nerve Root Evoked Muscle Action Potential (FREMAP)

Similar to the cochlear monitoring described previously, an intraoperative continuous nerve monitoring system is even utilized for the facial nerve. Following the conventional technology,[3,4] a special stimulant electrode (Patents: JP4303782, EP2229977) (Fig. 3.3) is set around the root exit zone (REZ) of the facial nerve, and an electrical stimulation with an intensity of 1–3 mA and a pulse width of 0.2 ms is given at 3-s interval. The advantage of this electrode is its shape and by deploying the silicone fin around the platinum electrode, the stability of the set electrode increases. Evoked electromyograms of the facial mimetic muscles (orbicularis oculi and oris muscle) are monitored. As stimulation is applied continuously onto the REZ of the facial nerve, we call the electric potential thus obtained as facial nerve root evoked muscle action potential (FREMAP).[5]

Placement of DNAP and FREMAP Electrodes

Retrosigmoid approach (RSA) is more suitable as an approach in the operation as the DNAP and FREMAP electrodes are set medially close to the brainstem (Fig. 3.4) at the foramen of Luschka and facial nerve REZ, respectively. However, retrolabyrinthine approach (RLA) is possible in case where the tumor is not fully blocking

Fig. 3.1: Position of dorsal cochlear nucleus (DCN) and the dorsal cochlear nucleus action potentials (DNAP) electrode. The DCN exists on the extension of the cochlear nerve of brain stem. The DNAP electrode is inserted into foramen of Luschka along the glossopharyngeal nerve

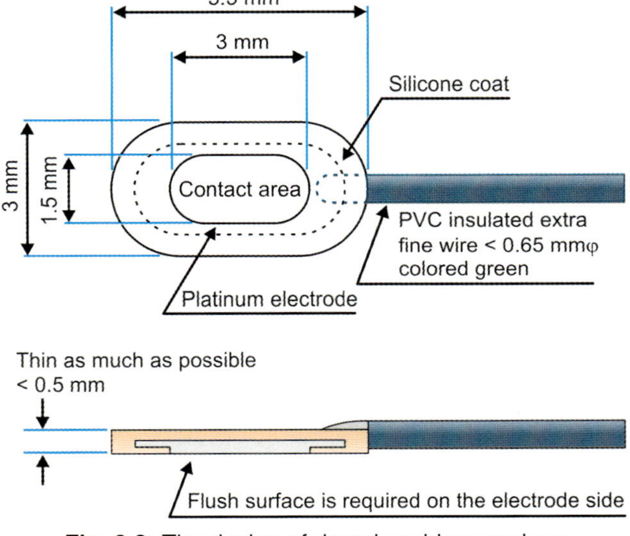

Fig. 3.2: The design of dorsal cochlear nucleus action potentials electrode

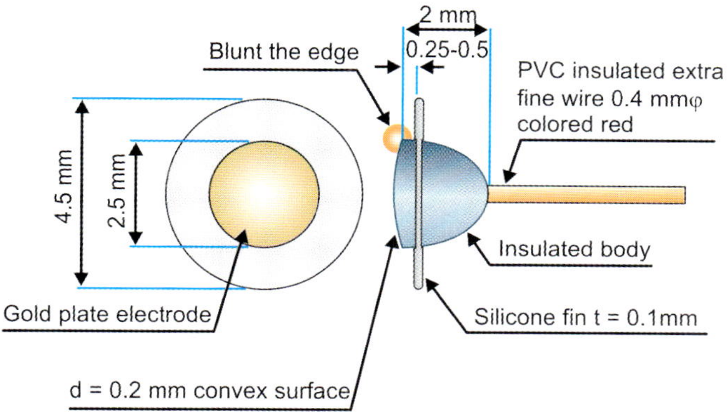

Fig. 3.3: The design of facial nerve root evoked muscle action potential electrode

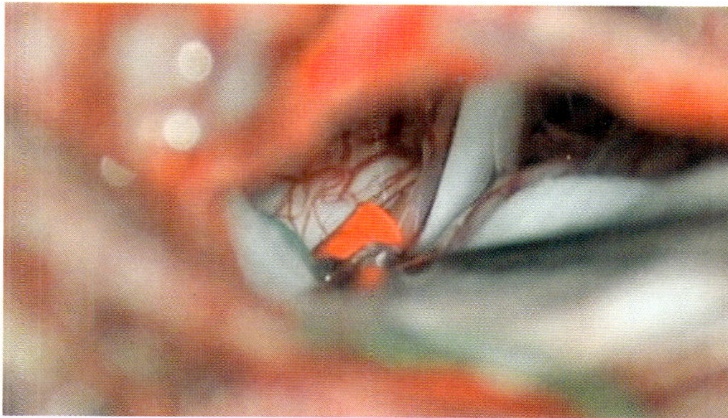

Fig. 3.4: A microscopic view of the setting of dorsal cochlear nucleus action potentials and facial nerve root evoked muscle action potential electrodes on the left side using a retrosigmoid approach

the fundus of the IAC. The size of craniotomy with the supine lateral position is small with the opening having a diameter of 25 mm. To facilitate the setting of the DNAP electrode it is designed in a teardrop shape with extention toward the caudal side.[3] The placement of the stimulant electrode should be done as early as possible in the operation, namely at the stage just after the dura mater is incised and the separation of arachnoids around the lower cranial nerves is sufficiently achieved. We normally first set the DNAP electrode and then the FREMAP electrode. In order to prevent the DNAP electrode and the attached cord from interfering in the surgical field, the electrode is inserted along the glossopharyngeal nerve, by drilling the craniotomy sufficiently inferiorly up to the condyle of the occipital bone in order to facilitate setting the DNAP electrode. Before opening the dura mater, the anesthetist is instructed to hyperventilate the patient to reduce the swelling of the cerebellum. It is of no exaggeration to say that this one step is the most important intervention for the hearing preservation operation as it facilitates the cerebrospinal fluid (CSF) to spurt out from the cistern and there is no need to use the retractor avoiding the unintended traction to the cochlear nerve. The dura mater is opened by incising it as an anteriorly based "U-shaped" flap and is sutured to the adjacent anterior soft tissue. To protect the cerebellum, we use Neuropatch (alternately, oxidized cellulose sheet can be used on the surface of the cerebellum and further covered with a neurosurgical cottonoid sheet). All the operation procedures are carried out over the Neuropatch or the neurosurgical cottonoid sheet. When the cistern around the lower cranial nerve is widely opened and the spurting of the CSF is obtained, the cerebellum spontaneously retracts toward the dorsal side and then a wide surgical field becomes available without using a retractor. After releasing the arachnoids in the caudal part of the craniotomy, the arachnoid around the REZ of the facial nerve at the brainstem and around the foramen of Luschka is removed to set the FREMAP and DNAP electrodes. The DNAP electrode is inserted along the superior margin of the glossopharyngeal nerve in front of the choroid plexus into the foramen of Luschka (Fig. 3.5). The FREMAP electrode is next adjusted over the REZ of the facial nerve just anterior to the vestibulocochlear nerve (Figs 3.4, 3.6 and 3.7).

There are cases where setting the DNAP and FREMAP electrodes becomes difficult owing to large acoustic tumors. For setting stable DNAP and FREMAP electrodes in such cases, opening the cerebello-medullary and horizontal fissures is very important. By doing so, the spontaneous cerebellum retraction is obtained and the operating space for setting up of the electrode becomes satisfactory. In such cases, the FREMAP electrode may not necessarily be set right on the REZ of the facial nerve. By exposing the glossopharyngeal nerve at the brainstem, if a part of the electrode could be set to touch the side of the brainstem on its ventral side, in most cases, enough data regarding FREMAP could be obtained. The minimum electrical current level may be raised and continuous stimulation is conducted at the minimum current level (normally between 1.5 and 2.5 mA) with stable maximum amplitude. As the area of the electrode is large, it is not dangerous even when the electrical current is raised to around 3 mA as the current density is small compared a needle-type stimulant probe, commonly used for facial nerve mapping as described later. However, there are cases where the shoulders move owing to the reaction of the accessory nerve caused by the strong electrical current. If the FREMAP amplitude does

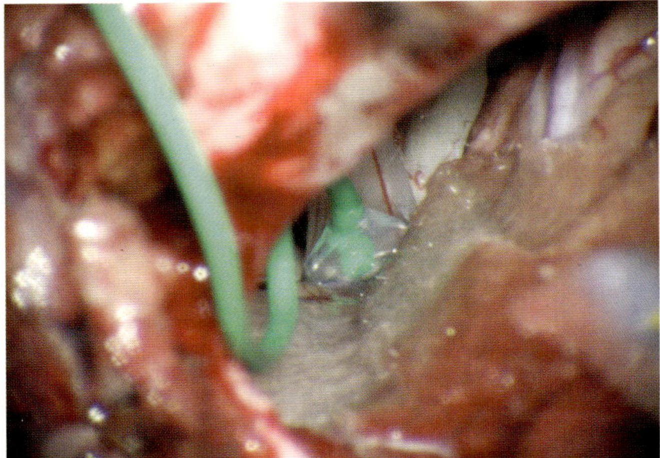

Fig. 3.5: A microscopic view of the setting of dorsal cochlear nucleus action potentials (DNAP) electrode on the left side. The DNAP electrode is inserted into the foramen of Luschka along the glosspharyngeal nerve

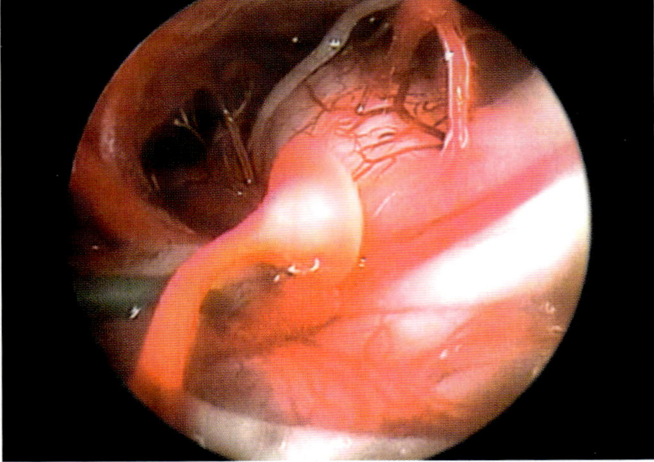

Fig. 3.6: A 30°-angled endoscopic view of the setting of dorsal cochlear nucleus action potentials (DNAP) and facial nerve root evoked muscle action potential (FREMAP) electrodes on the left side. The FREMAP electrode is on top of the REZ of the facial nerve. The DNAP electrode is set on its caudal side and the green cord extending from it could be observed

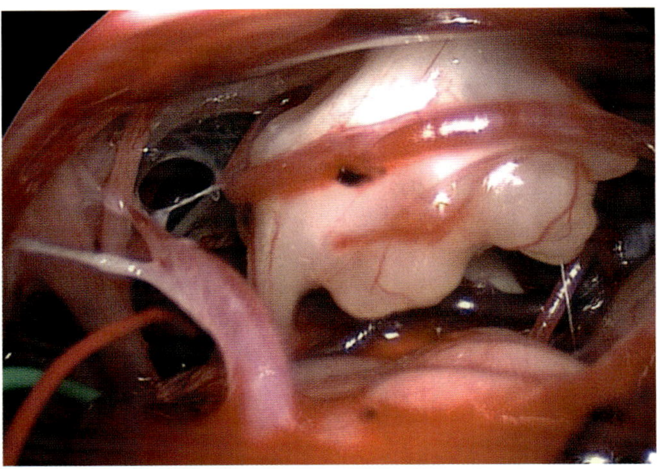

Fig. 3.7: A 30°-angled endoscopic view of the setting of dorsal cochlear nucleus action potentials (DNAP) and facial nerve root evoked muscle action potential (FREMAP) electrodes on the left side. The FREMAP electrode is on top of the REZ of the facial nerve. The DNAP electrode is set on its caudal side and the green cord extending from it could be observed

not stabilize without increasing the current, the position of the electrode needs to be changed. Actually, FREMAP could be monitored in most cases by raising the electrical current even when the electrode is partially displaced from the root of the nerve, but if the amplitude varies frequently it suggests that the electrode is completely detached from the REZ of the facial nerve, and the position of the electrode must be readjusted. If the electrode tends to get lifted from the side of the brainstem, use of a gelfoam to suppress the electrode could stabilize the FREMAP.

Depending upon the surgical technique, there could be a chance that the facial nerve gets damaged before the placement of the electrode. To avoid such incidences, we do not use the retractor at all. If the retractor needs to be used, greatest care is required, as the action to retract the cerebellum itself may cause damage to the acoustic-facial bundle. Similar to the cochlear monitoring, it is important to set the electrode from the caudal side. By doing so, the electrode and the cord attached to it will not interfere with the surgical field. However, there is a danger of serious accident if the cord of the electrode becomes trapped when drilling the IAC. The FREMAP electrode pulled out suddenly could potentially rip the artery such as the AICA apart and to avoid such mishap, we secure the cord of the electrode by suturing it to the dura mater inferiorly or to the muscle flap on the caudal side. The electrodes are set in their position while taking care to prevent contact to the tumor to a minimum.

CONTINUOUS COCHLEAR AND FACIAL NERVE MONITORING AND ITS SIGNIFICANCE

The details of the technique of dissecting the tumor from the facial and cochlear nerve are discussed later in the chapter on acoustic neuroma surgery. Intraoperative monitoring of these nerves begins by placing the respective electrodes as early as possible during the surgery. The initial stable amplitude of the FREMAP and DNAP potentials obtained is set as the base and is considered 100% (Figs 3.8 and 3.9). The surgical steps are performed by monitoring the level of DNAP and FREMAP to prevent them to fall below 40% and 65%, respectively. After the electromyographics (EMGs) of orbicularis oculi muscle and orbicularis oris muscle each are obtained stably, the maximum amplitude is set as 100% (Fig. 3.9) and the surgery, is conducted so that the amplitude during the surgery does not go below 65%. In case, it goes below 65% rapidly, there could be a possibility that the facial nerve may either be stimulated or damaged by the surgical manipulation in the immediate preceding step and the surgical manipulation must be stopped immediately. Even though the lowering of amplitude may be transient it is a sign of potentially dangerous manipulation. Ignoring it and continuing with the surgery could end up in a facial nerve paralysis after the surgery. In our experience, we noticed that when it goes lower than 30% it results in some kind of a permanent facial nerve paralysis. Therefore, even when the lowering of the amplitude is gradual, if it goes lower than 65%, all surgical manipulation should be stopped, recuperating treatment should be conducted (Figs 3.10 and 3.11), and one should wait for the amplitude to recover.[6] Sometimes surgical manipulations conducted near the facial nerve and not exactly over the facial nerve often lead to a lowering of the amplitude. In such cases, one should either change the area where the surgical manipulation is conducted or change the surgical procedure, and avoid continuing the same surgical manipulation at the same place. The facial nerve is relatively strong to endure surgical stress when compared with the cochlear nerve at the CPA, but to preserve the nerve function, it is helpful to pursue the surgical manipulation according to the information provided by the FREMAP monitoring.

There are many factors that cause the hearing loss and drop in DNAP potentials during acoustic neuroma surgery (Fig. 3.12), such as injury to cochlea or labyrinth or nerve damage due to adhesion between the tumor and the nerve, direction or the strength of the traction, methods of hemostasis and others. If the procedure could be stopped immediately, in most cases, the electrical potentials for DNAP and FREMAP recover within 30 min. It is important to patiently wait for the nerve to recover. It is important and

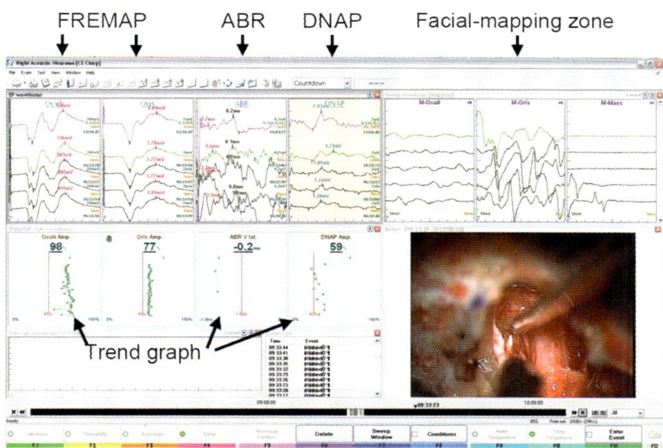

Fig. 3.8: Monitoring screen: The screen shows the images for intraoperative continuous facial (upper left) and cochlear nerve (upper right) monitoring. The various screens above show the free run waveform obtained from orbicularis oculi muscle and orbicularis oris muscle, waveforms of auditory brainstem response and dorsal cochlear nucleus action potentials (DNAP). The screens below show trend graph of percentage of amplitude of facial nerve root evoked muscle action potential (FREMAP) and DNAP as compared to that at the beginning of surgery. In the lower right is the image from the microscope showing dissection of acoustic neuroma

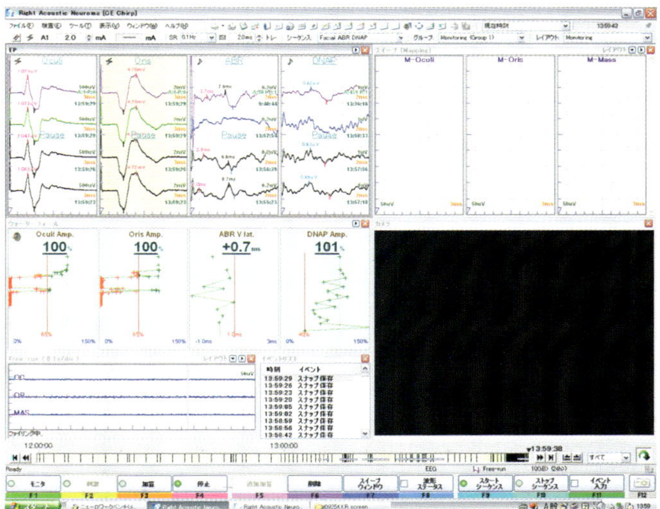

Fig. 3.9: Monitoring screen: The screen shows the images for intraoperative continuous facial (upper left) and cochlear nerve (upper right) monitoring. The various screens above show the free run wave form obtained from orbicularis oculi muscle and orbicularis oris muscle, waveforms of auditory brainstem response (ABR) and dorsal cochlear nucleus action potentials (DNAP). The screens below show trend graph of percentage of amplitude of facial nerve root evoked muscle action potential and DNAP as compared to that at the beginning of surgery

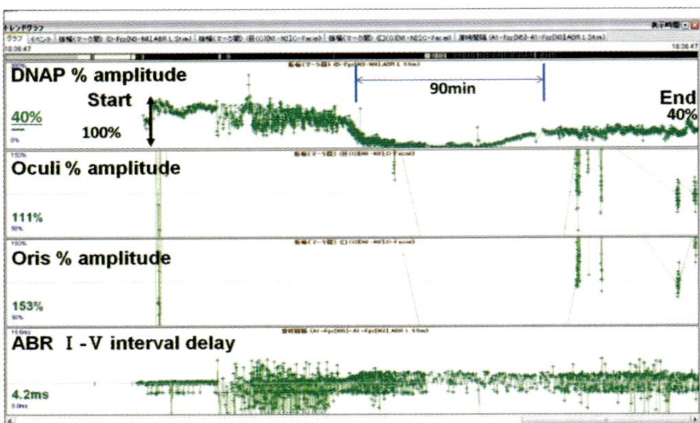

Fig. 3.10: Trend graph: dorsal cochlear nucleus action potentials (DNAP) amplitude percentage, orbicularis oculi muscle amplitude percentage, orbicularis oris muscle amplitude percentage and latency of auditory brainstem response (ABR) (I–V peak) are shown from the start to the end of monitoring with time. In this example, it could be understood that the DNAP amplitude became low and there was a 90-min standby in surgery and the surgery was resumed when its level recovered to above 40%

fundamental that the surgeon believes in the monitoring data obtained real time and be attentive in conducting the surgical procedure. If the amplitude level goes lower than the aforementioned numbers during the surgery, surgical procedures should be stopped immediately and one should wait till the potential recovers.[6] We call it recuperating therapy. This is to minimize the time of nerve damage and maximize the chance of recovery of nerve function. This is a new concept that we developed for nerve function preservation operation based on intraoperative continuous nerve monitoring. In vestibular neurotomy surgery, the decline in DNAP amplitude tends to be more or less transient, but in acoustic nerve tumor operation electrical potential is less likely to recover immediately.

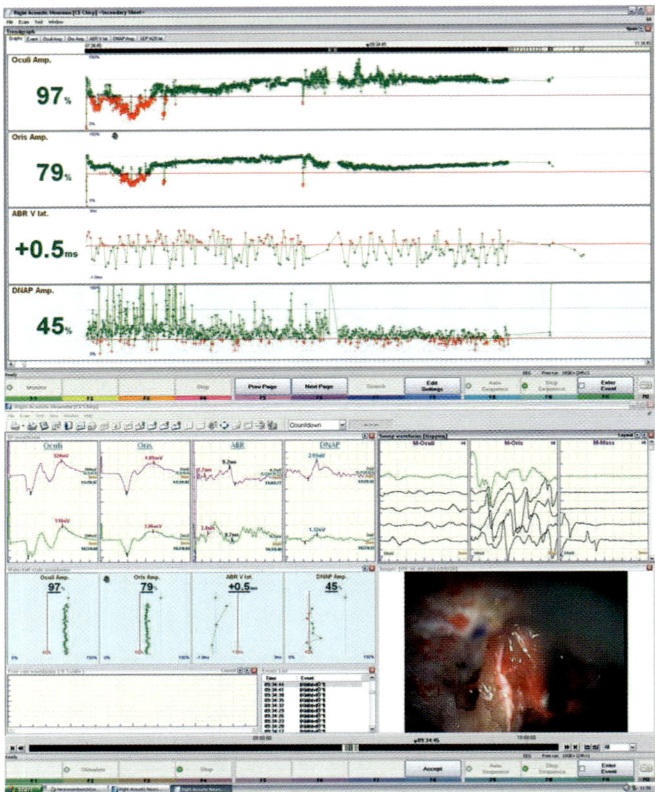

Fig. 3.11: Trend graph: Neuromaster Intraoperative Monitoring System MEE-1100 has dual screen, so we can see real-time monitoring of facial nerve root evoked muscle action potential (FREMAP), auditory brainstem response (ABR), dorsal cochlear nucleus action potentials (DNAP) and the trend graph at the same time during the surgery. Orbicularis oculi muscle amplitude percentage, orbicularis oris muscle amplitude percentage, latency of ABR (I–V peak) and DNAP amplitude percentage are shown from the start to the end of monitoring with time. In this example, it could be understood that the DNAP amplitude became low (45%) but was above 40%. Also seen is the facial nerve mapping on screen as well as in microscopic picture during acoustic neuroma dissection in the internal auditory meatus (IAM). The facial nerve mapping at 0.1 mA being conducted in the internal auditory canal (IAC) shows strong response even at 0.1 mA

COCHLEAR NERVE MAPPING BY USING DNAP ELECTRODE

We were able to obtain another revolutionary electrophysiological method by developing the DNAP electrode. Cochlear nerve mapping is a mapping (identification of nerve running position) done on vestibulocochlear nerve similar to the mapping that is being conducted by unconstrained stimulus to locate the probable site of the facial nerve. As shown in Figure 3.9, a single electrode stimulus with a weak electrical current (0.1–0.2 mA) is applied on the eighth cranial nerve. As it requires about 50 additions in order to obtain a stable wave profile, the stimulus probe should not be taken off from the stimulated part in less than 3 seconds. In order to prevent damage to the cochlear nerve a dull tip needle is used as the stimulus probe. In the CPA, the eighth cranial nerve, the cochlear nerve and the vestibular nerve runs as one nerve fascicle. But the wave profile recorded from the DNAP electrode by stimulating one of these two nerves distinguishes the difference between them. The running of the cochlear nerve can be identified using this information. The peak

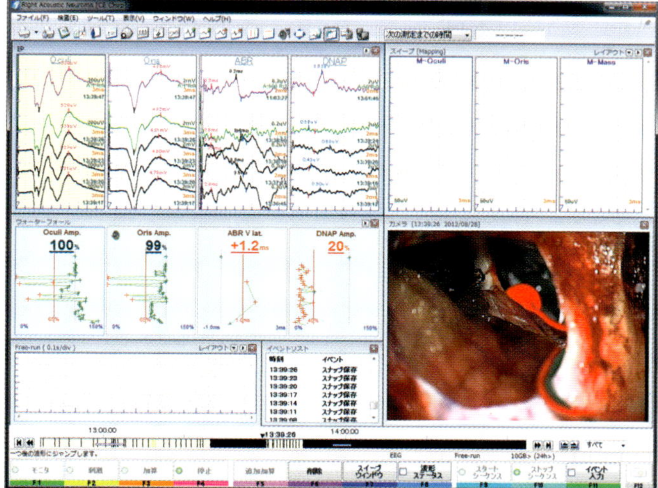

Fig. 3.12: Trend graph: dorsal cochlear nucleus action potentials (DNAP) amplitude percentage, orbicularis oculi muscle amplitude percentage, orbicularis oris muscle amplitude percentage and latency of auditory brainstem response (ABR) (I–V peak) are shown from the start to the end of monitoring with time. In this example, ABR latency got prolonged by 1.2 ms and the DNAP amplitude fell to 20% of the original. A 30-min standby in surgery was considered and the surgery was resumed when its level recovered to above 40%

observed at around 1 ms is obtained from either the cochlear nerve or the vestibular nerve; this information alone cannot distinguish from which nerve (cochlear or vestibular) the electrical potential is generated. But the peak observed at around 2 ms is seen only when the cochlear nerve is stimulated (Fig. 3.13). Thus, in case where two peaks are observed at around 1 and 2 ms, one can conclude that the cochlear nerve is running in the stimulated area (Fig. 3.13). The peak observed around 2 ms, which is delayed approximately 1 ms from the peak at around 1 ms, is hypothesized to be the time taken to travel through one synapse from its latent time. This is an electrical potential presumed to be coming from the superior olivary nucleus, which is the synapse next to the DCN, and we assume that this corresponds to the third wave of the ABR (Fig. 3.13).

This method is especially useful in an acoustic tumor surgery when the cochlear nerve is running on the surface of the tumor or the cochlear nerve is stretched and thinned and its boundary is difficult to observe. By strictly carrying out the cochlear nerve mapping and the facial nerve mapping prior to removing the tumor, the area to be removed safely can be predetermined. In vestibular neurotomy, the cochlear mapping becomes an equally important tool. The eighth cranial nerve at the CPA usually has the cochlear nerve fibers on the caudal side and the vestibular nerve fibers usually run on the rostral side. But it is known that there are a range of variations.[7] In a survey conducted after the vestibular neurotomy,[7] the ratio of unsuccessful complete neurotomy suspected based on these anatomical backgrounds was up to 15%. The exact cochlear nerve position can now be identified with the cochlear nerve mapping (Figs 3.13 and 3.14) and it became possible to conduct the vestibular neurotomy with higher certainty. Now the protocol is to first carry out the cochlear nerve mapping on the eighth cranial nerve and identify the cleavage line with the vestibular nerve. While observing the change in ABR and DNAP monitoring, only the vestibular nerve is gradually cut off. After the section, a mapping on the cross section is conducted and when it shows that some fibers of vestibular nerve remain, they are peeled off from the cochlear nerve and cut off.

FACIAL NERVE MAPPING

Facial nerve-monitoring method by unconstraint stimulation applied to a facial nerve using a monopolar stimulator nowadays is often called facial nerve mapping as it allows detecting the position of the facial nerve. Even before continuous facial nerve-monitoring technology appeared, it was reported[8,9] as an intraoperative monitoring technology and is currently the most prevalent facial nerve-monitoring method. Although there may be some differences among the stimulation instruments, if a response from the facial muscles of expression dominating the facial nerve could be obtained with stimulation of 0.1 mA, it means that the stimulation was right on top of the facial nerve. It shows that as the amount of the electrical current, where a response is obtained, gets higher, the distance to the facial nerve gets farther.[3] This technology is used in parotid gland surgery, middle ear surgery and in CPA surgery (especially in acoustic tumor surgery). Except where the facial nerve could be observed directly, prediction of the running of the facial nerve is made by first applying 1 mA stimulation. If a response is obtained at 1mA, the stimulation is continued with the amount of the electrical current gradually reduced and by doing so approximate distance to the facial nerve is assessed. If there is a response at 0.1 mA, it is determined that it is from the facial nerve itself (Fig. 3.15).

SPECIAL FEATURES OF DNAP/FREMAP MONITORING INSTRUMENT

For both the DNAP and the FREMAP measurements, intraoperative monitoring system MEE1200 (European

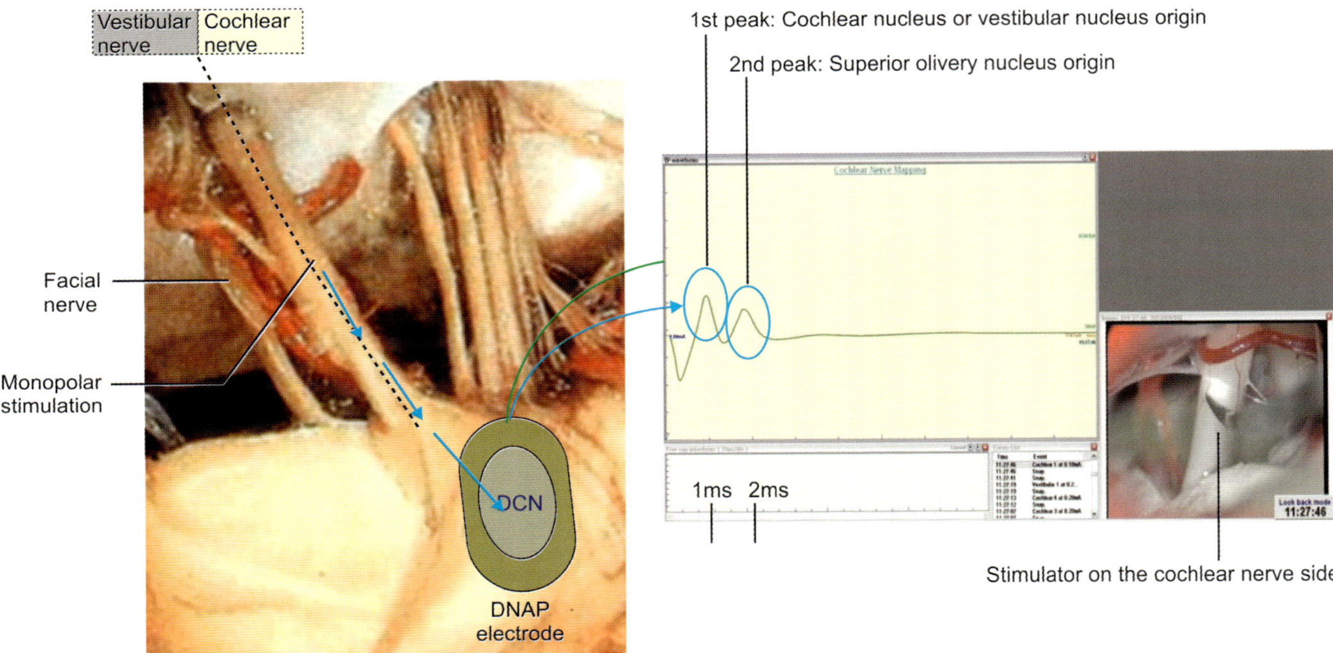

Fig. 3.13: Cochlear nerve mapping: On stimulation of the cochlear nerve two peaks are observed (blue circles) at around 1 and 2 ms

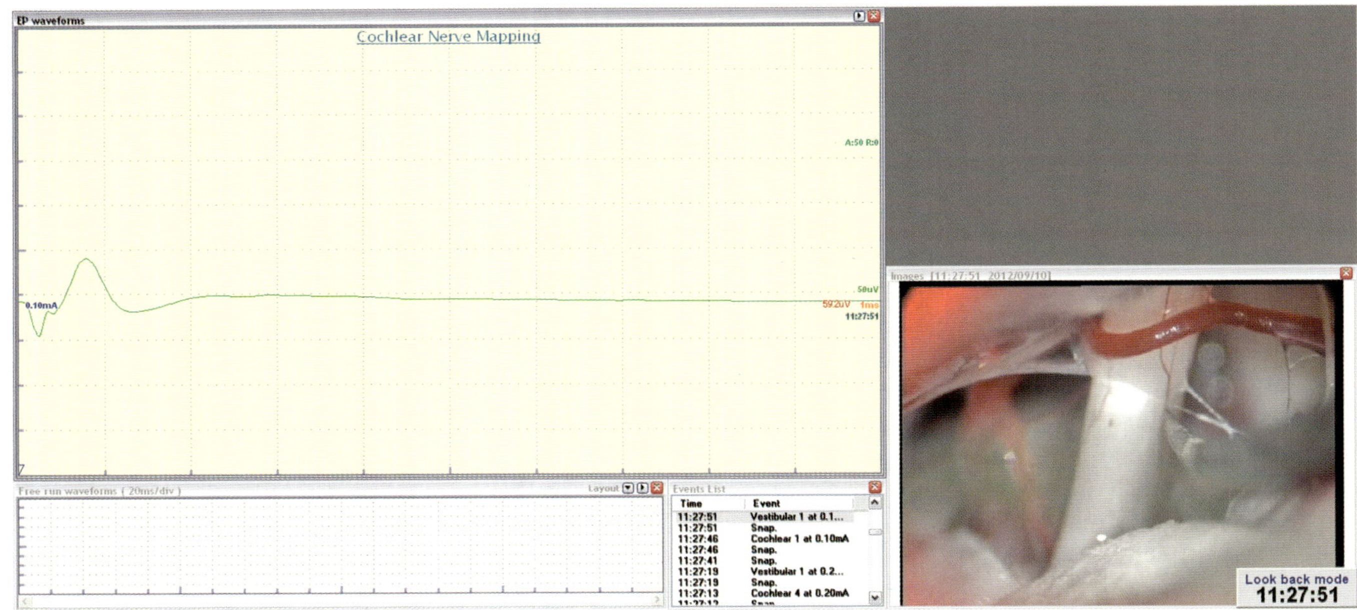

Fig. 3.14: Cochlear nerve mapping: On stimulation of the vestibular nerve only one peak is observed at around 1 ms

type designated MEE-1100) by NIHON KOHDEN is used (Fig. 3.16). By introducing the new DNAP and FREMAP monitoring instruments, it becomes possible to consolidate the monitoring and mapping functions of both the facial and the cochlear nerves (which were done previously with two instruments) in one instrument and display on one monitor, whereby decisions could be easily made by viewing all monitoring information at once (Fig. 3.8). In addition, as images from the operating microscope and endoscope are also displayed in the monitoring screen, it becomes another unique feature so that both the surgeon and the neurophysiologist in charge of the

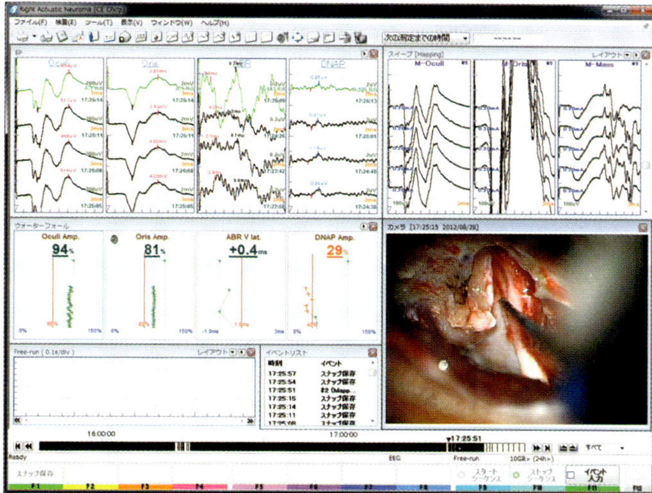

Fig. 3.15: Facial nerve mapping: Image on the right upper corner shows facial nerve mapping at 0.1 mA being conducted in the internal auditory canal (as seen in the microscopic picture). Strong response is obtained even at 0.1 mA, suggesting the stimulator to be on the facial nerve

monitoring could get hold of what was going on in the surgery at the same time. And by having dual display in the monitoring screen, it becomes possible to show in another screen the trend graph of the FREMAP, ABR and DNAP, enabling exactly which surgical practice gave the damage to the nerve when, where and of what kind (Fig. 3.11). The instrument is very useful to the surgeon as it gives feedback information not only during the surgery but even after.

CONCLUSION

The DNAP, FREMAP and cochlear nerve mapping are powerful tools in nerve function preservation operation. But it does not mean that just having them will allow a nerve function preservation operation. It goes without saying that for these tools to exert their force, knowledge of the basics of surgical procedure and clinical anatomy, having the technique to cope with various troubles and having the knowledge and experience to avoid them is indispensable. Today when medical litigations are increasing rapidly, the next generation surgeons have to acquire these operation techniques with extreme difficulty. The monitoring instrument described here will become a very valuable tool for the next generation surgeons. While there may be fewer actual cases, with the feedback from the monitoring surgery, the surgeon can learn more than what he experienced.

If the nerve function preservation rate increases under a new concept of monitoring-based surgery, the indications

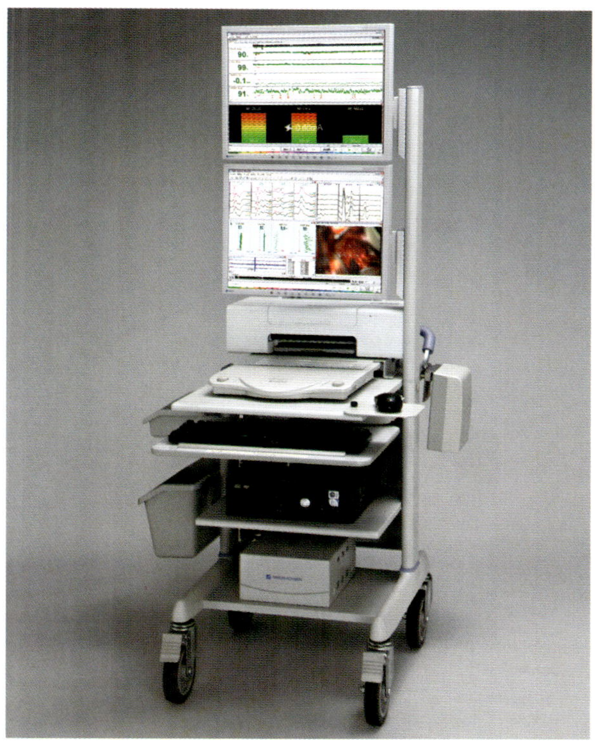

Fig. 3.16: Monitoring instrument: Neuromaster Intraoperative Monitoring System MEE-1100 made by NIHON KOHDEN

of acoustic tumor surgery should gradually change. We take a standby during the surgery if the electrical potential worsens, expecting that it recovers by changing the surgical procedure or the part to operate according to the nerve electrical potential obtained real time. If the hearing preservation is the major target, it is easier technically to preserve when the size of the tumor size is small. Even when the tumor is comparatively large, we try not to change the hearing class to what target we set prior to the surgery as far as DNAP could be measured. On the other hand, even though the tumor size may be small and the hearing class is good, there were cases where due to the status of the IAC the DNAP dropped suddenly and hearing preservation failed or the tumor could not be removed completely. The dilemma that a residual tumor increases the danger of a recurrence and a complete removal of the tumor increases the danger of a nerve function disorder makes the surgery of this benign tumor disease difficult. We have repeatedly discussed with many patients and their families about nerve function preservation and residual tumor. Through such discussions the conclusion we reached is "to operate depending on the numerical value given by intraoperative continuous nerve monitoring and finishing in a result which meets as much as possible what the patient requests." We came to the conclusion that the rate of tumor remnant and the level of nerve function preservation are something that the surgeon should not decide, and the surgeon operating on an acoustic tumor with the use of monitoring should take a position "to do his best during surgery believing the monitoring data and target the results according to the will of the patient." It could be considered right to take a view to wait and scan the small tumor that is not changing, but at the same time one has to repeatedly check and confirm how the patient would think in case the nerve function deteriorates even though the tumor may be small. We feel that today we have entered an era when the decision of whether to leave the tumor alone for a regular follow-up, have a monitoring surgery, or consider a gamma knife therapy should be exhibited to the patient and let the patient choose.

REFERENCES

1. Møller AR, Jannetta PJ. Monitoring auditory functions during cranial nerve microvascular decompression operations by direct recording from the eighth nerve. J Neurosurg. 1983;59:493–9.
2. Kileny PR, Niparko JK, Shepard NT, Kemink JL. Neurophysiologic intraoperative monitoring: Auditory function. Am J Otol. 1988;9:17–24.
3. Taniguchi M. Intraoperative monitoring for facial nerve preservation during acoustic neurinoma removal. Rinsho Noha. 1998;40(9):553–8.
4. Amano M, Kohno M, Nagata O, Taniguchi M, Sora S, Sato H. Intraoperative continuous monitoring of evoked facial nerve electromyograms in acoustic neuroma surgery. Acta Neurochir. 2011;53:1059–67.
5. Nakatomi H, Miyazaki H, Tanaka M, Kin T, Yoshino M, Oyama H, Usui M, Sano H, Okada M, Moriyama H, Kaga K, Saito N. Visualizing, tracking neural function with continuous direct brainstem evoked potentials and discriminating reversible injury by intraoperative extended recuperating treatment improved functional preservation in acoustic neuroma surgery. (Submitted to J Neurosurg).
6. Miyazaki H, Nakatomi H, Moriyama H. Minimally invasive keyhole retrosigmoid approach for vestibular schwannoma - Tear drop Euro coin burr hole technique. Otol Jpn. 2008;18(5):675-81.
7. Leveque M, Seidermann L, Tran H, Lanqaqne T, Chays A. Vestibular function outcomes after vestibular neurectomy in Meniere disease: can vestibular neurectomy provide complete vestibular differentiation? Auris Nasus Larynx. 2010;37(3):308–13.
8. Delgado TE, Buchheit WA, Rosenholtz HR, Chrissian S. Intraoperative monitoring of facial muscle evoked responses obtained by intracranial stimulation of the facial nerve: A more accurate technique for facial nerve dissection. Neurosurgery. 1979;4(5):418–21.
9. Møller AR, Jannetta P. Preservation of facial function during removal of acoustic neuromas. Use of monopolar constant-voltage stimulation and EMG. J Neurosurg. 1984;61:757–60.

Minimally Invasive Retrosigmoid Approach (MIRA)

4

INTRODUCTION

The first attempts to assess cerebellopontine angle (CPA) were made nearly a century ago by Fraenkel[1] et al. and Krause[2] separately in the early twentieth century for removal of tumors of CPA, especially acoustic neuroma. They described the suboccipital craniotomy to give a wide view of the posterior fossa and since then this approach has been the mainstay of access to this area by neurosurgeons. Cushing[3] popularized this operation, consisting of bilateral exposure of the posterior fossa, operating the patient in the prone position. It was Dandy,[4] who described the unilateral suboccipital approach in the seated position with considerable reduction in mortality rates. By tradition, the suboccipital approach was performed for large to giant acoustic neuromas without the illumination and magnification provided by the microscope. It consisted of a long straight incision extending well into the neck, elevation of the nuchal muscles from the posterior aspect and undersurface of the occipital bone, and removal of a large segment of the bone, extending laterally to the sigmoid sinus, medially to the midline, superior to the transverse sinus and inferior to the foramen magnum. Following opening of the dura, a segment of cerebellum was resected to gain access to the CPA, after which the tumor could be removed. This large opening and approach was required owing to lack of technology in the form of an operating microscope, inadequate lighting and instrumentation. With the advent of the operating microscope and improvement in anesthesia techniques, the suboccipital approach underwent many modifications, ultimately resulting in what has come to be called the retrosigmoid approach. With the progress in diagnostic imaging technology and audiological advances, early diagnosis for small acoustic neuroma and meningioma (that are often minimally symptomatic or totally asymptomatic) has become possible[5] and there has been an increase in chance when neurovascular conflict in CPA is diagnosed as the cause of a cranial nerve dysfunction. Minimally invasive functional surgery is demanded by the modern society for such benign pathologies of CPA. By functional surgery of CPA, we mean surgery performed to preserve functions of all the cranial nerves that are not already affected by the disease pathology with safety and minimal invasion. The minimally invasive retrosigmoid approach (MIRA) was first described by senior author, J Magnan, and his teachers Bremond and Garcin in 1974.[6,7] This approach involves a small curved incision, stopping well above the undersurface of the skull, no dissection of nuchal muscles from the occipital bone, a limited removal of bone behind the sigmoid sinus (around 2 cm in diameter), and no resection or mechanical retraction of the cerebellum. Minimally invasive functional surgery is less invasive with shorter postoperative recovery and is technically feasible for most of the surgeons[8] after obtaining training with cadaver models. This approach is also described as the "keyhole approach," with the motto of "smaller is safer" and not "smaller is better." At the same time, it should not be forgotten that CPA lesion surgery is an extremely delicate and challenging surgery, which has to be performed carefully with the goal of minimal complications and no residual disease. Since 1990, the MIRA has been performed by us by combining the use of an endoscope along with a microscope to achieve a safer, more reliable exploration through the keyhole retrosigmoid approach for CPA surgery. Since the early 1990s, there has been increasing literature[9–18] emphasizing the various advantages of using straight and angled endoscopes with videoendoscopic equipment in CPA surgeries for improved surgical exposure in this difficult-to-reach area. With its wide angle of illumination, the endoscope was able to provide a panoramic view of neurovascular structures in the CPA and to better understand their relationships with each other without the need for retraction or dissection of the cerebellum. Incorporating the use of videoendoscopy in the surgical armamentorium along with MIRA has made an important impact in reducing the morbidity of the CPA to a minimum. The rate of major complications during the past 40 years of our practicing this approach has been considerably low as compared to other more invasive conventional approaches. The combinations of endoscopes together with microsurgery provide accurate information and are now becoming indispensable for these operations with the goal toward functional surgery. We have been performing surgeries on various CPA lesions by applying this outstanding minimal retrosigmoid approach since 1974 with good results reported.[14–21]

INDICATION

By utilizing MIRA, a wide variety of CPA operations are performed as function-preserving surgery. The most common functional surgeries performed by this approach are as follows:

1. Microvascular decompression for hemifacial spasm, trigeminal and glossopharyngeal neuralgia, certain cochleovestibular disorders (based on a careful clinical, audiological and radiological assessment of the patient, on the onset, on the intensity, on the duration and frequency of the episodes, on the evolution and trigger factors and on psychophysical involvement).
2. Tumor removal of small and medium size progressively increasing acoustic neurinoma, CPA meningioma, epidermoid cyst, etc. where hearing preservation is possible.
3. Vestibular neurotomy for disabling refractory Meniere's disease with repeated dizziness attacks (based on the frequency of the vertigo episodes, on the degree of hearing impairment in the affected ear as well as the other ear and careful consideration of the patient's emotional state and his/her professional status).

BASICS OF LATERAL SKULL BASE SURGERY

Neurotologic surgery encompasses a wide range of procedures including many variations of presigmoid transpetrosal approaches and retrosigmoid approaches for resection of CPA tumors and functional surgery for cranial nerves. All such operations employ microsurgical techniques. The basic principles of neurotologic surgery are similar to any other surgery, but for the intricate anatomy and microscopic demands, there are high chances for compromise in the final results. Parfocal setup of operating microscope, appropriate use of magnification and binocular three-dimensional microscopic vision for depth perception improves safety and accuracy of the surgery. The safe use of the endoscope and its role cannot be understated and it takes a few sessions before optimal adaptation.

The successful lateral skull base surgeon must master the following three major categories of technical skills:

1. A complete and thorough knowledge of the anatomy of the temporal bone with associated skull base and CPA.
2. A system of incisions and approaches capable of producing excellent exposure.
3. A consistent method of dealing with surgical hemorrhage and closure technique with minimal cerebrospinal fluid (CSF) leak and wound complication.

ROLE OF CADAVER DISSECTION AND KNOWLEDGE OF TEMPORAL BONE AND CPA ANATOMY

Cadaveric temporal bone and lateral skull base dissection provides the platform to master the temporal bone and CPA anatomy as well as provides skills to utilize this knowledge to navigate around the entire temporal bone and CPA from one constant landmark to another. This ability to orient and navigate through the most intricate anatomy in the temporal bone and CPA provides the confidence to do the same in the diseased patients with minimal efforts and anxiety. Cadaveric dissection provides an opportunity to perform practically any procedure many times in the laboratory before transferring the acquired skills and knowledge to the operating room. Otologists are fortunate to be able to learn and increase the technical skill by cadaver temporal bone dissection. The temporal bone dissection lab setup should simulate the operation theater setup as closely as possible. One can begin temporal dissection by exploring the temporal bone anatomy by drilling it progressively to gain a three-dimensional orientation of the relations of various structures to each other, and especially with facial nerve. Once the general knowledge of the temporal anatomy is mastered, then each surgical approach should be practiced separately. Retrosigmoid approach is practiced in whole-head specimen (preferably after injecting different colored silicone in arteries and veins/sinuses of posterior cranial fossa). The hands-on experience with the videoendoscopic procedure on a cadaver infuses confidence to use the same in the operation theater. Practicing each surgical procedure repeatedly on a cadaver infuses surgical confidence, which is scanty in the early formative years and remains so if not mastered. Insufficient surgeons are made, not born. Poor habits translate into poor surgical results.

The secret of temporal bone and CPA surgery is in knowing the anatomical landmarks and how to use them. Sometimes this is difficult and from time to time even the most able surgeon will find himself temporarily disoriented. In such situations, one must go to another part of the surgical field, find a known landmark and then work back into the difficult area. One should treat the cranial nerves as a friend, not a foe. If you know where it is all the time, chances are little for it to be inadvertently damaged. Incomplete knowledge is the cause for fear and failures. Lastly, the knowledge of temporal bone and CPA anatomy cannot not be gained in a day or a week by attending a single workshop (we do not condemn workshops, it helps in getting initial orientation to the subject), but requires dissection for many hours a week for many months. All through his carrier the surgeon always learns something more while practicing in the anatomic laboratory.

IMPORTANCE OF GOOD EXPOSURE

One of the basic surgical principles is to obtain adequate exposure of the operative site. In the retrosigmoid approach surgery, this implies the place and type of incision one employs to gain access to the craniotomy site, the location and size of craniotomy based on constant landmarks such as the emissary vein and the digastric ridge, and complete relaxation of the cerebellum by hyperventilation to achieve this purpose. These maneuvers provide an excellent view of the contents of the CPA. Changing the height and tilt of the operating table and changing the angle of the microscope makes most areas of the CPA and internal acoustic meatus accessible. Finally, the use of 30°- angled endoscope is routinely used to improve the exposure and mapping of the contents of the CPA as per the requirement for various surgeries of CPA.

HEMOSTASIS DURING SURGERY

One of the main difficulties most amateur surgeons encounter in their first attempts at neurotologic surgery is the control of perioperative bleeding. It is frustrating to struggle to carry out a particular step of the surgery in a pool of blood. It is important to understand the concepts of maintaining hemostasis as this will significantly shorten the operative time and improve the final outcome. The basic concept is to control hemorrhage as it occurs and to prevent it whenever possible.

Local anesthesia (surface anesthesia and infiltration with 1% lignocaine with 1:100,000 adrenaline) as mentioned later has a vital role in maintaining hemostasis in soft tissue dissection for craniotomy. Local anesthetic infiltration precedes surgery by at least 10 min. Monopolar cautery is useful for the initial soft tissue dissection, but bipolar cautery helps to control bleeding in an atraumatic manner within the CPA as the electrical current passes between the two tips only and not through the whole body to the neutral electrode as in monopolar cautery. Reduce the power of bipolar coagulation when using directly overexposed dura/sinus and it is better to be conservative in the use of excessive cautery over the exposed dura as that can lead to a defect in the dura and subsequent CSF leak.

Diamond burr is very effective in controlling bleeding from small blood vessels in the bone. Rotating diamond burr can be placed over the bleeding bone with gentle pressure without irrigation to plug the bleeding vessel by bone dust. Bone wax may be required for the control of bleeding from larger blood vessels or the emissary vein under the bone. Bleeding from the emissary vein can be reduced by preventive bipolar cauterization before cutting it. In a large emissary vein, packing with a piece of oxidized cellulose (Surgicel) is usually required.

A controlled suction-irrigation cleans the operating field with saline solution. While using the bipolar cautery, the tips of the cautery probe are irrigated with saline to prevent generation of local heat and avoid adhesion between cautery tips and the soft tissue. Bipolar cautery is not safe to use at certain situations like bleeding from close proximity to cranial nerve or diffuse oozing without a pinpoint bleeder. In such cases a piece of Surgicel can be placed over the bleeding site with mild pressure from neurosurgical cottonoid.

Management of the accidentally injured lateral sinus or dehiscent jugular bulb consists of covering the defect immediately with a finger or cottonoid to prevent air embolism. It is then usually controlled by placing a piece of gelatin sponge (Gelfoam) or Surgicel over the venous rent and compressing it with a larger size of cottonoid. Extraluminal sealing of the defect with a large piece of Surgicel followed by mild pressure from neurosurgical cottonoid or bone wax (particularly if further drilling is required in same place) is occasionally required to control a much bigger tear. While controlling bleeding from the sinus, care should be taken to avoid packing with very small pieces of Surgicel to avoid its embolization in venous circulation. A few minutes spared for achieving hemostasis is rewarded as it prevents struggling later while working in the CPA for tumor removal or vascular decompression.

CLOSURE

Closure is particularly more important in intracranial surgery compared to other surgeries as postoperative CSF leak is the most commonly reported and potentially hazardous complication following craniotomy. The dura should be approximated tightly. We routinely fortify the closure with absorbable polyglactin-derived artificial Durapatch and fibrin glue. The accidentally opened mastoid air cells must be tirelessly pursued and sealed with bone wax and soft tissue. The subcutaneous and skin incisions are initially planned in opposite directions as discussed later to further strengthen the closure. The use of abdominal fat is mandatory in revision surgery or in combined presigmoid retrolabyrinthine and retrosigmoid approaches.

ROLE OF SYSTEMATIC TRAINING AND STANDARDIZATION OF SURGICAL STEPS

The present generation is lucky to be seated on the shoulder of giants, whose dedication, perseverance in research, innovation for better outcome and zeal of teaching new generations of neurotologists/neurosurgeons have given birth to the present era of excellence. The young neurotologists/neurosurgeons now have an option to carve a career in neurotology and should not miss the opportunity to train under such stalwarts in a systematic fashion. The importance of steady stepwise training for gaining surgical confidence under an expert surgeon cannot be understated.

The aspiring neurotologic surgeon should learn optimal techniques that can be adapted to a variety of patients and pathologic conditions. The repertoire should include a standard preparation, injection of local anesthesia, incisions, craniotomy/labyrinthectomy, exposure of CPA, and dissection and wound closure. It should be performed in a standardized manner to gain proficiency and speed. The compulsive application of each and every surgical step in a standardized pattern maximizes the chances of successful results and anything less is a compromise. Finally, mastering the neurotologic technique (like any surgical technique) requires discipline, dedication, knowledge, judgment and precision, and is achieved in that order.

SURGICAL PROCEDURE

Preoperative Patient Evaluation

Before surgery the patient has to be thoroughly evaluated for the disease pathology that has led to consideration for surgery and for the preoperative evaluation of the fitness for major surgery (retrosigmoid craniotomy and procedure as per the pathology) under general anesthesia.

The preoperative assessment of patient CPA pathology includes thorough history taking not only for confirming the diagnosis but also to assess the amount of psychological and physical disability caused by the symptoms to the patient. Complete ENT and neurological examination is performed. Preoperative elaborative audiological and vestibular evaluation is performed, especially in patients with acoustic neuroma, Meniere's disease and vascular compression syndromes involving the vestibulocochlear nerve. This includes pure tone audiometry (PTA), speech discrimination score (SDS), auditory brainstem responses (ABR) and videonystagmography (VNG). Radiological evaluation is a must in all the cases undergoing MIRA. For most of the lesions, magnetic resonance imaging (MRI), with or without gadolinium contrast, is the study of choice. Magnetic resonance imaging in both T1 and T2 three-dimensional Fourier transform (3DFT) sequences is the most effective method of delineating both the cranial nerves and the surrounding vascular structures in the CPA. The T2 is carried out using constructive interference in steady state (CISS) sequences.[22] Imaging of the CPA is done with serial thin slices of 0.4 mm thickness. The axial plane offers the most comprehensive and demonstrative images. Magnetic resonance imaging for acoustic neuroma reveals a filling defect in the CSF on T2 images and is brightly enhancing on postcontrast T1 images. Magnetic resonance imaging is performed to evaluate whether the tumor is intracanalicular or extra-axial, the initial size of the extra-axial part of the tumor (measured as maximum diameter as well as total volume of the tumor), whether it is progressively increasing in size on follow-up studies (for small intracanalicular tumors) and to know the relation of the tumor with the fundus of the internal auditory meatus (IAM).

Magnetic resonance imaging is able to reproduce the anatomy of the CPA and to demonstrate the presence of a neurovascular conflict in vascular compression syndromes using the T2 CISS sequences with serial thin slices. It also eliminates other potential causes of vascular compression syndromes such as a tumoral process or multiple sclerosis. To confirm the diagnosis of vascular compression syndromes, the single presence of a neurovascular contact is not sufficient. Several radiological criteria are required, with some variability regarding the cranial nerves involved. These criteria are illustrated below. Common criteria include a perpendicular contact between the vascular loop and the cranial nerve, visualized along two different perpendicular planes, and a distortion of the nerve or other neural structures. For the facial nerve, the location of the conflict at the root exit zone (REZ) of the nerve and the distortion of the brainstem at this level are additional criteria. The most common offending vessels in the hemifacial spasm are the posterior inferior cerebellar artery (PICA) and a dolicho vertebral artery. For the trigeminal nerve, the reduction in diameter is an additional criterion. The most common offending vessel is the superior cerebellar artery (SCA), but in 20% of cases, a venous structure (aberrant trigeminal vein) might be the cause of the conflict, and it is visible only on T1 with gadolinium. For the auditory nerve, we expect to see displacement of the nerve with a certain distance between the facial and cochlear nerves, with an imprint on the nerve and reduction in its diameter, and with brainstem distortion caused by the vascular structure at the level of the REZ of the cochlear nerve.

Once the diagnosis is confirmed, the patient is informed about the various treatment options available. Most of the pathologies discussed in this book are functional disorders leading to poor quality of life and are usually not life threatening. The patient is explained about the surgical procedure and its associated risks, anesthesia risks, expected outcome and anticipated recovery time. The postoperative care and follow-up plans are discussed. It should be an informed choice of the patient to demand surgery.

The progressive increase in life expectancy and improved quality of life, typical of industrialized countries, has exposed neurotologists to an increasing number of requests for surgery by elderly patients. Meniere's disease and the neurovascular conflicts of the CPA are undoubtedly a disabling disorder for elderly patients, which produce a worsening of their quality of life and are an obstacle to their permanence in working and social life. Progress in otoneurosurgical techniques with the introduction of endoscopic procedures, improvements in anesthesia techniques, and the increasingly widespread use of intraoperative nerve monitoring devices have made it possible to expand the range of elderly patients eligible for surgery on whom the retrosigmoid approach allows for very low invasiveness and a reduction in operating time and morbidity.[22] The remaining life expectancy, associated general health and the diminished capacity to equilibrate postoperatively are age-related factors that are to be considered. The major advantage of the minimally invasive posterior fossa approach is its safety in the elderly population above 70 years of age.[22] It is even easier to perform MIRA in the elderly due to the cerebellum atrophy.

Once the decision for surgery is made, the routine preoperative work-up including the hematological and radiological evaluation, consultation with the anesthetist and further work-up for any associated chronic disease is completed by the concerned consultant. Proper control of diabetes and hypertension is ensured. Patients taking anticoagulation medicines are informed to stop the medicines 1 week before the procedure after consent from the treating internist. The patient is routinely given preoperative anxiolytics and the hair cleaned with antiseptic shampoo the evening and the morning before surgery.

Operation Theater Requirement and Setup

Neurotologic surgery requires substantial institutional infrastructure in the form of a well-equipped operation theater, intensive care unit (ICU), preferably an in-house imaging unit with facilities of computed tomography (CT) scan and MRI, and most of all, well-trained paramedical staff. The operation theater must be large enough to easily accommodate all the gadgets required for the neurosurgical intervention. The normal armamentarium of the neurotologist includes an operating microscope, a surgical drill, a monopolar and bipolar cautery, an ultrasonic aspirator and a cranial-nerve monitoring unit apart from the anesthetic requirements for neuroanesthesia. The ICU should be equipped with monitors and personnel trained to deal with postoperative complications. The paramedical staff includes a consistent team of scrub nurses solely for neurotologic surgery, personnel trained in intraoperative monitoring including monitoring of the cochlear nerve, and a postoperative rehabilitation team.

The operative room setup that we prefer is shown in Figures 4.1 to 4.5. The surgeon sits on the side of the patient's head and the microscope is placed opposite the surgeon. The scrub nurse is seated beside the head of the patient and the surgical instrument trolleys are placed on top of the patient's head. The anesthetic setup and the anesthetist are always at the foot end of the patient. The electrophysiological monitoring setup is situated on the foot end of the patient beside the anesthetist. The drill, ultrasound aspirator and cautery units are located on the lower part of the operation table, preferably on the same side as the surgeon. The endoscopic trolley with light source, camera and video monitoring, and recording system are located beside the operating microscope on the opposite side of the patient. We prefer to have the foot pedals of suction and the drill to be in the surgeon's control (Fig. 4.6), and leave the control of the bipolar cautery for the scrub nurse to operate. We always prefer to use the suction foot control for the amount of suction to be transferred to the operating field as it has the potential to cause maximum damage during CPA surgery, if not utilized judiciously.

Anesthesia

All the patients are seen by the anesthetist at least 2 days prior to surgery. A detailed anesthetic history is taken and investigations studied. Any prior comorbid condition and ongoing medicines are noted and consultation with the appropriate consultant planned, if necessary. A preoperative intravenous antibiotic (1.0 gm cefazolin) is administered and intravenous midazolam is used for premedication half an hour before intubation. Routine monitoring of multiple parameters is done including blood pressure, pulse and respiratory rate, oxygen saturation and capnography. In patients requiring tumor removal by MIRA, urinary catheterization is performed after intubation to facilitate urine output monitoring. We do not use central venous line and arterial line in all our patients as a routine and they are considered only in special cases. After preoxygenation, induction is accomplished with thiopental, propofol and sufentanyl. The short-acting muscle relaxant, atracurium, is avoided or is used only initially to facilitate laryngoscopy and endotracheal intubation. The action of the muscle relaxant wears off by half an hour and is not repeated further to facilitate facial nerve monitoring. The patient is put on mechanical ventilation and normocarbia maintained. As the surgeon is about to begin craniotomy and expose the dura, the patient is hyperventilated to obtain a hypocapnia (in the range of 24–26 mmHg), which helps spontaneous cerebellar retraction to diminish the intracranial pressure before opening the dura. This step allows an easy penetration in the CPA without the use of a cerebellar retractor. The progress in neuroanesthesia makes it unnecessary to use lumbar puncture and mannitol 20% infusion to help spontaneous cerebellar retraction. Hyperventilation is not required after opening the posterior cisterna. Profound and balanced anesthesia is maintained by the complementary use of analgesics, hypnotics and neuroleptics (continuous intravenous perfusion of propofol and su/remifentanyl and inhalational isoflurane). Finally, the emergence from anesthesia should be smooth and should avoid extreme blood pressure fluctuations and coughing. The patients are extubated in the operation theater and shifted to a step down unit for observation overnight.

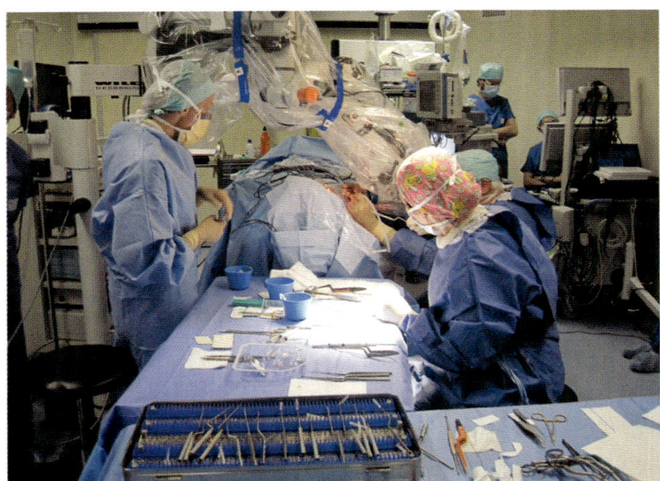

Fig. 4.1: The operation theater setup during microscopic part of surgical procedure

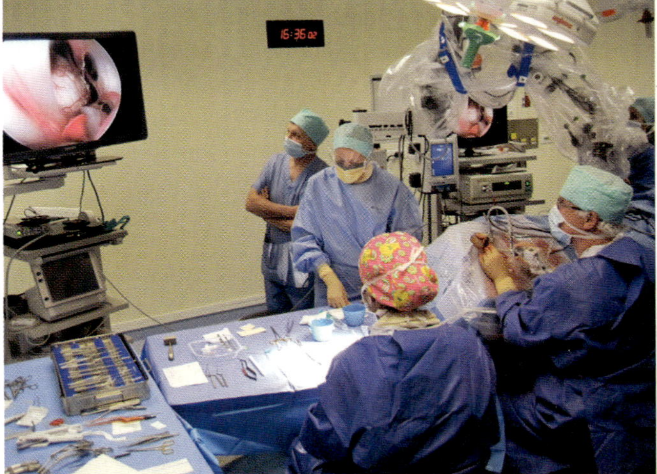

Fig. 4.2: The operation theater setup during endoscopic part of surgical procedure

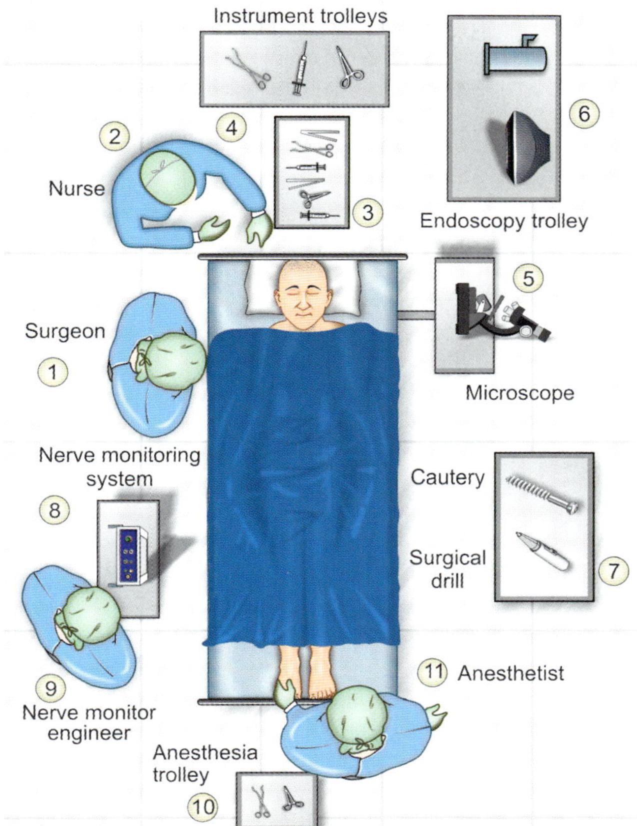

Fig. 4.3: The diagrammatic picture showing operation theater setup: 1. Surgeon; 2. Nurse; 3 and 4. Instrument trolleys; 5. Microscope; 6. Endoscopic screen with trolley for camera, recording system etc.; 7. Extra trolley for surgical drill, cautery etc; 8. Nerve monitoring system; 9. Nerve monitor engineer; 10. Anesthesia trolley; 11. Anesthetist

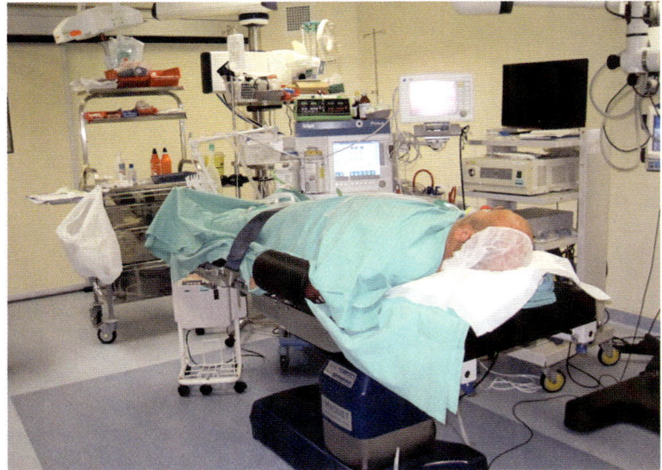

Fig. 4.5: Supine "otologic" position is preferred by us in retrosigmoid as well as presigmoid approach

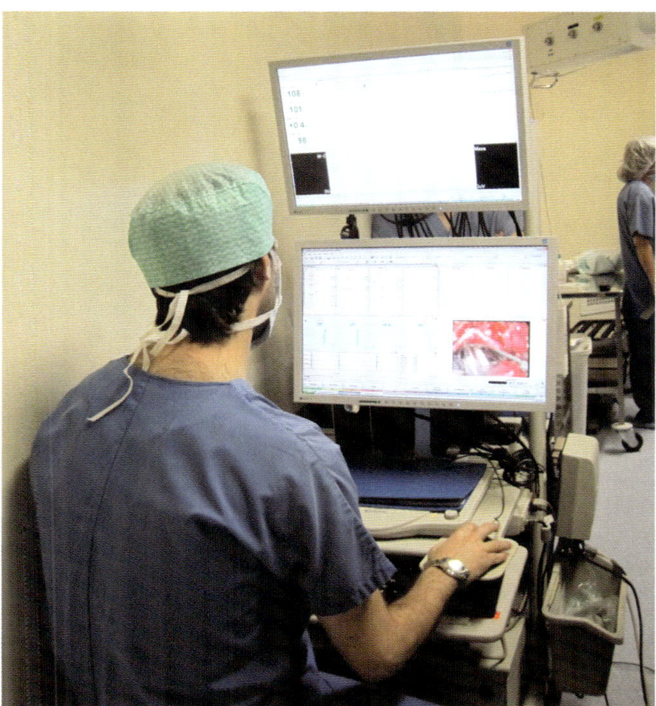

Fig. 4.4: Nerve monitoring system in use during the surgery

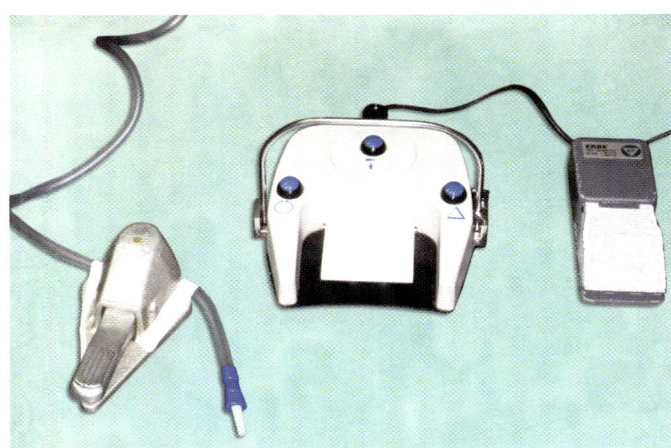

Fig. 4.6: Foot pedals of suction and drill are in surgeon's control

Patient's Preparation and Position

All the procedures of CPA by retrosigmoid as well as combined presigmoid/retrosigmoid approach are performed by us in the supine position (Fig. 4.5). The patient is laid on a gel sheet to prevent any pressure sores on bony contact areas due to prolonged surgery. The patient is placed in the supine position and the head is elevated by around 15° by putting it on "donut" (Figs 4.7 to 4.9). Additional elevation of the head up to 30° may be required

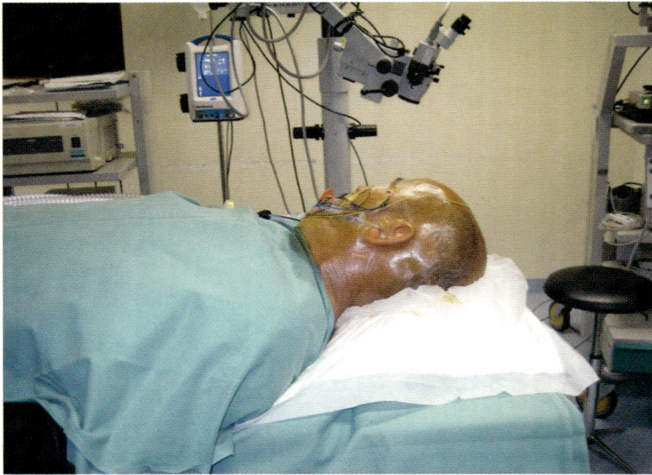

Fig. 4.7: The head of patient is elevated by around 15° by putting it on "donut." The head of obese patient (with short neck and large shoulders) is elevated by around 30° by putting some extra padding formed by rolled bedsheet under the donut. Correct position of head after adequate flexion and rotation toward opposite side

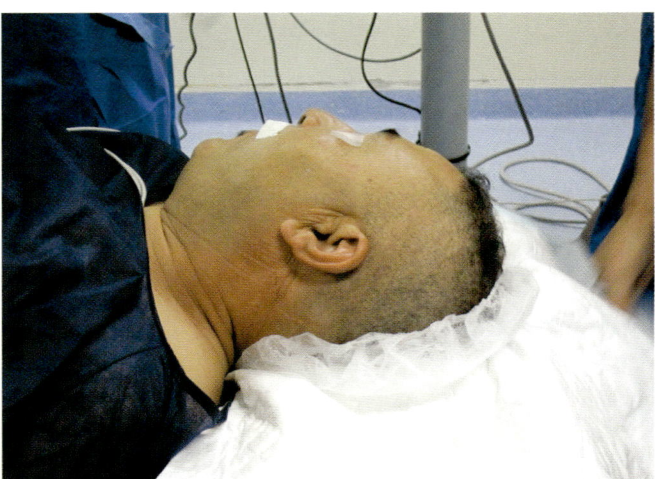

Fig. 4.8: Incorrect position of head due to inadequate flexion

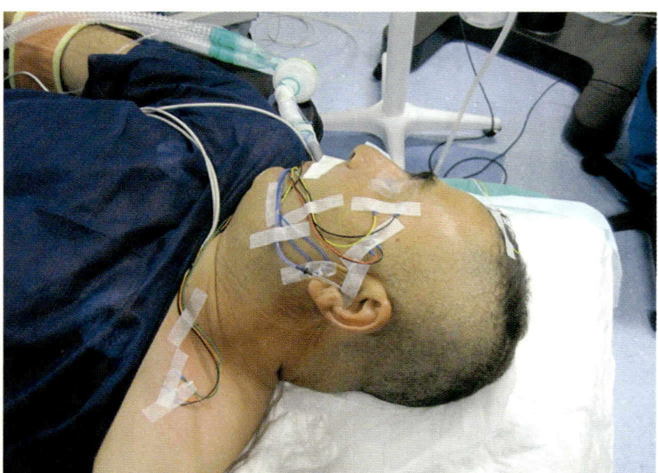

Fig. 4.9: Incorrect position of head due to inadequate rotation of the head

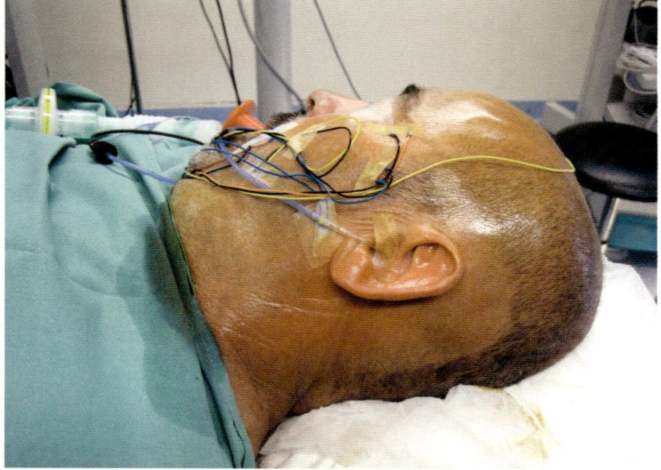

Fig. 4.10: The insert earplugs and electrodes for facial and cochlear function monitoring are inserted. The post auricular hairs are shaved about 1 inch above the pinna and 2 inch behind the posterior hair line. The local area is finally prepared with 10% betadine solution and methylated alcohol. The surgical site after final preoperative preparation

for fat patients with short neck and large shoulders, and is achieved by putting additional sheets under the donut (Fig. 4.7). The head is turned to the opposite side such that the operative site is facing upward. The head is preferred in slightly flexed position over the contralateral shoulder (Figs 4.7 to 4.9). To protect the face, the forehead of the healthy side may be fastened with a gel sheet, without pin fixation of the skull.

The insert earplugs and electrodes for facial and cochlear function monitoring are inserted as discussed in Chapter 3 (Fig. 4.10).

Preparation of the surgical site is important to limit colonization of skin by commensal bacteria. The surgical site with adjoining hair is cleaned with betadine scrub. The post auricular hairs are shaved about 1 inch above the pinna and 2 inch behind the posterior hair line (Fig. 4.10) with electrical clipper. The local area is finally prepared with 10% betadine solution and methylated alcohol (Fig. 4.10). The surgical site is draped with sterile, nonabsorbent, self-

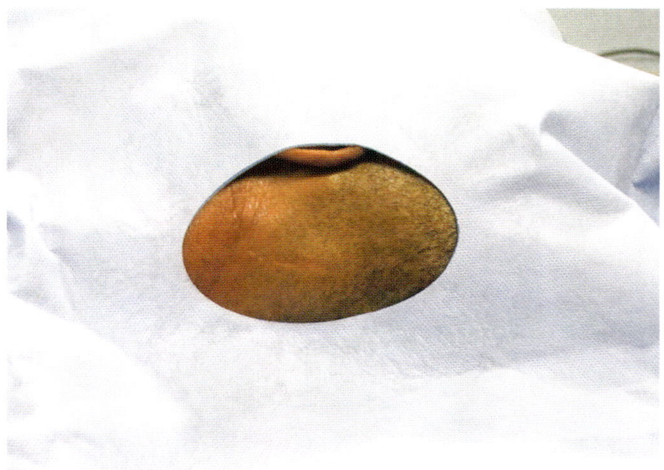

Fig. 4.11: The surgical site is draped with sterile, nonabsorbent, self-adhering barrier drapes with precut aperture

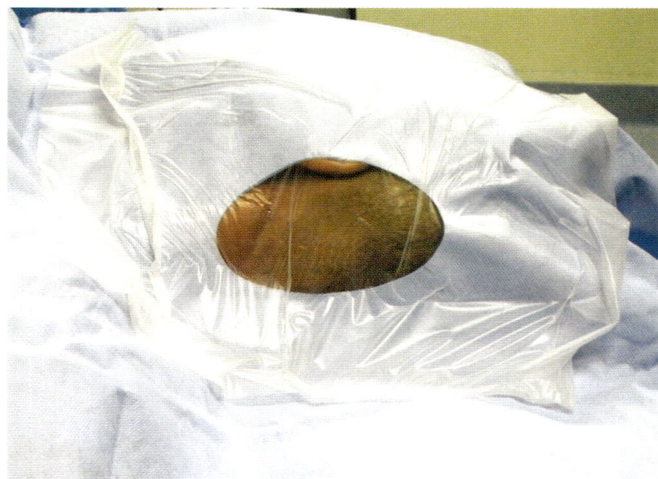

Fig. 4.12: A wide-field adhesive drape is applied over self-adhering barrier drapes with precut aperture

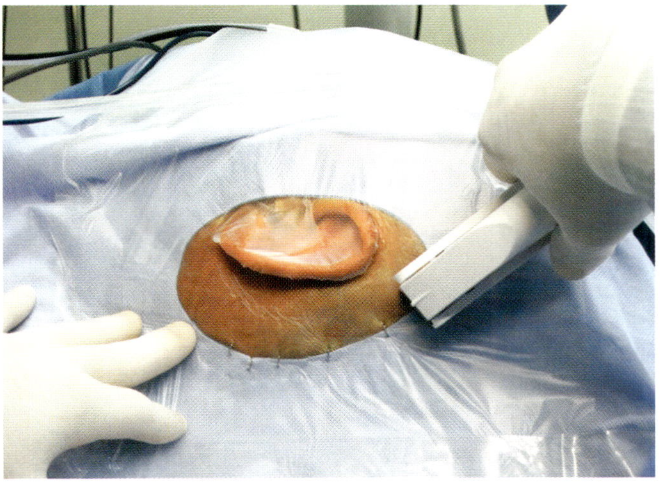

Fig. 4.13: The posterior margins of the surgical field along with adhesive drapes are fixed with sutures or staplers to prevent detachment of drape from the skin

adhering barrier drapes with precut aperture and a wide-field adhesive drape is applied over it (Figs 4.11 and 4.12). The posterior margins of the surgical field are fixed with sutures or staplers to prevent detachment of the drape from the skin (Fig. 4.13). A separate pouch is attached over the head side of patient for placing various handheld devices like suction cannula, monopolar and bipolar cautery, drill, facial and cochlear nerve stimulators. A separate plastic pouch is also attached to collect irrigation fluid with a provision for suction.

Key Points

- By having a standard protocol of the same position in all the procedures, it eases the preoperative preparation.
- If the right side is the operating side, as the right shoulder will restrict the surgeon's right arm movement, it is necessary to take sufficient care in setting the head position.

Incision

The incision in retrosigmoid craniotomy procedure with a minimally invasive approach is performed as given below.

The first line is designed by backward extension along the so-called Frankfurt plane (plane that extends from the lateral canthus of the ipsilateral eye to the superior margin of the external auditory canal). The line thus runs from the upper edge of the lateral canthus of the operating side above the external auditory canal (Figs 4.14 and 4.15). The second line runs tangential to the mastoid tip along the posterior margin of the mastoid meeting the first line (Figs 4.14 and 4.16). The first line marks the probable position of the transverse sinus and the second line marks the position of the sigmoid sinus (Fig. 4.17). A 2 cm diameter keyhole is drawn just below and behind the point where the two lines cross (Figs 4.18 and 4.19). This keyhole is the tentative position for retrosigmoid craniotomy.

At this juncture, 5–7 mL of local anesthetic agent with adrenaline (1% lignoicane with 1:100,000 adrenaline) is injected along the proposed line of incision to achieve hemostasis during incision and soft tissue dissection (Fig. 4.20).

For skin incision, draw an arc 6 to 8 cm in length with the convex side toward the back around 1 cm behind the circle for keyhole craniotomy, starting on the superior line and ending at a position one finger behind the oblique line (Fig. 4.18). After initial skin incision with

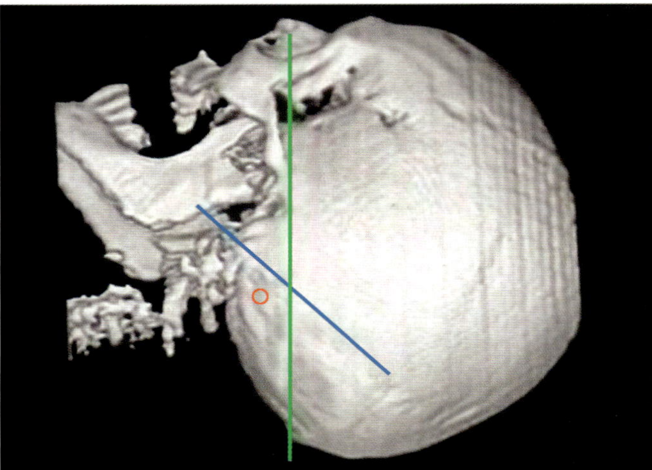

Fig. 4.14: Diagrammatic picture showing the landmarks used for making the incision. "Frankfurt" plane (plane that extends from the lateral canthus of) marks the horizontal line thus runs from the upper edge of the lateral canthus of the ipsilateral eye to the superior margin of the external auditory canal. The second line runs tangential to the mastoid tip along the posterior margin of the mastoid meeting the first line. The first line marks the probable position of transverse sinus and the second line marks the position of the sigmoid sinus. The red dot suggests the approximate position of the emissary vein

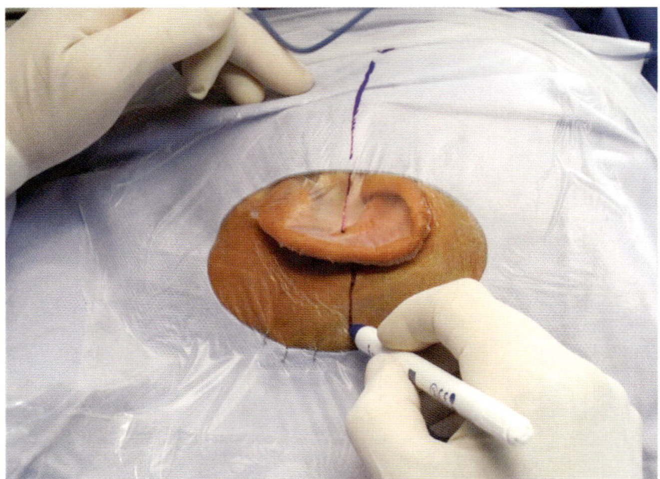

Fig. 4.15: Marking of "Frankfurt" plane that extends from the lateral canthus of ipsilateral eye to the superior margin of the external auditory canal

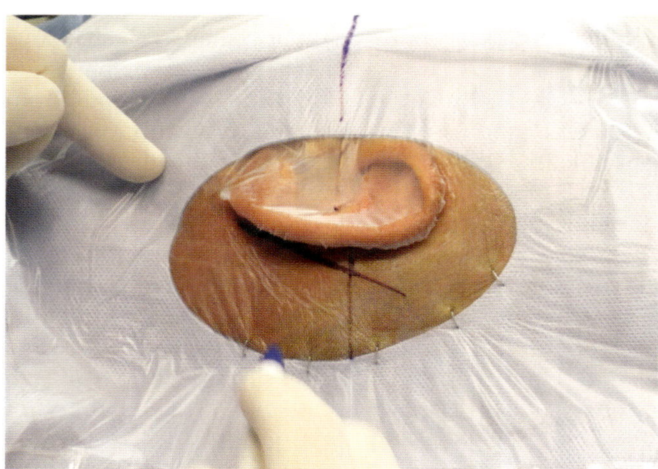

Fig. 4.16: The second line runs tangential to the mastoid tip meeting the first line to make an angle of around 120°

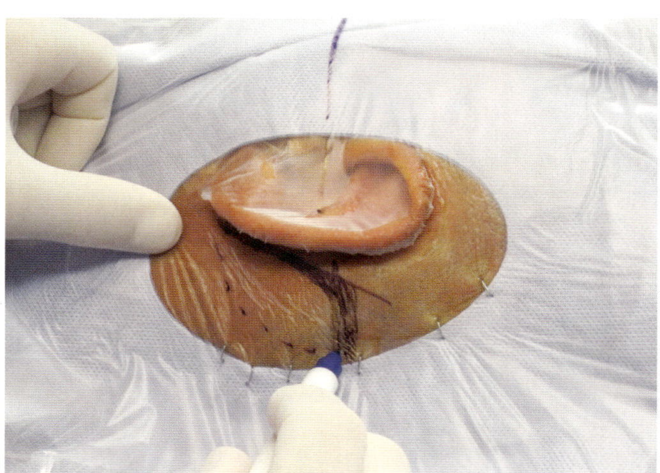

Fig. 4.17: The first line marks the probable position of transverse sinus and the second line marks the position of the sigmoid sinus

23 number knife (Figs 4.21 and 4.22), an anteriorly based skin and subcutaneous tissue flap is elevated with monopolar cautery up to the anterior oblique line (Figs 4.23 and 4.24). The anteriorly based skin-subcutaneous flap may be secured anteriorly to the drape with a suture, if required. After elevating the anteriorly based skin-subcutaneous tissue flap (Fig. 4.25), the muscle-periosteal incision is kept with a monopolar cautery 2 inch anterior to the skin incision (starting anterior to the oblique line landmark) with the convex side toward the front (Fig. 4.26) to raise the posteriorly based musculoperiosteal flap (Fig. 4.27). The muscle-periosteal incision and the skin incisions are "stair-stepped" (placed in reverse directions, the former being posterior-based and the latter being anterior-based) to fortify the closure for prevention of postoperative CSF leak. The posteriorly based musculoperiosteal flap is raised from the underlying mastoid bone by monopolar cautery (or periosteal elevator) till one encounters the exit of the emissary vein posteroinferiorly (Fig. 4.28). Care is taken not to injure the emissary vein while doing so. The emissary vein is cauterized with bipolar forceps to shrink

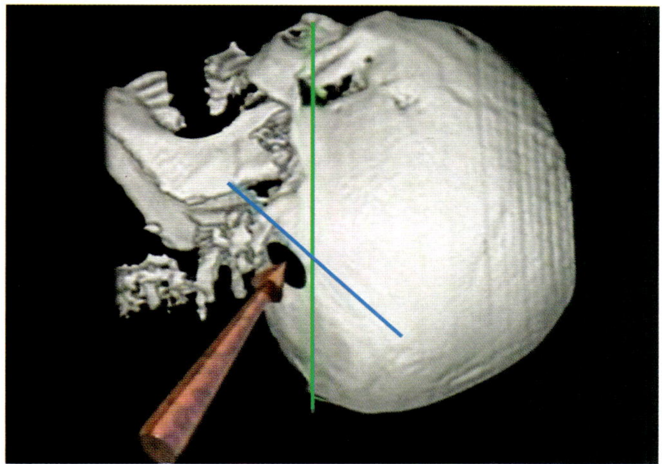

Fig. 4.18: Diagrammatic picture showing the site for craniotomy and its relation to landmarks used for making the incision

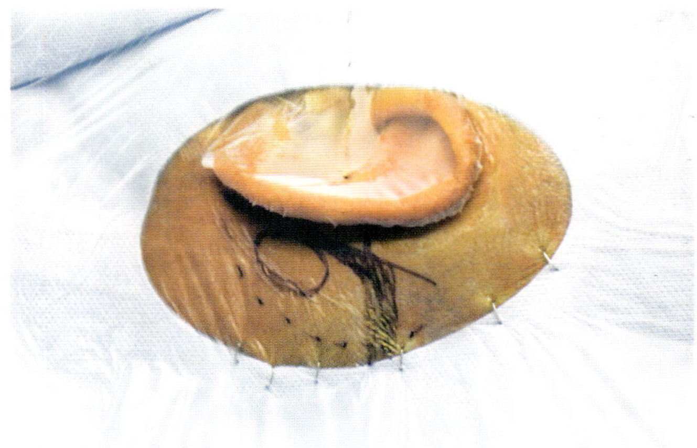

Fig. 4.19: A 2 cm diameter keyhole is drawn just below and behind the point where the two lines cross. This keyhole is the tentative position for retrosigmoid craniotomy

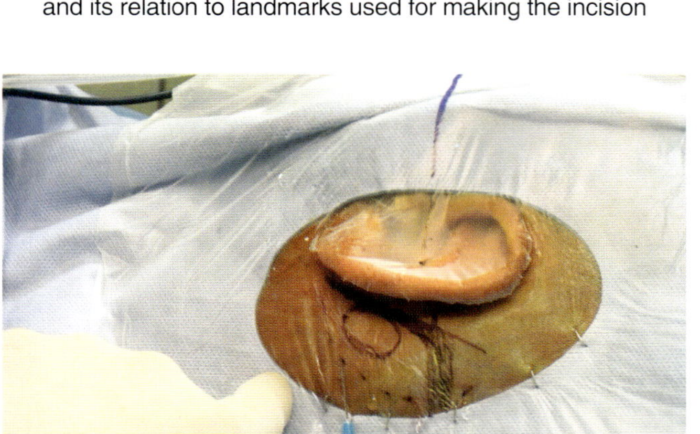

Fig. 4.20: Injection of local anesthetic with adrenaline along the proposed line of incision and under the periosteum of the bone at the craniotomy site

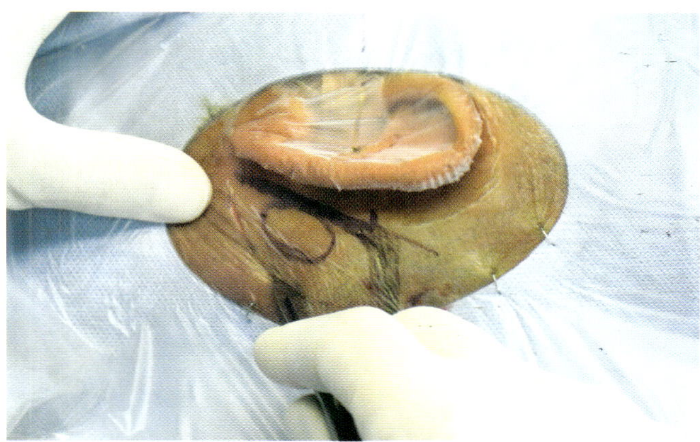

Fig. 4.21: Initial skin incision with 23 number knife along an arc 6–8 cm in length with the convex side toward the back around 1 cm behind the circle for keyhole craniotomy, starting on the superior line and ending at a position one finger behind the oblique line

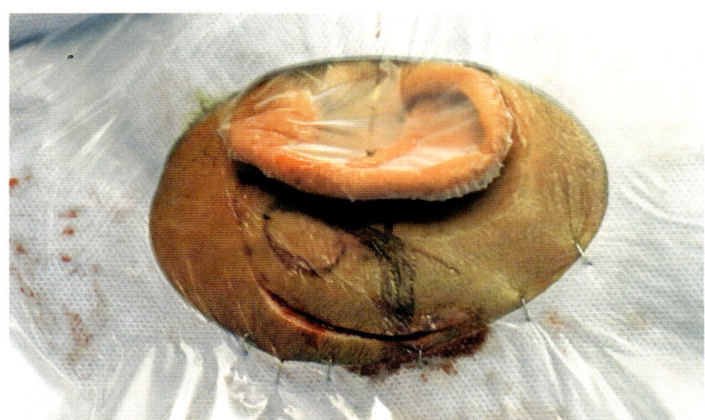

Fig. 4.22: Initial skin incision

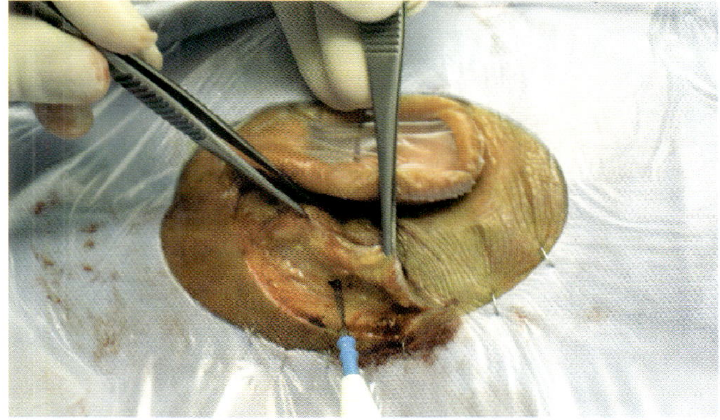

Fig. 4.23: An anteriorly based skin and subcutaneous tissue flap is elevated

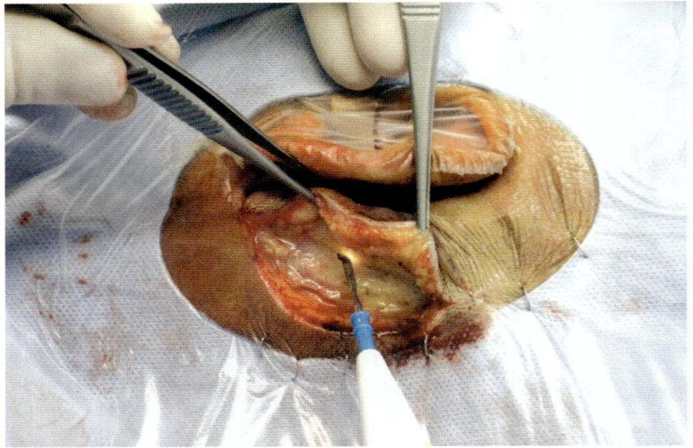

Fig. 4.24: The anteriorly based skin-subcutaneous flap is raised anteriorly up to the anterior oblique line drawn on the skin that marks the tentative location of sigmoid sinus

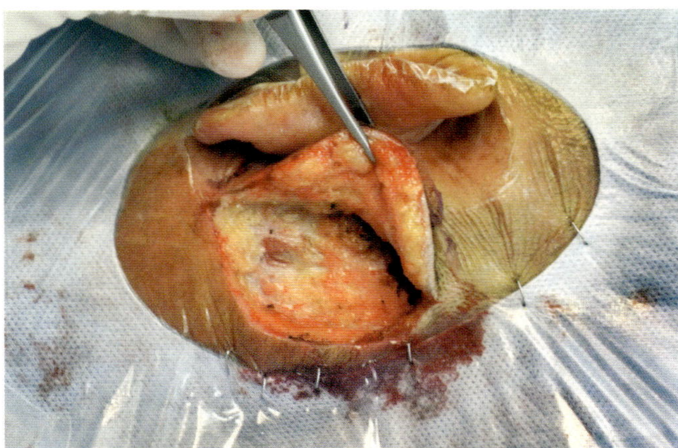

Fig. 4.25: The anteriorly based skin-subcutaneous flap

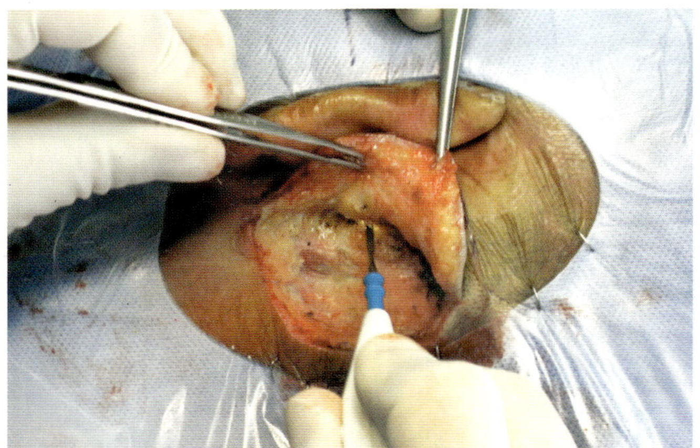

Fig. 4.26: The musculoperiosteal incision is kept with a monopolar cautery

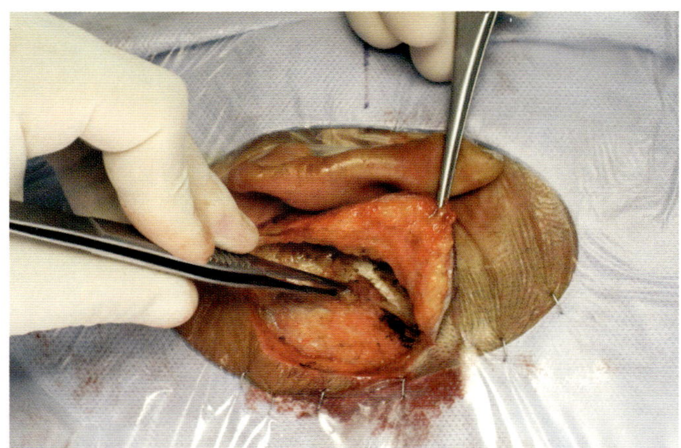

Fig. 4.27: The posteriorly based musculoperiosteal flap is raised

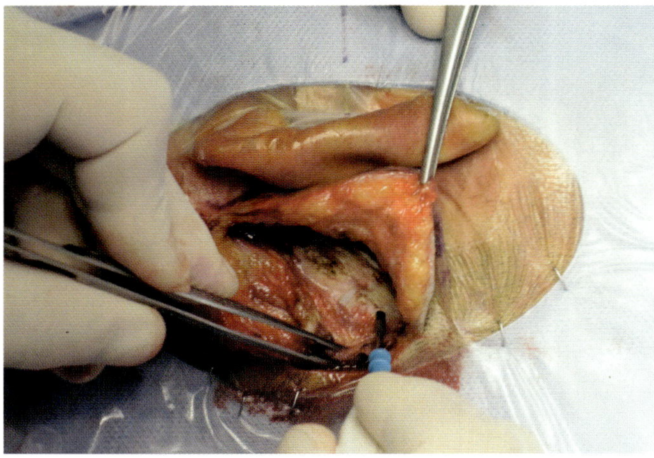

Fig. 4.28: The emissary vein is delineated during dissection and elevation of posterior musculoperiosteal flap

it substantially in the case of a large vein or to completely seal it in the case of a small vein. The coagulated emissary vein is divided with monopolar cautery and any bleeding from it is stopped by plugging it with bone wax or Surgicel (Figs 4.29 and 4.30). The digastric ridge is exposed posteroinferiorly and is an important landmark for the site of craniotomy (Figs 4.29 and 4.30). After exposing the bone surface sufficiently, the scalp flap is retracted forward and the periosteal flap along with occipital muscles is retracted backward by placing a self-retaining mastoid retractor, taking care that the positioning of retractor does not constrict the approach (Figs 4.29 and 4.30).

Craniotomy

After exposing the bone surface, the anesthetist is reminded to begin hyperventilating the patient

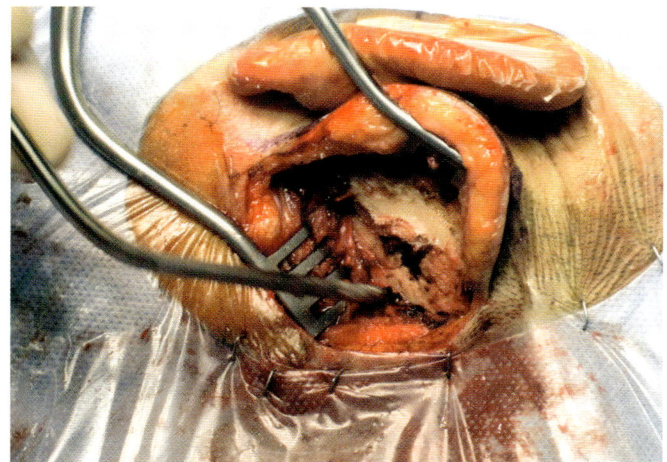

Fig. 4.29: The emissary vein is cauterized with bipolar forceps. Bleeding from emissary vein is plugged with Surgicel. The digastric ridge is an important landmark for the site of craniotomy. The subcutaneous flap is retracted forward and periosteal flap along with occipital muscles is retracted backward by placing a large self-retaining mastoid retractor

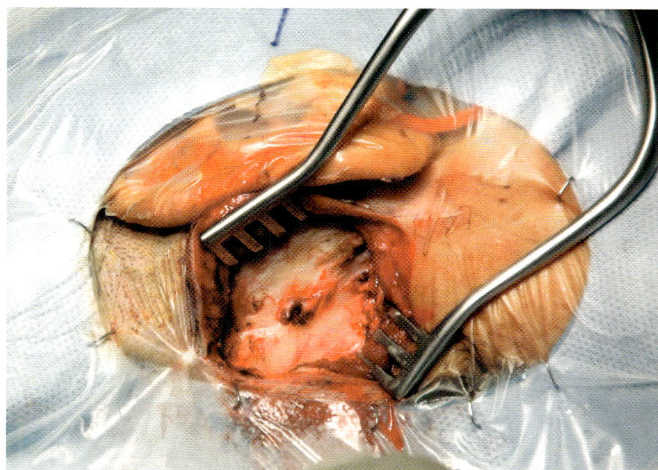

Fig. 4.30: The mastoid emissary vein and digastric ridge is an important landmark for keyhole retrosigmoid craniotomy

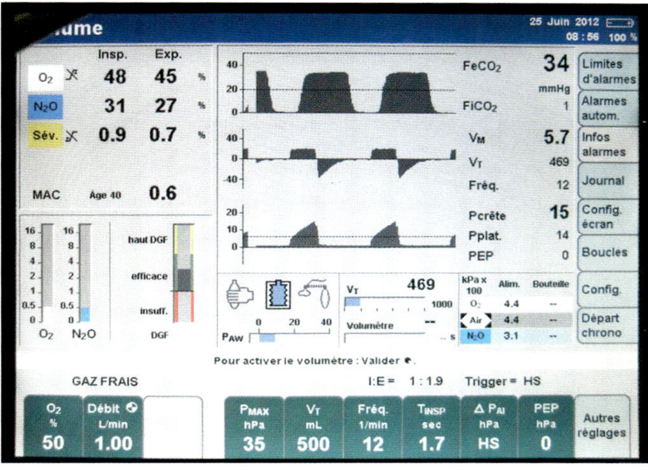

Fig. 4.31: Before initiating drilling for craniotomy the $FeCO_2$ with normal rate of ventilation is around 34–35 mmHg

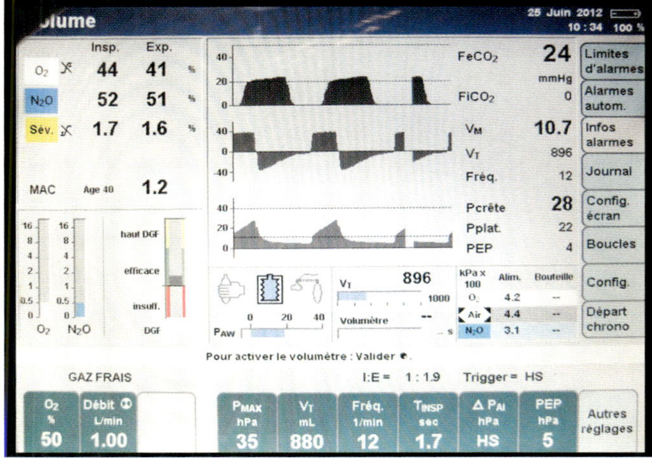

Fig. 4.32: The target $FeCO_2$ before entering the cistern magna is less than 25 mmHg and is achieved by hyperventilation for 15–20 min

to achieve hypocapnia up to 25 mmHg (Figs 4.31 and 4.32). The site for keyhole craniotomy is planned with the mastoid emissary vein as an important landmark (Fig. 4.33). The bone removal for retrosigmoid craniotomy begins around the emissary vein keeping it in the center as a marker. The posterior part of the digastric ridge is also an important landmark (Fig. 4.33) and drilling is extended up to the ridge. The bone drilling is initially carried out using large cutting bur (6 or 7 mm size). A limited irrigation is performed at this stage, so that the dry bone dust thus created can be collected in a bowl for use later. The drilling is continued in a circumferential manner around the emissary vein, preserving an island of bone around for use later (Fig. 4.34). The diamond bur is used as one proceeds close to the dura medially and the sigmoid sinus anteriorly (Fig. 4.34). Circular craniotomy, 15 mm to maximum of 25 mm in diameter (Fig. 4.35), centered on the emissary vein is followed up to the posterior margin of the sigmoid sinus. The emissary vein may bleed while drilling around it and needs to be plugged with Surgicel. When the operation reaches the posterior fossa dura and the posterior margin of the sigmoid sinus it is advisable to use the microscope

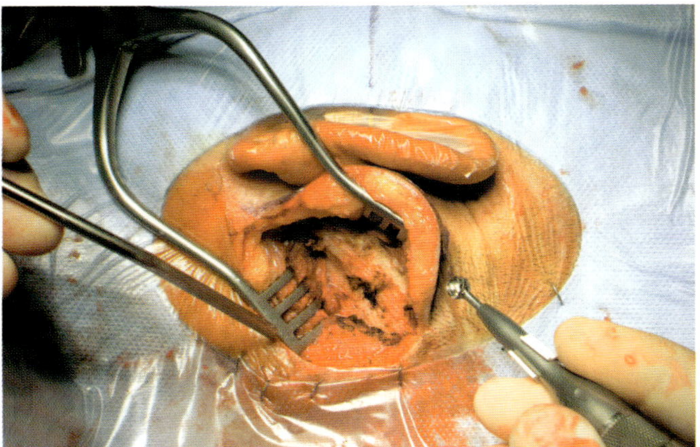

Fig. 4.33: The bone removal for retrosigmoid craniotomy begins around the emissary vein, which is the most constant landmark. The posterior part of digastric ridge is also an important landmark and drilling is extended up to the ridge. The bone drilling is initially carried out using large cutting bur

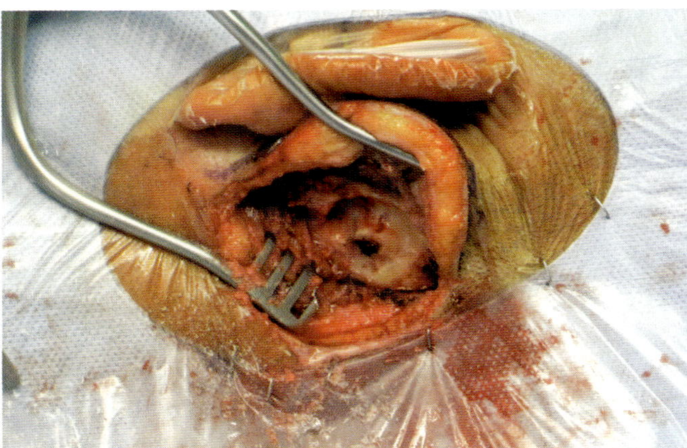

Fig. 4.34: The drilling is continued in circumferential manner around the emissary vein, preserving an island of bone around later

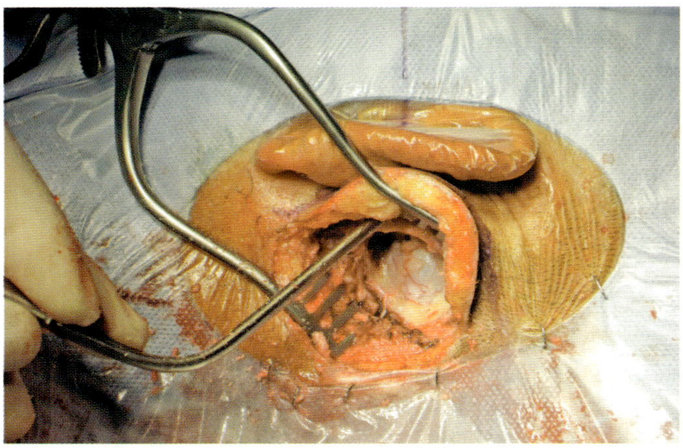

Fig. 4.35: The final picture of circular craniotomy, 20–25 mm in diameter

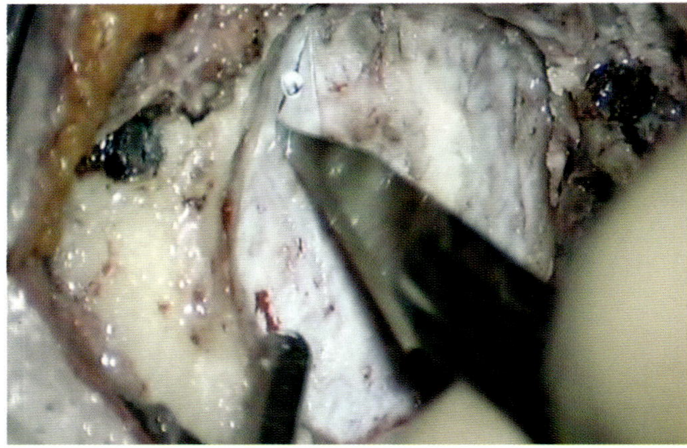

Fig. 4.36: The retrosigmoid dura is incised to make an anteriorly based U-shaped flap attached anteriorly along the sigmoid sinus. The incision begins with a small knick in the dura posterior to sigmoid sinus using an 11 number surgical knife

for further steps. After securing sufficient hemostasis, the retrosigmoid dura is incised to make an anteriorly based U-shaped flap attached anteriorly along the sigmoid sinus. The incision begins with a small knick in the dura posteriorly using a 11 number surgical knife (Figs 4.36 and 4.37) and the incised dura is lifted from the underlying cerebellar surface using a hook or blunt tissue forceps (Figs 4.38, 4.39 and 4.40) to prevent injury to underlying blood vessels. The incision is then extended visualizing the underlying cerebellum and the blood vessels over it to make the U-shaped flap based anteriorly on the sigmoid sinus. The dural flap is retracted anteriorly by either suturing it with the soft tissue anteriorly (Figs 4.41, 4.42 and 4.43) or by fixing it anteriorly over the craniotomy bone with fibrin glue. Perisigmoid mastoid air cells are often exposed while exposing the retrosigmoid dura. It is important to obliterate all the opened-up mastoid air cells with bone wax (Figs 4.39 and 4.40) to prevent CSF leakage. There could be minor injury to the sigmoid sinus, which is controlled with bipolar cautery or Surgicel as discussed earlier.

Once the dural flap is secured, the surgeon changes his microscopic view so that he is now viewing the inferior part of the dural opening at the anteroinferior petrosal surface of cerebellum (Fig. 4.43). Once sufficient cerebellar relaxation is achieved, a fine neurosurgical cottonoid or Neuropatch

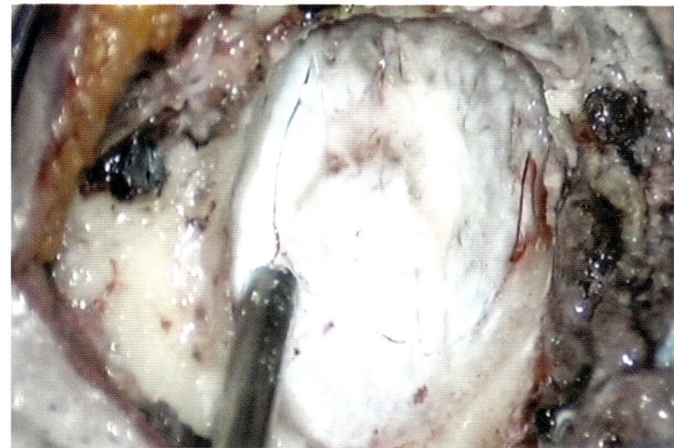

Fig. 4.37: The retrosigmoid dura is incised to make an anteriorly based U-shaped flap attached anteriorly along the sigmoid sinus

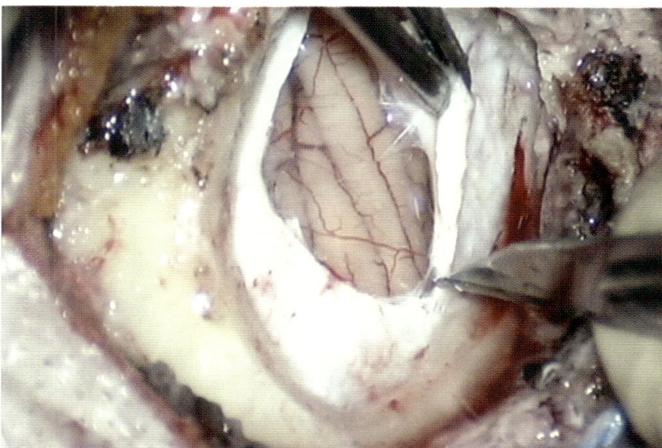

Fig. 4.38: The incised dura is lifted from underlying cerebellar surface using a blunt tissue forceps to prevent injury to underlying blood vessels

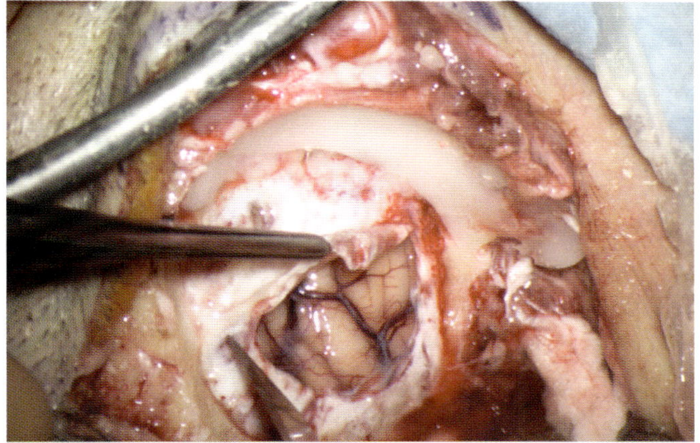

Fig. 4.39: The perisigmoid mastoid air cells exposed due to drilling of craniotomy are obliterated with bone wax to prevent cerebrospinal fluid leakage. A dural flap is elevated using an 11 number surgical knife

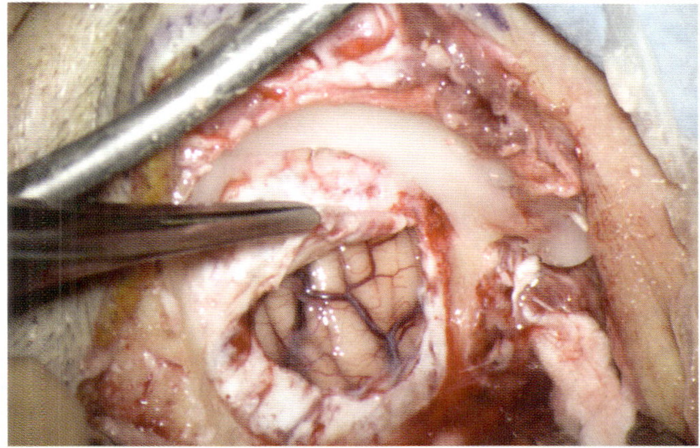

Fig. 4.40: The incised dura is lifted from underlying cerebellar surface using a blunt tissue forceps to prevent injury to underlying blood vessels

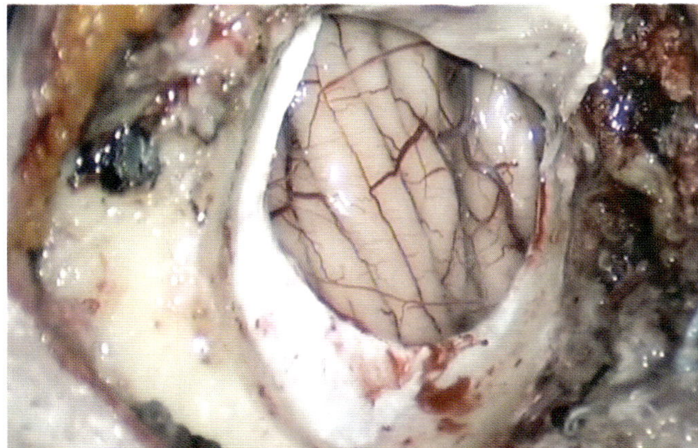

Fig. 4.41: The U-shaped dural flap based anteriorly on sigmoid sinus. The dural flap is retracted anteriorly by suturing it with the subcutaneous tissue anteriorly

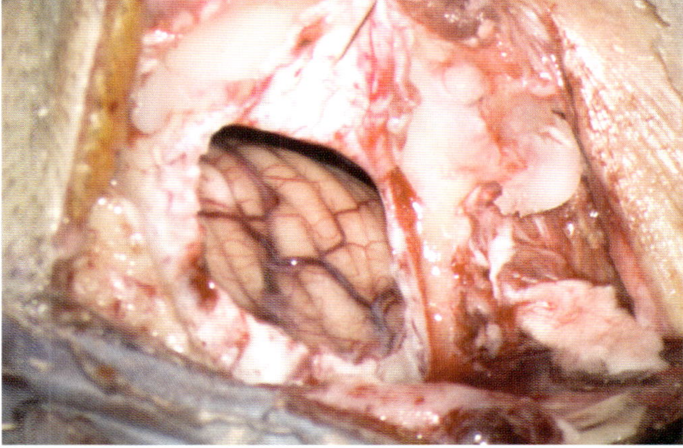

Fig. 4.42: The U-shaped dural flap based anteriorly on sigmoid sinus. The dural flap is retracted anteriorly by suturing it with the subcutaneous tissue anteriorly

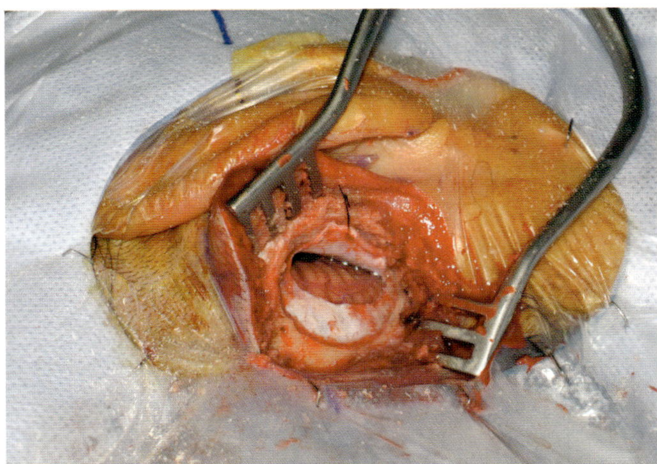

Fig. 4.43: The nonmicroscopic view of the craniotomy showing the size and relations of the craniotomy. The surgeon changes his microscopic view toward the inferior part of the dural opening at the inferior petrosal surface of cerebellum to open cistern magna

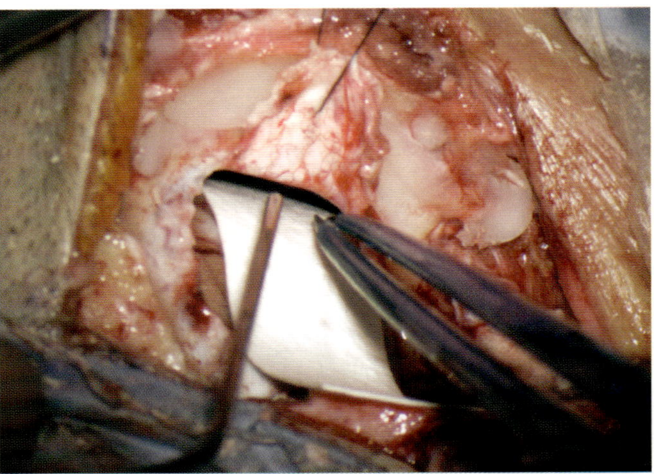

Fig. 4.44: A 1.5 cm wide by 5 cm long fine neurosurgical cottonoid or Neuropatch is placed over the cerebellum to protect it from injury. A safe surgical corridor between the petrosal surfaces of temporal bone and cerebellum is opened by sliding the Neuropatch along the cerebellum with bipolar forceps to enter the posterior cisterna magna

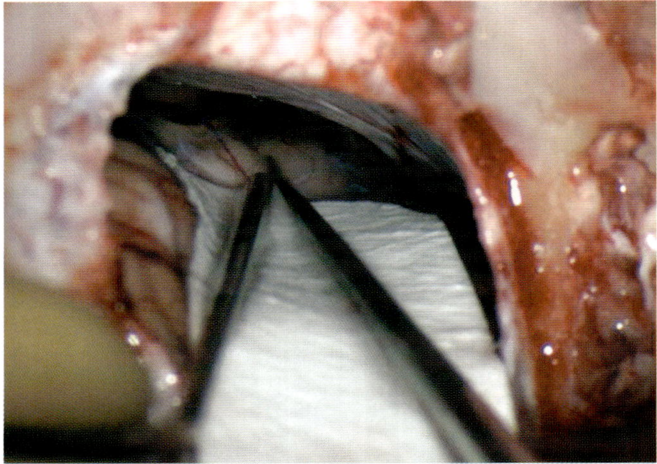

Fig. 4.45: The arachnoid layer is opened using dissection with blunt probe or bipolar forceps to enter in the subarachnoid space at the level of lower cranial nerves

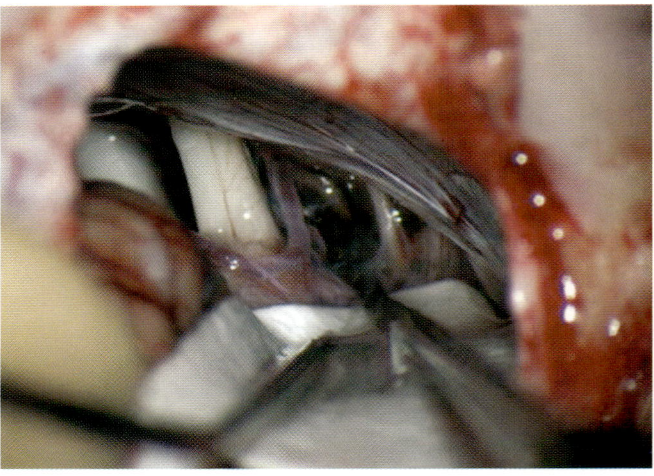

Fig. 4.46: Spontaneous cerebellar retraction as the cerebrospinal fluid is drained gives adequate space to perform surgery without any cerebellar retractor. The arachnoid layers are dissected with sharp and blunt dissection using bayonet scissors and elevators to expose the contents of CPA

(1.5 cm wide by 5 cm long size) is placed over the cerebellum to protect it from injury while introducing the instruments during subsequent steps (Figs 4.44 to 4.53 right sided CPA). A fine blunt bayonet-shaped bipolar forceps is slided gently along the cottonoid with the suction canula through a safe surgical corridor between the petrosal surfaces of the temporal bone and the cerebellum to enter the posterior cisterna magna (Fig. 4.44) at the level of the lower cranial nerves. The arachnoid plane of the cisterna magna is fenestrated with bayonet bipolar forceps or blunt probe (Fig. 4.45). The CSF draining into the wound is cleared with suction. Wait for the complete spontaneous cerebellar retraction as the CSF dries up. Once sufficient cerebellar relaxation is achieved, no brain retractor is necessary (Fig. 4.46). At this juncture, it is necessary to lift the height of the table so that one can see the contents of the CPA along the line of the craniotomy (Fig. 4.47). Under microscopic examination, the arachnoid draping the CPA and its

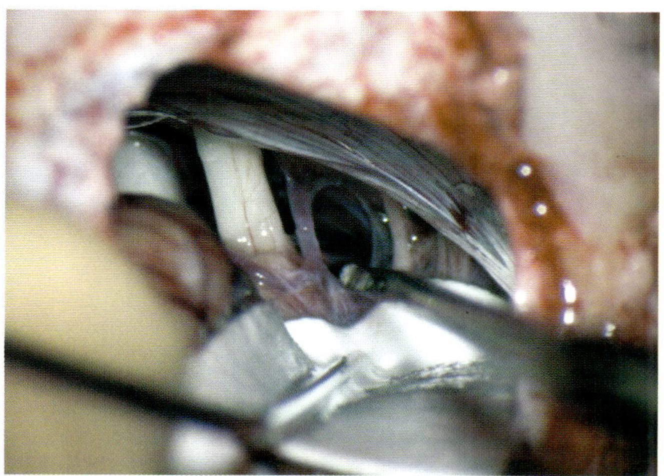

Fig. 4.47: Diagrammatic picture showing the position of the surgeon and the height of the table before and after craniotomy

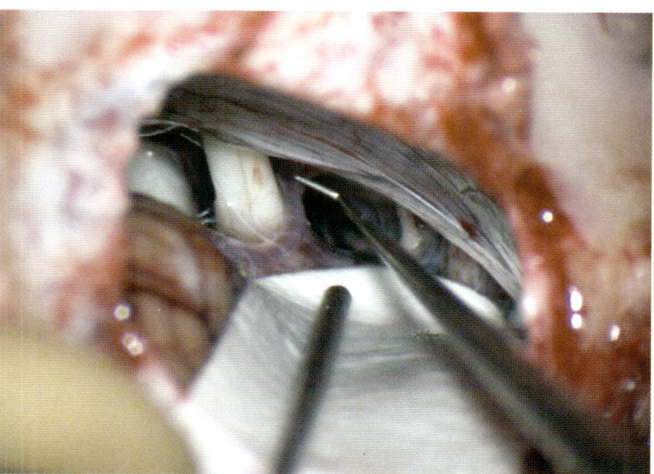

Fig. 4.48: The arachnoid layers are dissected around acousticovestibular nerve bundle and lower cranial nerves with blunt dissection using bayonet right angled probe to expose the contents of CPA

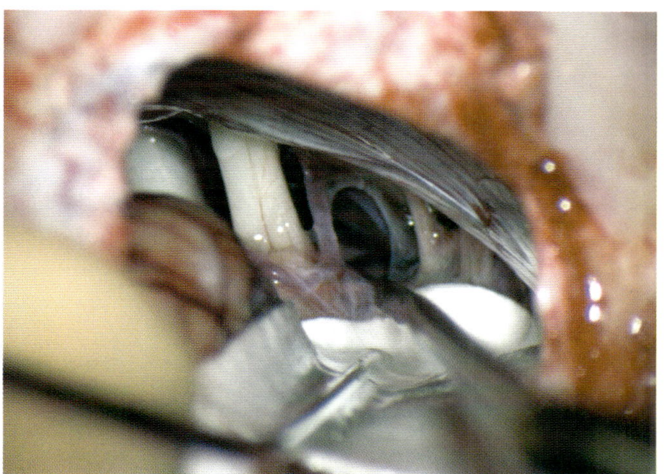

Fig. 4.49: The arachnoid layers are dissected around acousticovestibular nerve bundle and lower cranial nerves with blunt dissection using bayonet elevator to expose the contents of CPA

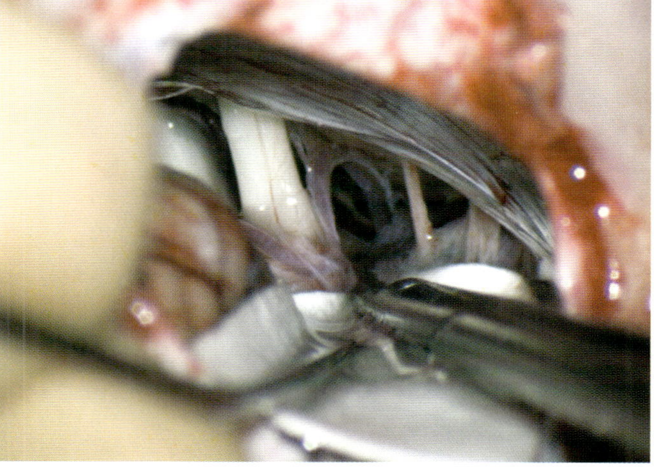

Fig. 4.50: The arachnoid layers are dissected around acousticovestibular nerve bundle and lower cranial nerves with sharp dissection using bayonet scissors to expose the contents of CPA

contents are opened initially with a smooth, blunt bayonet-shaped probe (Fig. 4.48). Under direct vision, the arachnoid layers are dissected with a smooth, blunt bayonet-shaped probe (Figure 4.48) and bayonet scissors (Figs 4.49, 4.50 and 4.51) to expose the lower cranial nerves initially followed by vestibulocochlear bundle and the trigeminal nerve along with their accompanying blood vessels. If the small arterioles in the arachnoid are in the field of dissection, they are coagulated with bipolar cautery before cutting with scissors. Care should be taken to avoid damage to the venules entering into the tentorium draining the superior surface of the cerebellum. If it bleeds, it is coagulated with fine bipolar cautery forceps. However, sometimes it may retract into the tentorium and plugging with Surgicel followed by pressure with cottonoid is required in such cases. The major arteries of the CPA are often projecting into the subarachnoid space and care should be taken not to injure them while opening the arachnoid. It is essential that the arachnoid is completely denuded from all the structures of the CPA to ease the surgery and endoscopy in the CPA. At this juncture the vision is shifted from the microscopic picture to the endoscopic apparatus.

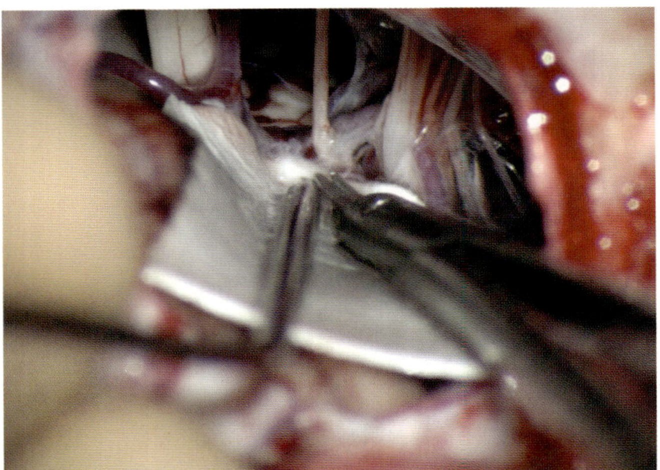

Fig. 4.51: The arachnoid layers are dissected around acousticovestibular nerve bundle and lower cranial nerves with sharp dissection using bayonet scissors to expose the contents of CPA

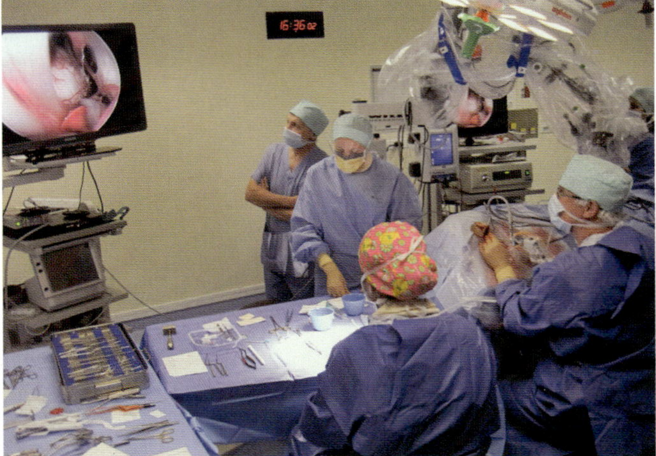

Fig. 4.52: Conversion from microscope to endoscope is carried out maintaining the strict asepsis. The autoclaved endoscope with sterile disposable draping of videoendoscopic attachments should be brought in the surgical field, while the microscope is temporarily pushed aside

- Care is taken when removing bone over the dura, especially in the elderly patient when the dura is more friable.
- A cutting bur may be used initially, but the diamond bur is safer once the dura is close.
- Dura and cerebellar tissue are always kept wet to avoid dessication of the tissue, which makes it more friable and susceptible to infection.
- It is mandatory to change the height of the table once the dura is opened and CSF drained, permitting further dissection in the CPA under direct vision.

CPA Endoscopy

Despite the illumination and magnification offered by the operating microscope, it has distinct limitations. The operator can visualize structures only directly ahead and is unable to see around structures. The 30°-angled endoscope is a valuable and indispensable optical device to overcome this disability as it permits us to observe the blind spot by "looking around the corner", which even a panoramic search with a microscope cannot visualize. If one has a good knowledge of the maneuverability of endoscopes, it should be possible to get more critical information by simply "avoiding a blind spot created by surgical microscope." It is a very effective device in obtaining reliable information in a short time without moving either the microscope positions or the head positions of the patient and thus reduces the length of the surgical procedure. Thus, adjunctive complementary use of endoscopes and microscopes is of tremendous help, and improves safety and accuracy as well as avoids the need for excessive cerebellar retraction, particularly in microvascular decompression and CPA tumor removal by MIRA.

The autoclaved endoscope with sterile disposable draping of videoendoscopic attachments should be brought in the surgical field while the microscope is temporarily pushed aside. This conversion from microscope to endoscope and vice versa is carried out maintaining the strict asepsis and should not be a problem once the operative staff is accustomed to the procedure (Fig. 4.52). The endoscope should be inserted cautiously by gradually advancing it along the Neuropatch or neurosurgical cottonoid. Care should be taken to avoid contact with adjacent nerves and vessels. The endoscope is held with both hands (Fig. 4.53) to not make contact with the surrounding nerves and vessels in the CPA while inserting it and to be sure for a safe and accurate insertion. More specifically, for operating on the right side, it is important to hold and control the weight of the camera with the left hand and guide the endoscope with the right hand (Fig. 4.53), and vice versa for operating on the left side (Fig. 4.54). The endoscope is soaked in warm saline before inserting into the CPA to avoid fogging of the lens. The endoscope should be inserted slowly along the Neuropatch or neurosurgical cottonoid (Fig. 4.55). At the beginning of CPA endoscopy a long piece of cottonoid is placed near the lower cranial nerves (Fig. 4.55). During endoscopy, the tip of the endoscope can be cleared by

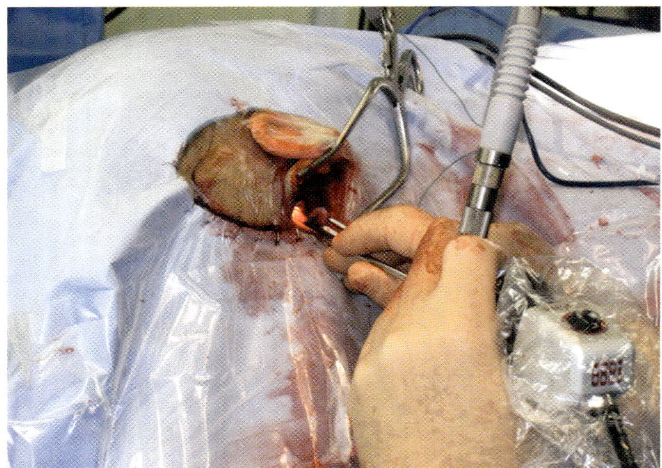

Fig. 4.53: The endoscope should be always held with both hands. For surgery on right side, the camera is controlled with left hand and the endoscope is held with right hand

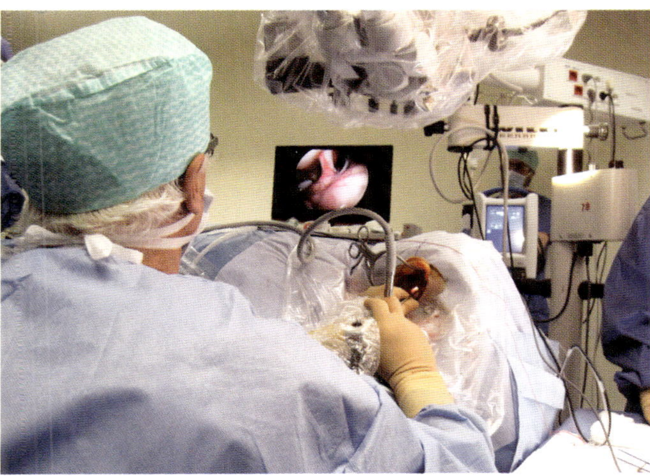

Fig. 4.54: For surgery on left side, the camera is controlled with right hand and the endoscope is held with left hand

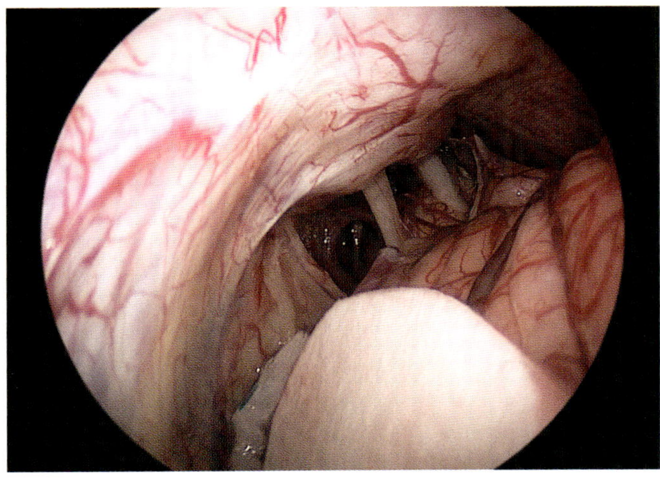

Fig. 4.55: The endoscope is inserted along the Neuropatch (left CPA). A long piece of cottonoid is placed near the lower cranial nerves at the beginning of CPA endoscopy

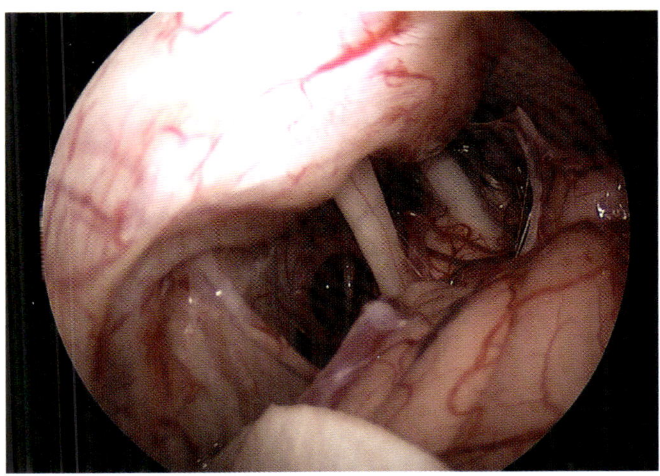

Fig. 4.56: Initially the 30° endoscope is placed with the angled view inferiorly toward cerebellum. The first pass of CPA endoscopy just at its entrance giving a wide panoramic picture of contents of CPA with vestibulocochlear nerve in center, lower cranial nerves inferior to it and trigeminal nerve superior to it

touching this piece of cottonoid placed near the lower cranial nerves to defog it so that one does not need to bring out the endoscope every time it fogs.

As a 30°-angled endoscope has a sharp front edge compared to a 0° endoscope and this makes it difficult to see the inserting direction directly, it is important to keep in mind that this inserting process could have a potential risk of damaging the normal tissues.

It is also necessary to avoid heating damage to nerves and vessels by the prolonged contact of the tip of the endoscope at the same spot.

The initial mapping of CPA is performed in all the surgeries of CPA by MIRA in the same manner to provide the general information about the relationship of various contents of CPA with each other. The mapping includes three passes, each performed with 30°-angled endoscope, first angled downward toward the cerebellum (Figs 4.56 to 4.64 left sided CPA) and later angled upward toward the IAM (Figs 4.65 to 4.68 left sided CPA). The first pass is just into the CPA giving a wide panoramic picture of the contents of the CPA (Fig. 4.56) with vestibulocochlear nerve in the center, the lower cranial nerves inferior to it and

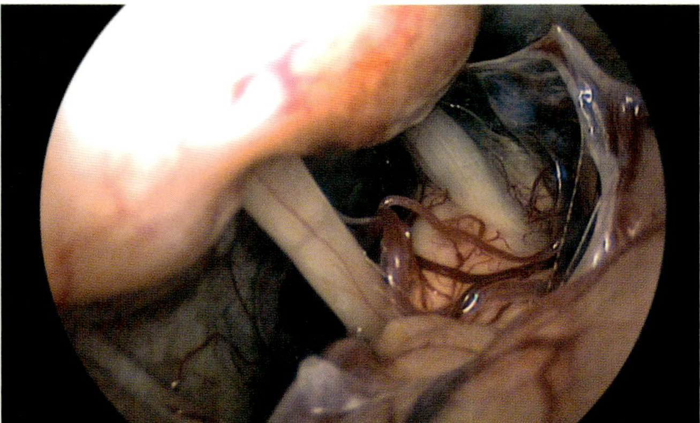

Fig. 4.57: The endoscope advances closer to vestibulocochlear nerve in center, trigeminal nerve superior to it

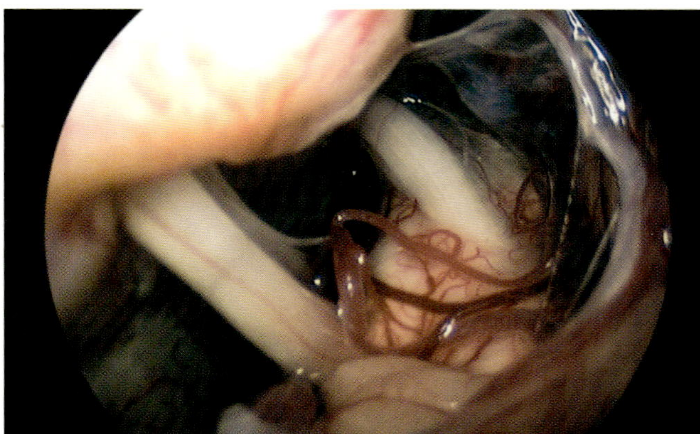

Fig. 4.58: The second pass of CPA endoscopy superior to the vestibulocochlear nerve to visualize the trigeminal nerve, the Dandy vein (cerebellar vein) and the facial nerve

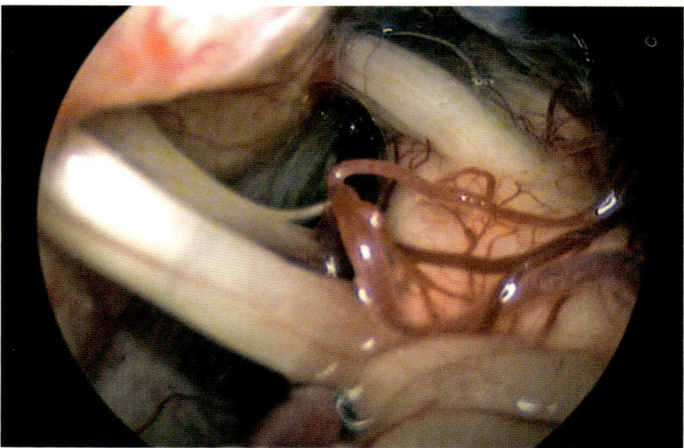

Fig. 4.59: The second pass of CPA endoscopy showing the facial nerve entering in the anterosuperior part of porus

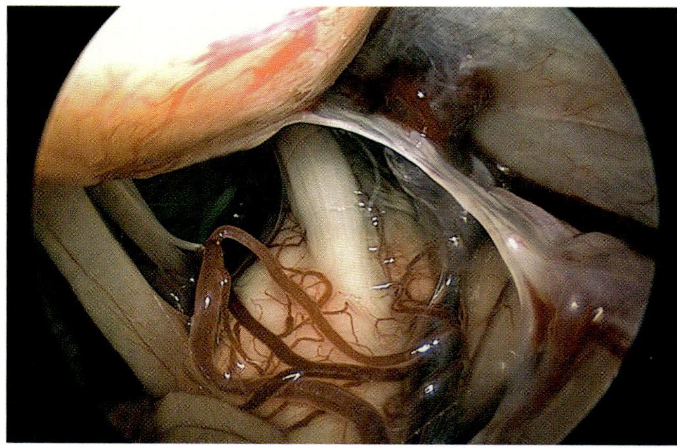

Fig. 4.60: The second pass of CPA endoscopy superior to the vestibulocochlear nerve to visualize the trigeminal nerve, the Dandy vein (cerebellar vein) entering into superior petrosal sinus and the abducent nerve

the trigeminal nerve superior to it. The second pass is by carrying the endoscope superior to the vestibulocochlear nerve to visualize the Dandy vein (cerebellar vein) entering into the superior petrosal sinus, the trigeminal nerve entering the Meckel's cave and the abducent nerve entering the Dorello's canal (Figs 4.57 to 4.60). The facial nerve is seen entering in the anterior part of porus (Fig. 4.60). The courses of the anterior inferior cerebellar artery (AICA) and SCA are seen in the background. The third pass is inferior to the vestibulocochlear nerve to visualize the facial nerve anteroinferior to the vestibulocochlear nerve at the root entry zone at the lateral part of the pontomedullary junction (Figs 4.61 to 4.64). Also seen are the glossopharyngeal, vagus and spinal accessory nerve entering the jugular foramen, PICA and usually the vertebral artery. The view of the porus, Meckel's cave and jugular foramen is much better with the endoscope angled upward (Figs 4.65 to 4.68).

The endoscope and the microscope are used intermittently in different surgeries at different steps. The specific advantages of using the endoscope for particular surgeries are delineated in brief below and will be discussed in detail in the respective chapter.

ENDOSCOPE-ASSISTED MICROSURGERY

Acoustic Neuroma Surgery

The surgery is performed targeting total removal of the tumor, while trying to preserve the hearing and facial nerve function as best as we can. The 30°- angled endoscope is of

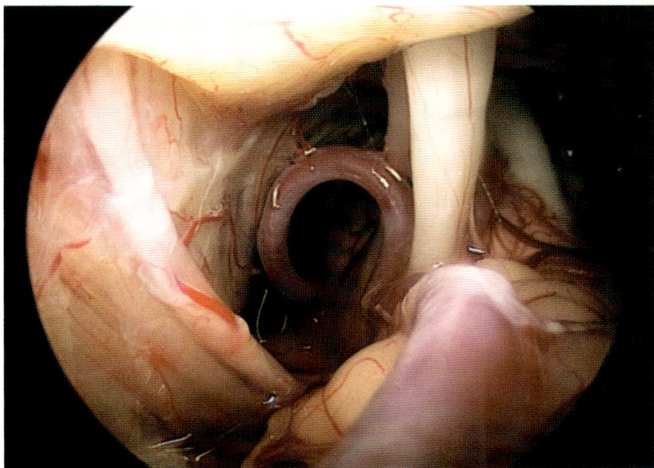

Fig. 4.61: The third pass of CPA endoscopy inferior to the vestibulocochlear nerve and superior to the lower cranial nerves to visualize the facial nerve anteroinferior to the vestibulocochlear nerve at the root entry zone at the lateral part of pontomedullary junction. Also seen in the background is abducent (VI) nerve

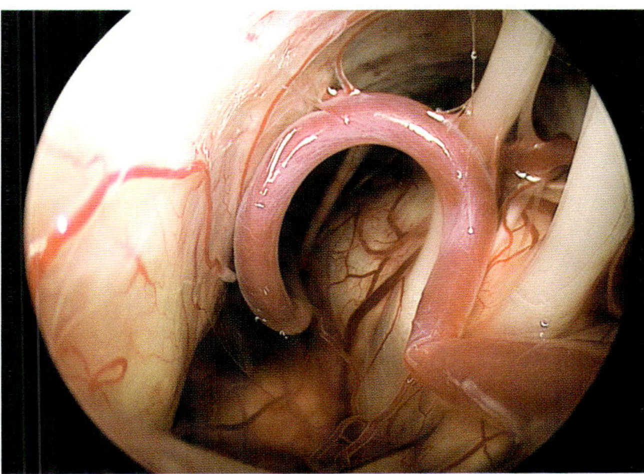

Fig. 4.62: The third pass of CPA endoscopy inferior to the vestibulocochlear nerve and superior to the lower cranial nerves to visualize the facial nerve, predominant AICA (giving rise to both AICA and terminating as PICA), and also seen in the background is abducent (VI) nerve

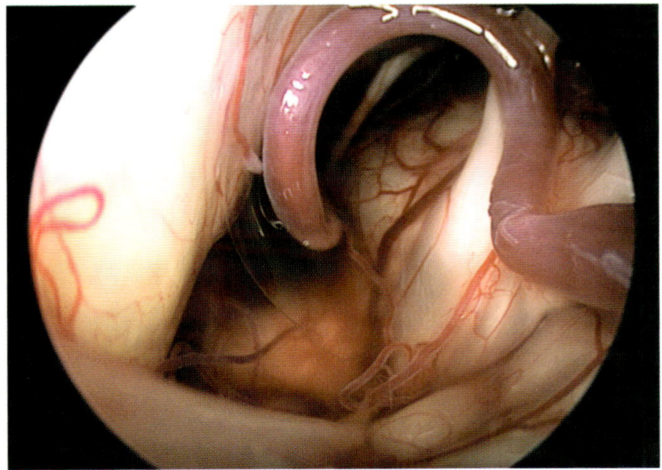

Fig. 4.63: The third pass of CPA endoscopy inferior to the vestibulocochlear nerve and superior to the lower cranial nerves to visualize the facial nerve anteroinferior to the vestibulocochlear nerve at the root entry zone at the lateral part of pontomedullary junction

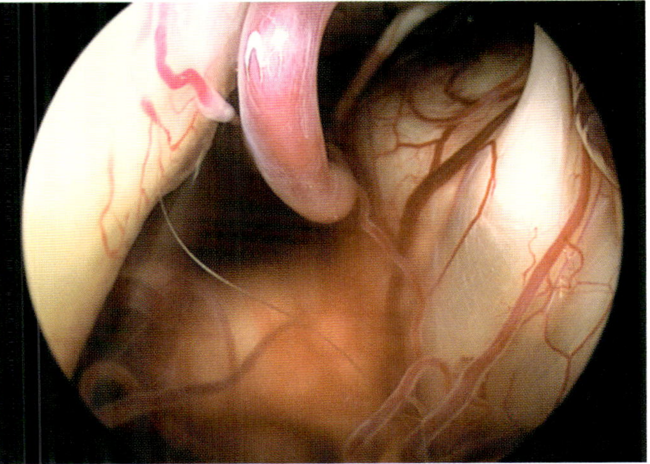

Fig. 4.64: The third pass of CPA endoscopy inferior to the vestibulocochlear nerve and superior to the lower cranial nerves to visualize the area of foramen of Luschka, which is usually filled with cerebrospinal fluid originating out of later

potential help to map the position of the tumor with regard to the facial nerve and AICA and its branches (especially internal auditory artery or labyrinthine artery), to assist removal of the lateral part of the acoustic tumor from the fundus of the internal auditory canal (IAC) without any neurovascular injury, which is difficult to visualize with a microscope alone.

Microvascular Decompression for Hemifacial Spasm and Trigeminal Neuralgia

The 30°- angled endoscope offers a panoramic view to identify the neurovascular conflict and the course of the offending vessels. The vision is particularly difficult with the microscope especially at the root entry zone site

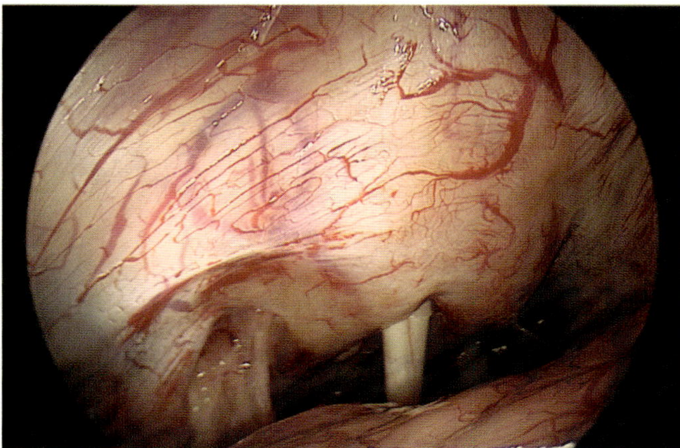

Fig. 4.65: After completing all the three passes while the endoscope was pointing inferiorly toward cerebellum, the endoscope is now rotated 180° to have superior view toward the porus end of vestibulocochlear nerve in center, inferiorly jugular foramen with entry of lower cranial nerves into it and superiorly the trigeminal nerve

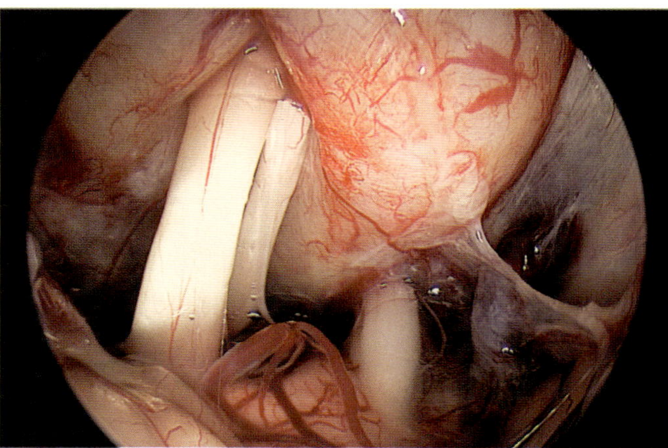

Fig. 4.66: Closer view of porus with vestibulocochlear nerve occupying its posterior part and facial nerve occupying its anterosuperior quadrant

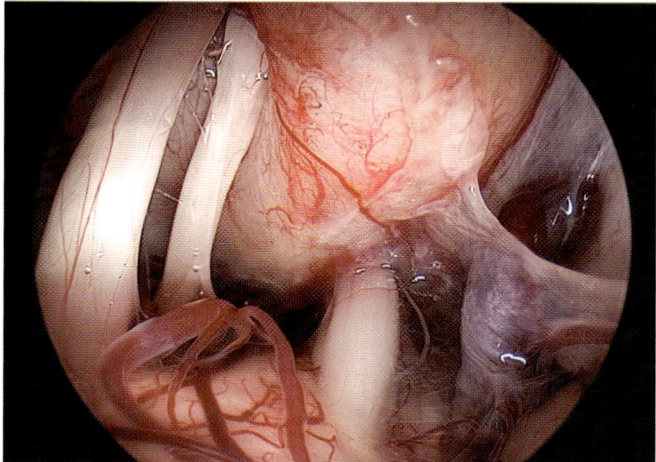

Fig. 4.67: The second pass of CPA endoscopy superior to the vestibulocochlear nerve to visualize the trigeminal nerve entering the Meckel's cave, the Dandy vein (cerebellar vein) entering into superior petrosal sinus and the vestibulocochlear nerve and facial nerve in porus

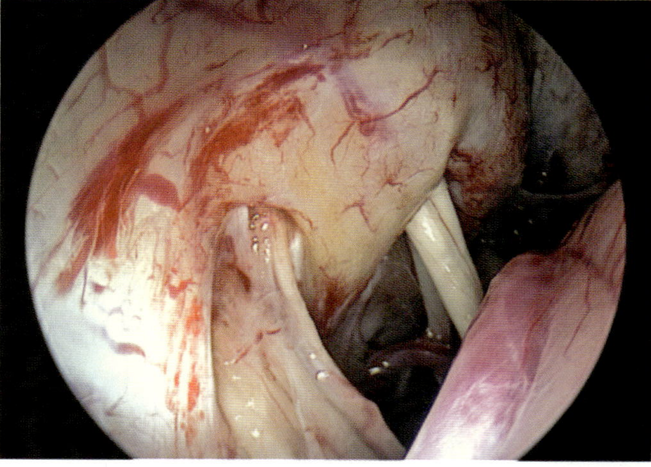

Fig. 4.68: The third pass of CPA endoscopy inferior to the vestibulocochlear nerve showing the glossopharyngeal, vagus and spinal accessory nerve entering the jugular foramen

of facial nerve as it is hidden by the flocculus and the vestibulocochlear nerve. Similarly, the vision of Meckel cave entrance requires endoscopic procedure. The endoscope is again used to confirm the final position of the Teflon sponge after performing the microvascular decompression.

Vestibular Neurotomy

With the endoscope, we can identify the exact three-dimensional position of the vestibulocochlear and facial nerve with regard to each other and with AICA as the vestibular nerve is intimately related to the nervus intermedius, facial nerve and AICA. The endoscope is useful to observe the position of the facial nerve.

Closure

At the end of the surgery, all the cottonoids are removed from the CPA and the same is confirmed with the scrub nurse, who keeps the tally. The hemostasis is once again confirmed. Before closing the dura completely, the

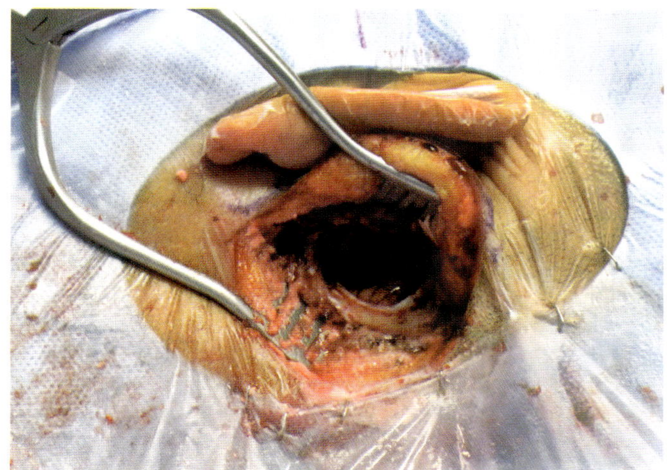

Fig. 4.69: At the end of procedure, the CPA is filled with physiologic saline at body temperature

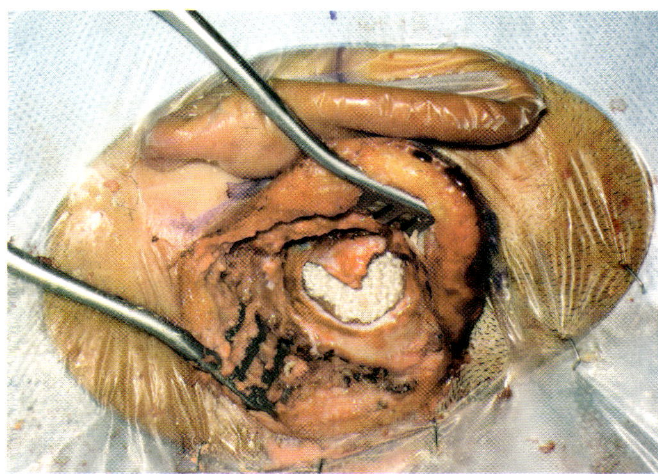

Fig. 4.70: A circular disc of Durapatch (Ethilon, Johnson & Johnson) is prepared with its size slightly larger than the defect of craniotomy. The Durapatch disc is gently glided through the defect such that the entire defect over the cerebellum is snugly covered

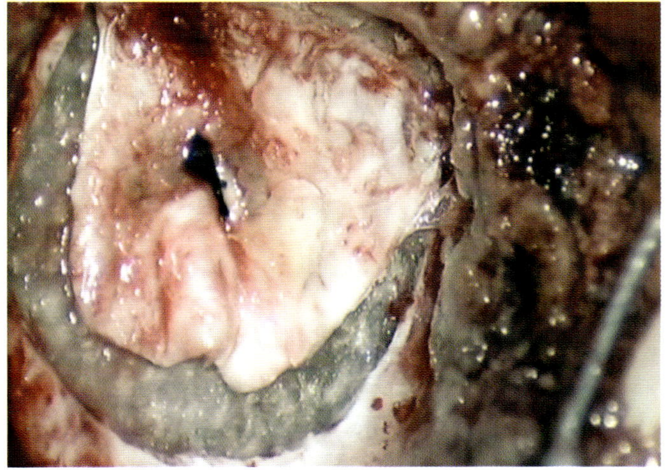

Fig. 4.71: The disc is sutured from its center to the center of dural flap with 5-0 silk on atraumatic needle

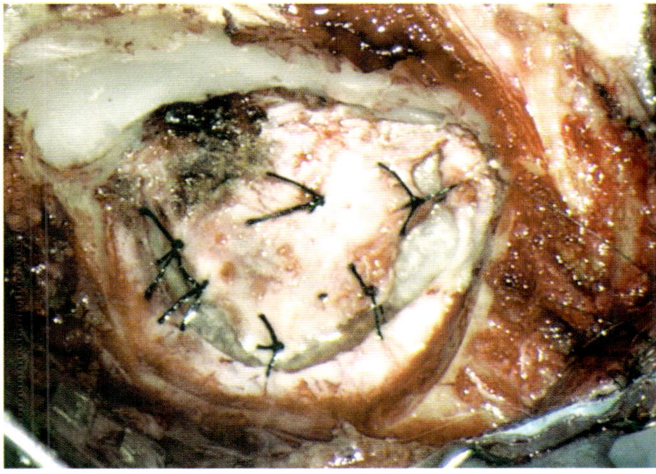

Fig. 4.72: The edges of dura mater over the craniotomy defect are sutured using 5-0 silk sutures (microscopic view)

CPA is filled with physiologic saline (Fig. 4.69) at body temperature to exclude air from CPA as much as possible, as it can cause postoperative pneumocephalus as well as headache. We prepare a circular disc of Durapatch (Ethilon, Johnson & Johnson), whose size is slightly larger than the defect of craniotomy (Fig. 4.70). The Durapatch is made of absorbable polyglactin and has two surfaces: the inner one supposed to line the cerebellum is coated with hydrophobic material so that the CSF does not get absorbed into it. The Durapatch disc is gently glided through the defect such that the hydrophobic side of the disc is placed toward the cerebellum (Fig. 4.70). The disc is sutured from its center to the center of the dural flap with 5-0 silk on atraumatic needle (Fig. 4.71). The incised dura mater is then sutured meticulously using 5-0 silk sutures with atraumatic needle (Figs 4.72 and 4.73). Occasional gaps between sutures are covered by pieces of muscle or subcutaneous fat and then covered by a fibrin glue layer to get a tightly sealed closure (Fig. 4.74). All the mastoid cells are reconfirmed to be obliterated by

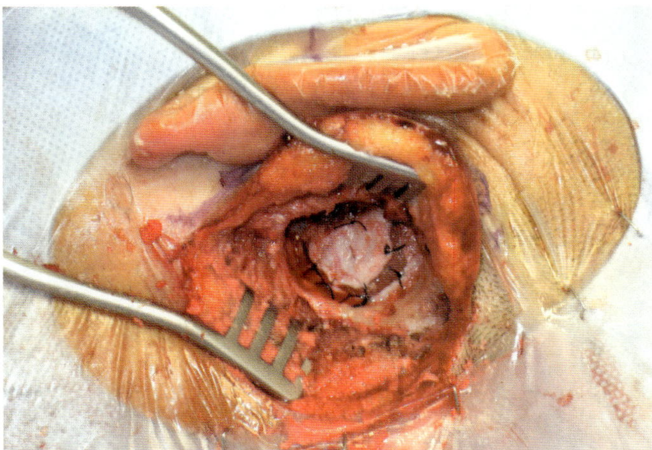

Fig. 4.73: The edges of dura mater over the craniotomy defect are sutured using 5-0 silk sutures

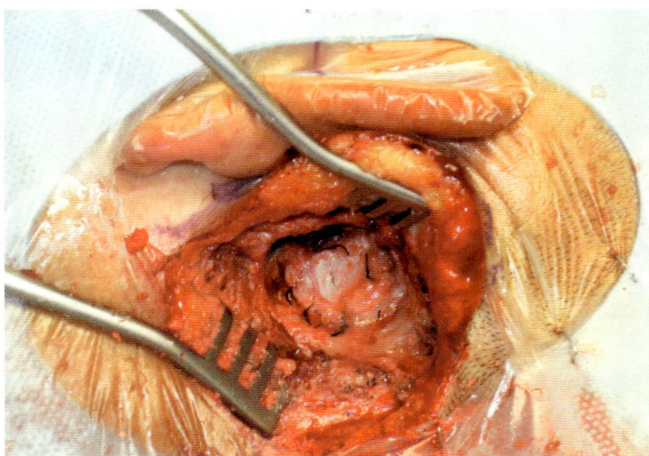

Fig. 4.74: Occasional gaps between sutures are covered by pieces of muscle and then covered by a fibrin glue layer in order to get a tightly sealed closure

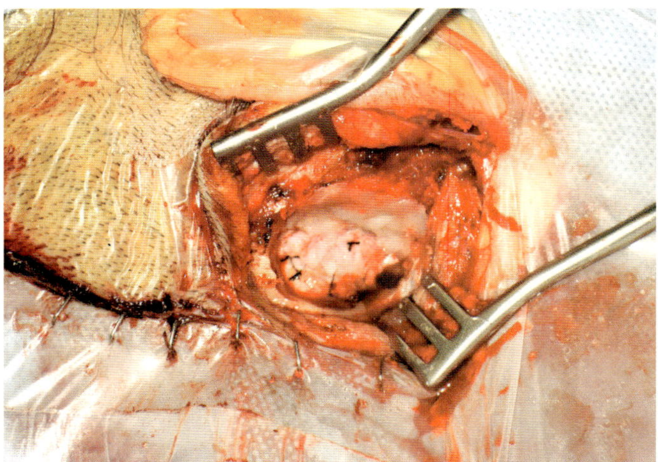

Fig. 4.75: The retrosigmoid air cells are again checked and additionally reinforced and sealed with bone wax to prevent cerebrospinal fluid leak through this route

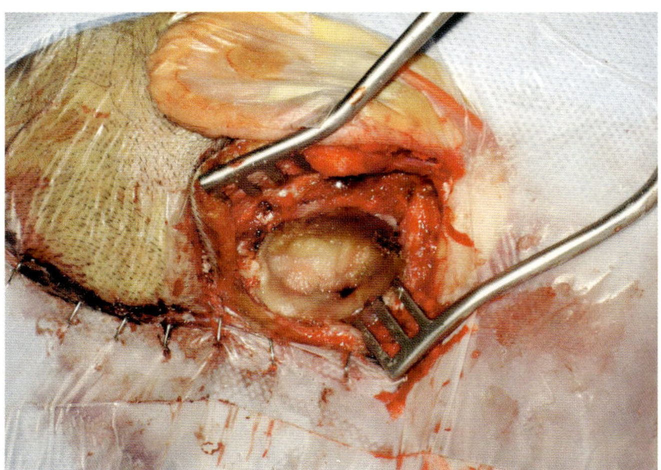

Fig. 4.76: The dura at the craniotomy site is covered by a piece of Surgicel

bone wax (Fig. 4.75). The dura at the craniotomy site is covered by a piece of Surgicel (Fig. 4.76). The bone dust collected initially while drilling the craniotomy is mixed with fibrin glue to make a bone paste that gets solidified in a circular plate shape (Fig. 4.77). This circular bone paste is used to cover the craniotomy site for closure (Fig. 4.78). An additional layer of adipose tissue/Surgicel can be used. The anteriorly based musculoperiosteal flap is sutured with the subcutaneous tissue at its incision site with 2-0 prolene on cutting needle (Figs 4.79 to 4.81). The subcutaneous layer is also sutured with 2-0 prolene (Fig. 4.82) and finally the skin incision is closed with 3-0 Nylon (Fig. 4.83). A mild pressure dressing is given over the wound site for 5 days (Figs 4.84 and 4.85).

POSTOPERATIVE CARE

The patients are monitored in the step down unit overnight and then shifted to normal hospital rooms the next day morning. Prophylactic compression stockings are recommended in patients with high risk for deep vein thrombosis. Early mobilization of the patient reduces the risk for deep vein thrombosis and patients are encouraged

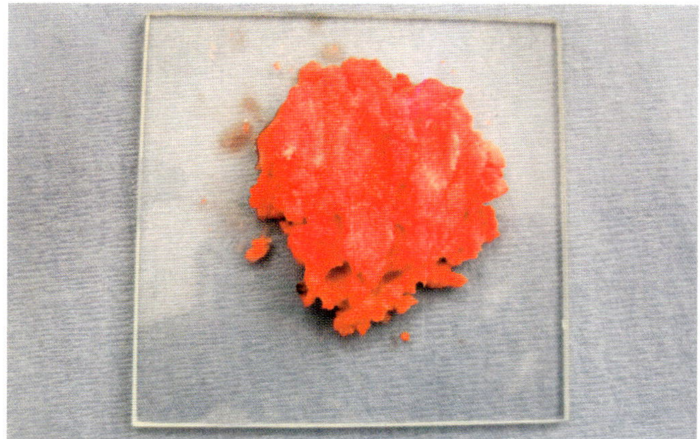

Fig. 4.77: The bone paste is prepared by mixing the bone dust collected initially with fibrin glue and is solidified in a circular shape bone paste

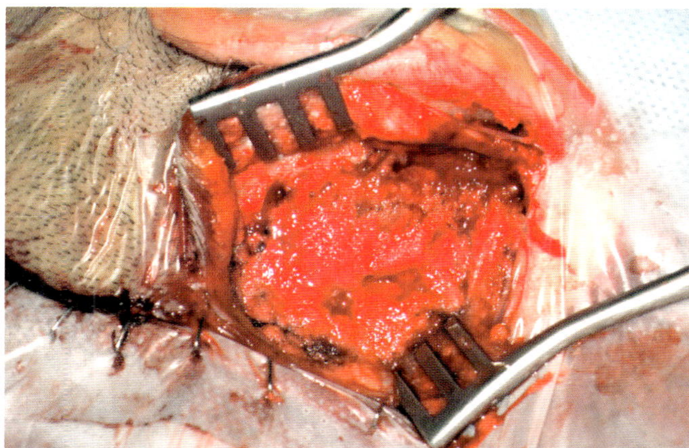

Fig. 4.78: The circular bone paste is used to cover the craniotomy site for closure

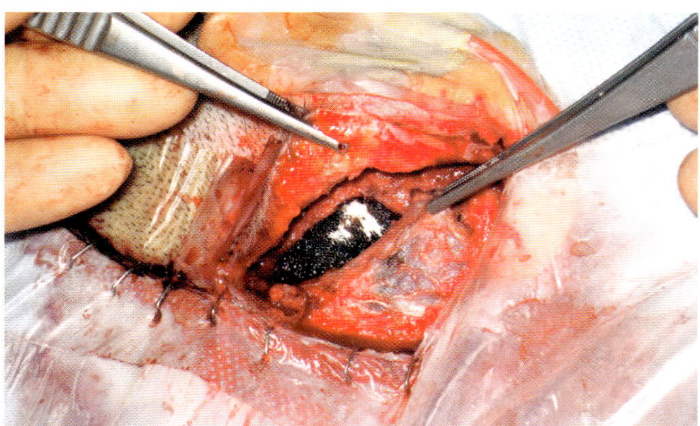

Fig. 4.79: The posteriorly based musculoperiosteal flap is sutured with anterior margin of subcutaneous flap to give "step ladder" pattern of closure to further prevent cerebrospinal fluid leak in postoperative period

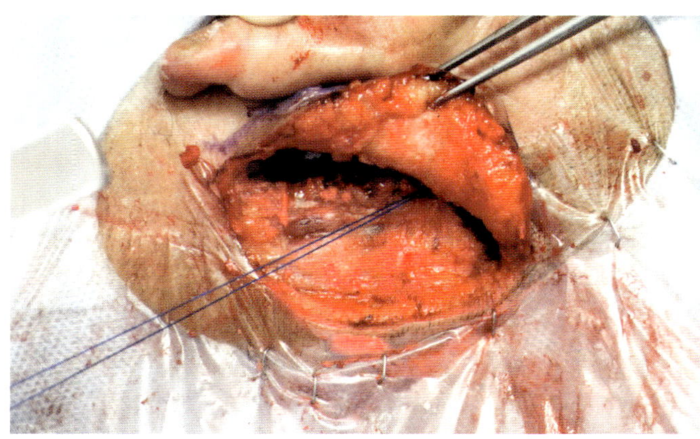

Fig. 4.80: The posteriorly based musculoperiosteal flap is being sutured with anterior margin of subcutaneous flap by 2-0 prolene on cutting needle

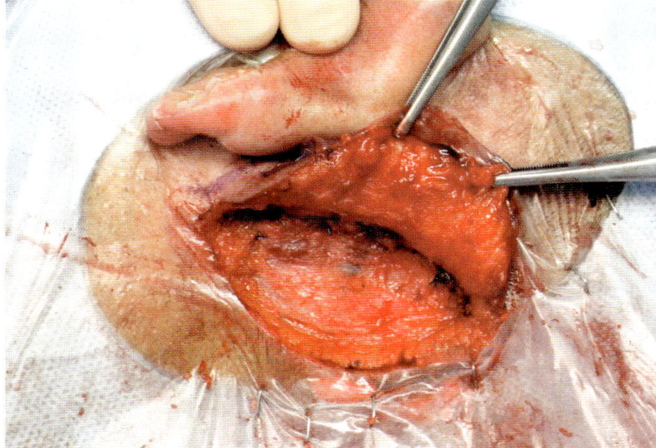

Fig. 4.81: The posteriorly based musculoperiosteal flap is sutured with anterior margin of subcutaneous flap by 2-0 prolene on cutting needle

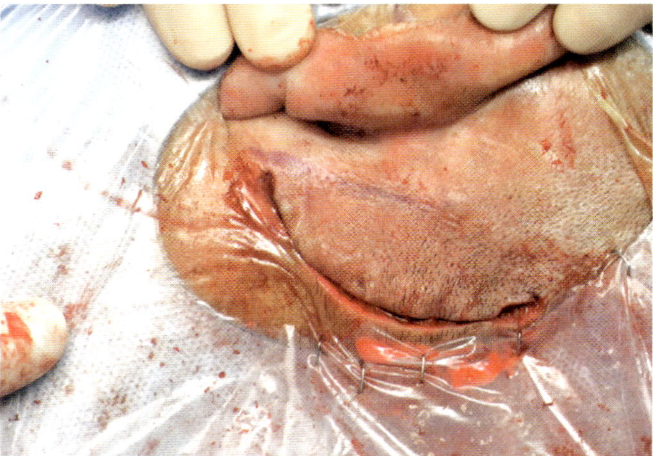

Fig. 4.82: The subcutaneous layer is also sutured with 2-0 prolene

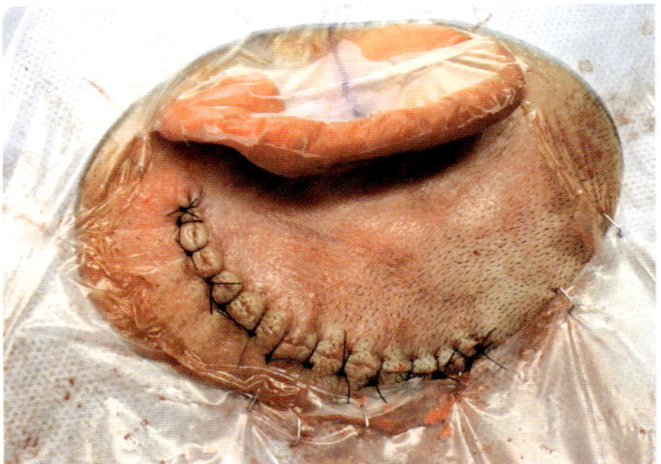

Fig. 4.83: The skin incision is closed with 3-0 Nylon on cutting needle

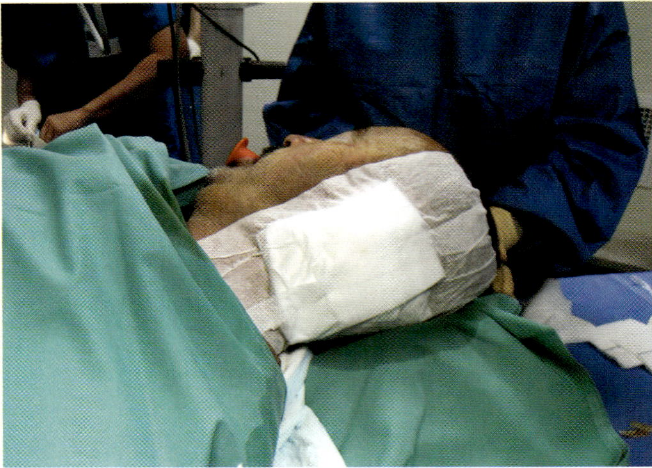

Fig. 4.84: Sterile dressing is given over the wound site

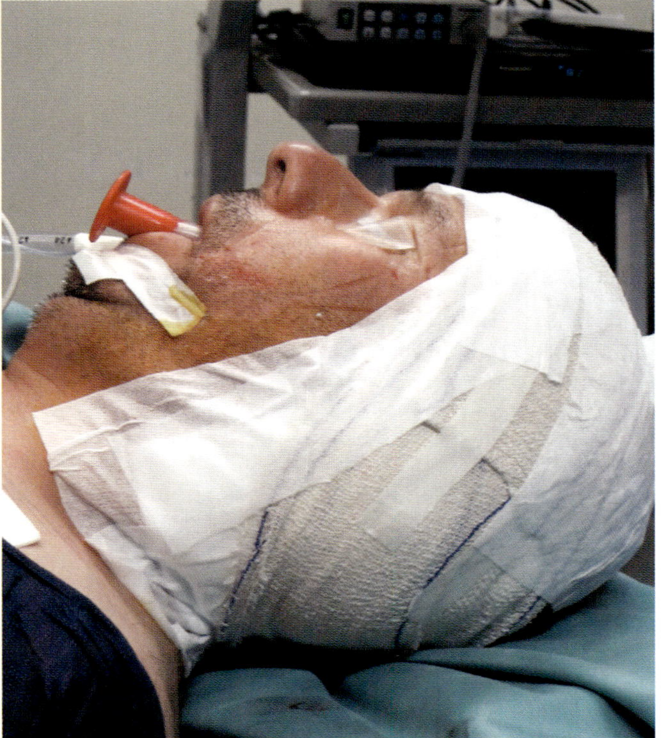

Fig. 4.85: A mild pressure dressing is given over the wound site for 5 days

to be out of bed the day after surgery. Postoperative medicines include intravenous antibiotics, analgesics and antiemetics for 4 days. The patient is discharged on the sixth postoperative day and is asked to return to the clinic 1 week later for suture removal. Most of the patients return to work after a month of surgery.

POSTOPERATIVE COMPLICATIONS

Cerebrospinal Fluid Leak

Despite taking all the precautions the postoperative CSF leak does occur in 3% of our patients who undergo MIRA. The management of CSF leak depends on the site of leak. The CSF leak from the wound is less common owing to multiple layers of closure and is usually mild and requires placing extra sutures over the site of leak, pressure dressing, elevation of head end and bed rest. However, if the CSF leak does not stop with these suggestions, we do not wait for long and do not recommend lumbar puncture and drainage for the belief that it increases the chances of meningitis and prolongs the hospital stay. We prefer to take the patient back to the operating room and reopen the wound, find the site of leak and obliterate it with free muscle graft or abdominal fat along with fibrin glue to seal the site permanently.

CSF otorhinorrhea is more common than the leak from the wound. It is usually due to failure on the part of the surgeon to seal all the mastoid air cells around the craniotomy site or at the site of opening the IAM for acoustic neuroma surgery. In nonacoustic tumor surgery patients, the wound is opened from the same incision and the perisigmoid air cells resealed with muscle and bone wax. In cases of acoustic neuroma or any procedure requiring drilling of IAM through MIRA, the skin and subcutaneous incision is extended to perform cortical mastoidectomy and all the perilabyrinthine cells are sealed, and the aditus and antrum blocked with muscloperiosteal plug, and mastoid filled with free fat grafts harvested from the abdomen. The eustachian tube and the middle ear are generally not plugged to avoid conductive hearing loss.

Meningitis

Meningitis is now a rare complication. Though the incidence of meningitis was 0.3% in the initial period, we did not have any incidence in the past 10 years. However, if the diagnosis of meningitis is confirmed with or without obvious CSF leak, the broad spectrum empirical intravenous antibiotics are started and later changed if required, based on culture sensitivity reports.

Wound Complications

Wound dehiscence is uncommon in neurotologic surgery. Dehiscence is usually involving the lower sutures and is most likely associated with CSF leak. There may be associated infection. The wound is addressed immediately with local debridement followed by resuturing. The cause of the associated CSF leak is addressed simultaneously. Pressure dressing is applied and dressing reevaluated daily for at least 5 days.

Headache

Though headache is often mentioned as one of the most common and debilitating complication of retrosigmoid approach, our patients usually did not complain of persistent refractory long-term headache. The headache was more common in the suboccipital approach probably due to adhesions between the dura and the occipital musculature, entrapment of occipital nerve in the scarred muscles or due to muscle spasm itself. In MIRA, as the occipital and upper cervical muscles are not exposed, there is virtually no incidence of headache.

Intracranial Hemorrhage

Intracranial hemorrhage is an acute emergency and is usually diagnosed within the first 24–48 h. We have had this complication twice in the past 40 years in more than 2000 patients. It occurs due to inadequate hemostasis during surgery or due to postoperative hypertension. Any suspicion of intracranial hemorrhage due to signs of raised intracranial pressure (delayed wake up, loss of consciousness, modifications of vital data) or focal neurologic deficits should be promptly followed up with CT scan, which confirms the diagnosis. It is difficult to evacuate the CPA hematoma caused by retrosigmoid approach by the same route as the increased intracranial pressure, and the hematoma will push the cerebellum out to herniate in the dural opening. So, it is preferable to perform the translabyrinthine approach, evacuate the hematoma and achieve hemostasis. For this reason, in the past, it was recommended to use a combination of retrosigmoid with transmastoid presigmoid approaches.

Cerebellar Edema

It presents similar to intracranial hemorrhage and requires CT/MRI for confirmation of diagnosis. Treatment includes head-end elevation of bed, corticosteroids and mannitol. If there is associated hydrocephalus, ventriculostomy is indicated.

Brainstem/Cerebellar Infarction

It usually occurs due to vascular insult (either due to cerebellar arteries or major vein/sinus occlusion) during surgery. It may be due to division, compression, coagulation or vasospasm of the artery. Cottonoids soaked in papaverine is applied topically to the artery if there are signs of vasospasm during its manipulation in tumor surgery or during microvascular decompression. If there is division or coagulation of the artery (the most common being AICA), it presents as a variable amount of infarction of pons and cerebellum depending upon the injury to either the main trunk (fatal AICA syndrome) or one of the terminal branches (generally favorable prognosis). A focal neurological deficit is present and the diagnosis is confirmed by MRI. Neurological assistance is taken for further management. We have never had a case of fatal AICA syndrome in our experience.

Cranial Nerve Injury

Facial paresis (partial weakness) or delayed facial palsy is treated conservatively with corticosteroids and facial physiotherapy. If the facial palsy is immediate and complete but with a certain anatomical continuity and a positive facial nerve stimulation (at 0.2–0.5 mA) at the end of the procedure, conservative therapy is pursued with good prognosis. If there is acute transaction of the nerve in the CPA and end-to-end anastomosis is not always possible (as usually is the case in facial neuroma), facial hypoglossal anastomosis is performed immediately or in the early postoperative period. Depending on the estimated time of recovery of eye function, temporary or permanent tarsorrhaphy or lid loading surgery is performed. Care is taken to maintain lubrication of cornea to prevent exposure and keratitis.

In patients with tenth cranial nerve palsy due to injury during surgery, there is dysphonia, dysphagia and aspiration of fluids. If the injury is complete and unrecoverable, Type I thyroplasty is performed with arytenoids adduction. If there is neuropraxic injury due to stretching of the nerve, conservative management with fat injection of vocal cord is performed.

Venous Embolism

Venous embolism occurs when the major venous structures remain open due to injury with subatmospheric pressure within the venous structure. It is possible after injury to the sigmoid sinus, jugular bulb, emissary vein or occasionally diploic bone spaces. The chances for venous embolism are higher in the sitting position due to higher subatmospheric pressure. It is rare in the supine position. Although, when there is injury to the sinus or jugular bulb, it is immediately covered with finger or cottonoid till the bleeding is controlled. If the embolism is suspected (fluctuating blood pressure and churning murmur in heart), the patient is shifted to the left lateral position with slight head low position and venous catheter inserted up to the right atrium to evacuate the air embolus.

The type of complications that occurred during MIRA in our experience and their frequency is summarized in Table 4.1.

CONCLUSION

The surgical management of CPA pathologies has undergone tremendous advances during the past four decades. This is all due to untiring efforts of outstanding neurotologists/neurosurgeons throughout the world, and the use of advanced microsurgical instruments, operative microscope and videoendoscopic setup, intraoperative monitoring and obviously advances in neuroanesthesia. Long-term experiences in neurotologic surgery with sincere postoperative follow-up and critical analysis of failures and appropriate modifications have made the procedure much simplified and standardized to get optimal facial nerve outcomes and serviceable hearing. Now we are in a position to achieve facial nerve preservation with considerable constancy and preservation of preoperative hearing in substantial number of patients with small to medium acoustic tumors. Nowadays more emphasis is on the refinement of steps in the methods of intraoperative cochlear monitoring for optimization of functional hearing level. In addition, the morbidity after functional CPA surgery, such as vestibular neurotomy and microvascular decompression is close to zero, except due to an unpredictable accident.

In this book, we intend to present our technique of endoscope-assisted microscopic microvascular decompression procedures, vestibular neurotomy and tumor removal performed using a keyhole MIRA. As these are surgical treatments of functional disorders, it is needless to say that any complications are not acceptable. At the same time, minimally invasive surgery must be promoted by reducing the surgical risk and the surgical cost. To perform the most accurate and safe surgery, we confirm that the endoscope represents an indispensable complementary help. It is required for the surgeon to be knowledgeable about the anatomy of the skull base and have good training of both endoscopic and microsurgical procedures.

Table 4.1 Summary of complications in our cases using MIRA

Complications	*Frequency/rate*
CSFL	3.0%
Meningitis	0.2%
Wound complication	3.0%
Headache	< 1%
Intracranial hematoma	2/2000
Cerebellar edema/infarction	0
Venous embolism	0

REFERENCES

1. Fraenkel J, Hunt J, Woolsey G, et al. Contributions to the surgery of neurofibroma of the acoustic nerve with remarks on the surgical procedure. Ann Surg. 1904; 293–319.
2. Krause E. Zur Freilegung der Linteren, Felsenbeinflache und des Kleinhirns, Beitr 2. Kline Chir 1903; XXXVII:728–64 (Upright).
3. Cushing H. Tumors of the nervus acusticus and the syndrome of the cerebellopontine angle. Philadelphia: WB Saunders; 1917.
4. Dandy WE. Results of removal of acoustic tumors by the unilateral approach. Arch Surg. 1941;42:1026.
5. Casselman W, Kuhweide R, Deimling M, et al. Constructive interferences in steady state 3DFT MR imaging of the inner ear and cerebellopontine angle. AJNR. 1993;14:47–57.
6. Bremond G, Garcin M, Magnan J, Bonnaud G. L'abord à minima de l'espace ponto-cérébelleux. Cah ORL. 1974;19:443–60.
7. Bremond G, Garcin M. Microsurgical approach to the cerebellopontine angle. J Laryngol Otol. 1975;89:237–48.
8. Gerszten P, Clyde B, McLaughin M, Jho H. Criteria on which to judge all minimally invasive neurosurgical techniques. Pittsburg: Joint International Congress on Minimally Invasive Techniques in Neurosurgery and Otolaryngology; 1995.
9. Magnan J, Chays A, Caces F, et al. Apport de l'endoscopie de l'angle ponto-cerebelleux par voie retrosigmoide. Ann Otolaryngol Chir Cervicofacial. 1993;110:259–65.

10. O'Donoghue G, O'Flynn P. Endoscopic anatomy of the cerebellopontine angle. Am J Otol. 1993;14:122–5.
11. McKennan K. Endoscopy of the internal auditory canal during hearing conservation acoustic tumor surgery. Am J Otol. 1993;14:259–62.
12. O'Donoghue G, Greengrass S, Magnan J. Endoscopy in otology and otoneurosurgery. Adv Otolaryngol Head Neck Surg. 1994;8:43–67.
13. Magnan J, Chays A, Lepetre C, Pencroffi E, Locatelli P. Surgical perspectives of endoscopy of the cerebellopontine angle. Am J Otol. 1994;15:366–70.
14. Magnan J, Caces F, Locatelli P, Chays A. Hemifacial spasm: endoscopic vascular decompression. Otolaryngol Head Neck Surg. 1997;117:308–14.
15. Magnan J, Sanna M. Endoscopy in neuro-otology. Stuttgart, New York: Thieme; 1999
16. Badr-el-Dine M, EL-Garem HF, Talaat AM, Magnan J. Endoscopically assisted minimally invasive microvascular decompression of hemifacial spasm. Otol Neurotol. 2002;23:122–8.
17. Magnan J. The value of endoscopy in otology and neuro-otology. Otol Jpn. 2003;13(3);163–73.
18. Miyazaki H, Deveze A, Magnan J. Neuro-otologic surgery through minimally invasive retrosigmoid approach. Endoscope-assisted microvascular decompression, vestibular neurotomy, and tumor removal. Laryngoscope. 2005;115(9);1612–7.
19. Magnan J, Bremond G, Chays A, Gignac D, Florence A. Vestibular neurotomy by retrosigmoid approach: technique, indications, and results. Am J Otol. 1991;12:101–4.
20. Magnan J, Deveze A, Miyazaki H, Canani FB. Cerebellopontine angle surgery by the retrosigmoid approach: our experience in elderly patients. Mediterr J Otol. 2005;1:1–7.
21. Guevara N, Deveze A, Buza V, Lafont B, Magnan J. Microvascular decompression of cochlear nerve for tinnitus incapacity: pre-surgical data, surgical analyses and long-term follow-up of 15 patients. Eur Arch Otorhinolaryngol. 2008;265(4):397–401.
22. Girard N, Poncet M, Caces F, Tallon Y, Chays A, Martin-Bouyer P, Magnan J, Raybaud C. Three dimensional MRI of hemifacial spasm with surgical correlation. Neuroradiology. 1997;39(1):46–51.

5 Vestibular Neurotomy by Minimally Invasive Retrosigmoid Approach

INTRODUCTION

Menière's disease has been the most incapacitating of the peripheral causes of the vertigo because of its paroxysmal nature, severe intensity and relatively longer duration along with associated vegetative symptoms like nausea and occasional vomiting. A single episode of vertigo leaves the patient both physically and mentally drained and apprehensive of the next episode. Though majority of patients are lucky to have control over these symptoms within 2–5 years (spontaneous remission is estimated to be between 50 and 70%),[1] not all of them are so fortunate. The tragedy with many patients with chronic Menière's disease is that the prophylactic medicines do not work in a considerable number and the acute episode occasionally arrives without an impending warning when the patient is alone or performing an activity that can cause injury to the patient and others. As the patients are not able to predict the next episode, over the time, they avoid such events and activities and become sedentary workers and socially dependent. This whole event leaves the patient with deep psychological trauma. The patient desperately needs the treatment option that is predictable in results, causes permanent relief in vertigo and prevents further loss of hearing. Most of the symptoms of chronic peripheral vertigo, especially Menière's disease, are persistent because of their inherent partially ablative nature disallowing normal central compensation. Also, any treatment causing incomplete or temporary vestibular ablation/suppression has considerable chances of recurrent/residual disease. The successful treatment options for severe incapacitating vertigo with permanent relief with hearing preservation have therefore always aimed at complete ablation. The ablation of hearing for the treatment for vertigo of Menière's disease is considered injudicious unless it is an end-stage disease with profound hearing loss. Therefore, the best option is selective complete vestibular ablation with preservation of hearing. The vestibular compensation is at its best with complete ablation of unilateral vestibular inputs. The therapeutic options for achieving selective unilateral complete vestibular ablation are chemical ablation of the vestibular hair cells with intratympanic gentamicin therapy or surgical ablation of selective vestibular nerve fibers by various hearing preservation approaches.

Both of these treatments have gained the confidence of patients and treating physicians in the past few decades. There is considerable literature available now presenting us the advantages and disadvantages of both.[2–15] The advantages of intratympanic gentamicin therapy are its being office procedure; it avoids the physical and mental trauma, such as the consequences of surgery like hospital stay and its associated morbidity and the cost. Initial regimens to achieve this were very intensive in nature giving multiple injections in a day for multiple days. This resulted in complete vestibular ablation but with profound hearing loss in more than 30% of patients.[16] The newer weekly "titrated" regimens lead to fewer rates of hearing loss while achieving near total ablation.[17] However, studies show that over the time the hair cells regrow[18] and considerable number of patients require further treatment due to recurrence of symptoms or not getting permanent cure. Recent comparative studies of both the treatments[19–22] nicely summarize the current scenario. "Although vestibular nerve section and transtympanic gentamicin are both acceptable treatment options for vertigo associated with Menière's disease, gentamicin causes a higher level of hearing loss related to treatment and vestibular nerve section has higher vertigo control rates."[22] We maintain that intratympanic gentamicin plays an important role in the treatment of the vertigo associated with Menière's disease. Although hearing is likely to be at greater risk with this treatment than with vestibular nerve section, there are many situations in which this risk is acceptable. In patients who are at risk for operative complications because of concomitant medical problems, gentamicin treatment offers an alternative that eliminates anesthetic risk and potential risk associated with postoperative complications. In some patients the pretreatment hearing in the affected ear may be so poor that aural rehabilitation is impossible and therefore damage to remaining hearing is inconsequential. Also, there are a group of patients who have serious apprehension about undergoing surgical intervention and are willing to accept the moderate increase in risk to remaining hearing to avoid an operative procedure.

Vestibular neurotomy is considered the reference treatment of intractable vertigo accompanying Menière's disease. Compared to endolymphatic duct surgery and intratympanic gentamicin injections, vestibular neurotomy had proved to be the best treatment in terms of vertigo control and hearing preservation.[22] The minimal invasive posterior fossa retrosigmoid approach[2,3] allows to preserve hearing with a near zero rate of serious complication. If the vestibular nerve section is complete, there is a total vestibular deafferentation[23] with complete areflexia at the caloric test. Selective vestibular nerve section by minimally invasive retrosigmoid approach (MIRA) gives permanent relief from rotatory vertigo in more than 95% of cases with excellent hearing preservation rates. It requires admission in the hospital only once and does not require repeated procedures lasting for many weeks. The vestibular compensation begins immediately postop and most patients are fit to resume work in 4–8 weeks. The hearing preserving selective vestibular nerve section can be performed by retrolabyrinthine, retrosigmoid or middle cranial fossa approach. While all the three options have advantages and disadvantages,[2,24-26] they give similar results for vertigo control and hearing preservation.

Our choice for selective vestibular nerve section is MIRA. It was Dandy[27,28] who first recognized that selective neurotomy of the vestibular nerve was possible via the posterior fossa, and performed 607 neurotomies in 587 patients with Menière's disease between 1924 and 1946. Aubry and Ombredanne[29] reportedly used the same suboccipital craniotomy and vestibular nerve section as early as 1935 in France. However, the morbidity and mortality associated with this surgery prevented it from gaining widespread acceptance. Vestibular nerve section fell into obscurity until being resurrected by the new microsurgical procedures popularized by House[30] in the 1960s. After Fluur and Tovi,[31] who published the microsurgical intracranial technique to cut the vestibular nerve, Bremond et al.[32,33] described in 1974 a minimally invasive approach through a keyhole retrosigmoid craniotomy. However, the operation was not much popularized until Millen and Meyer,[34] and then Silverstein et al.[35,36] stressed the advantages of this surgical procedure. It is now confirmed that retrosigmoid vestibular neurotomy provides certain and safe access to the vestibulocochlear nerve in the cerebellopontine angle,[2,3] and led to the concept of minimally invasive otoneurosurgery.[37]

PATHOPHYSIOLOGICAL BASIS FOR VESTIBULAR NEUROTOMY

The principle of vestibular neurotomy is to produce a total loss of afferent input from the offending vestibular periphery (most common being Menière's disease). Vestibular neurotomy seeks to stabilize inner ear function in the pathologic and fluctuating Menière's disease ear by the help of this remarkable plasticity of the central vestibular system composed of cerebellum and brainstem called vestibular compensation. Vestibular compensation can be defined as a central complex process involving multiple sensory substitution mechanism leading to restoration of posture and equilibrium after asymmetries in peripheral vestibular afferent activity. Vestibular compensation will relieve peripheral vertigo in most instances, provided the lesion is stable. Fundamental research dealing with an experimental model of neuroplasticity has carefully described the vestibular compensation process occurring after unilateral lesion of the peripheral labyrinth or the vestibular nerve since its original description by Flourens in 1824. Acute compensation occurs within first few days to provide relief from intense vertigo and vegetative symptoms by the inhibitory action of cerebellum ("cerebellar clamp") over both vestibular nuclei. However, it is common to have motion-induced vertigo/disequilibrium until chronic compensation is achieved. To relieve the motion-induced vertigo/disequilibrium, the cerebellar clamp has to be slowly released and replaced by symmetric activity of both vestibular nuclei and their accurate response to the head, postural and eye movements. This is achieved by stimulus to the ipsilateral affected vestibular nuclei from the contralateral normal vestibular system provided the ipsilateral affected side has stable afferent inputs. These adjustments by contralateral vestibular nuclei are quick and reasonably accurate and are enhanced by early head and body movements (vestibular rehabilitation exercises). Vestibular neurotomy has proven to be an effective procedure for relieving vertigo in intractable Menière's disease with a constant success rate over 95%.

INDICATIONS FOR VESTIBULAR NEUROTOMY

The most common indication for selective vestibular neurotomy is incapacitating unilateral Menière's disease with bothersome disability. Thorough investigation in the form of pure tone and speech audiometry, videonystagmography and magnetic resonance imaging, is must to confirm the diagnosis and access the level of hearing. The surgical indication relies on the patient's will after informed consent on the procedure and the alternative therapies. The duration of disease, frequency and severity of attacks, hearing status in the affected ear and profession of the patient are important criteria to guide for the decision and type of surgery. The perception of disability varies from one patient to the other and we leave it on the patient to decide the character of incapacitating disorder and the time of further intervention.

The goal of vestibular neurotomy is to control disabling vertigo while preserving hearing in patients with Menière's disease who are unresponsive to maximal medical treatment or have persistent vertigo following a failed endolymphatic sac procedure/intratympanic gentamicin. Although, vestibular neurotomy can be summarized as surgery for Menière's disease, such a surgical procedure can be offered to any patient, with recurrent vertigo of peripheral origin. These include vestibular injuries that are clearly peripheral in nature like posttraumatic labyrinthine fistula with good residual hearing (or occasionally poststapedotomy disabling vertigo with good hearing) or infective as in recurrent vestibular neuronitis/labyrinthitis) refractory to medical management. Although advanced age alone is not a contraindication for vestibular nerve section surgery, perioperative risk for medical and anesthetic complications should be taken into consideration. The process of vestibular compensation is considered to be slower in elderly patients due to associated visual and proprioceptive anomalies. This has not been confirmed in our experience. Elderly patients are less demanding and therefore their recovery is more than enough for their daily activities. The decision-making in bilateral Menière's disease is much more difficult and the status of contralateral hearing and vestibular function should always be assessed before performing any ablative procedure for treatment of Menière's disease. The initial survey by Perez et al.[38] to study the natural history of Menière's disease and to assess the development of contralateral symptoms showed highly variable figures from 2% to 78% in the literature. However, Perez et al. found the rate of involvement of the contralateral ear to be less than 5% after 2 or more years of follow-up. In our study group, bilateral disorder occurred in 1.7% of cases in the postoperative period after having vestibular neurotomy for initial unilateral disease (four cases within 5 years and one case after 10 years). This trend of reduced rate of contralateral disease in patients operated by vestibular neurotomy needs to be confirmed by a still longer follow-up and in several large series, but it still represents an important positive fact.

SURGICAL TECHNIQUE

The patient preparation, position, type of anesthesia, incision and the retrosigmoid craniotomy is discussed in Chapter 4, Surgical Approach. A 15-mm circular craniotomy is performed behind the sigmoid sinus and the dura opened. The cerebellum is allowed to retract spontaneously by assisted hyperventilation followed by draining of cerebrospinal fluid (CSF) after the opening of cistern magna. The cerebellar surface is protected from injury by a strip of Neuropatch/cottonoid to avoid injury to adjoining structures and obtain a safe corridor within which to operate. This surgical space has a safe corridor formed by the posterior surface of the petrosal bone anterosuperiorly and a protected cerebellar surface posteroinferiorly that is maintained spontaneously without the need for retractors.

Under the operating microscope with 250 mm focus, the arachnoid surrounding the acousticofacial nerve bundle is dissected away completely exposing the VII–VIII complex from its origin up to its entrance into porus. The vestibulocochlear nerve is visualized at the depth of around 55 mm from the anterior margin of craniotomy. The entrance of the vestibulocochlear and facial nerves into the porus acousticus provides their unquestionable identification (Fig. 5.1). The origin of the vestibulocochlear nerve and its medial 3–5 mm at the lateral pontomedullary junction is usually covered by the flocculus. Within the vestibulocochlear nerve, the vestibular fibers are more superior (rostral) and close to the trigeminal nerve, (Fig. 5.2) and the cochlear nerve is inferior (caudal) and close to the lower cranial nerves (Fig. 5.3). The vestibular

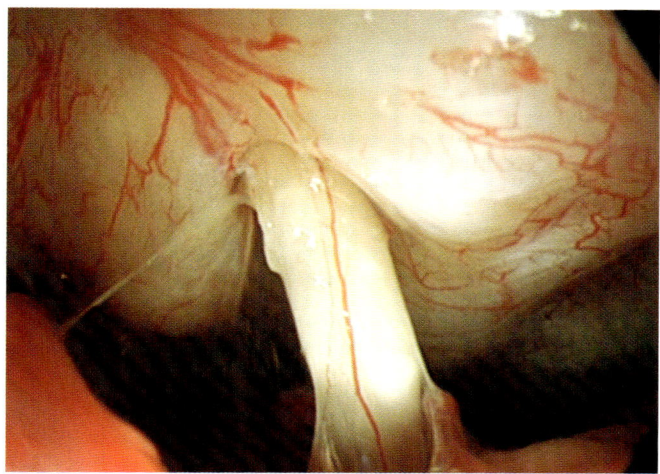

Fig. 5.1: Endoscopic picture showing the acousticofacial nerve bundle crossing through the middle of the cerebellopontine angle and its entrance in the internal auditory canal provides its sure identification. There is always an intervestibulocochlear cleavage plane in its cisternal course to the porus and is often marked by a small blood vessel running over this cleavage plane

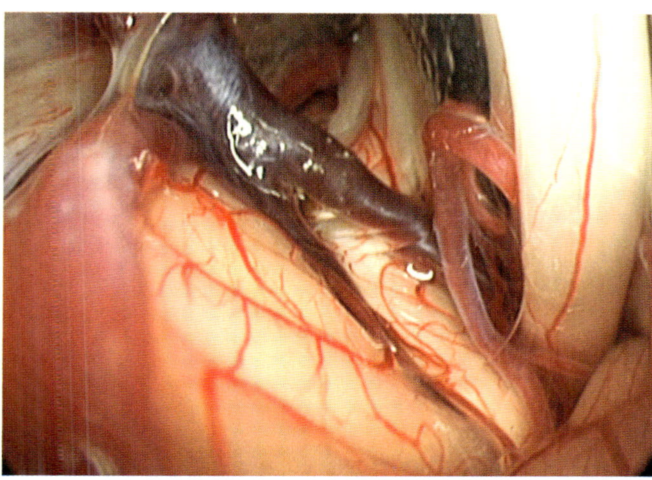

Fig. 5.2: Endoscopic picture showing the vestibulocochlear nerve with the vestibular nerve fibers being more superior (rostral) and close to the trigeminal nerve

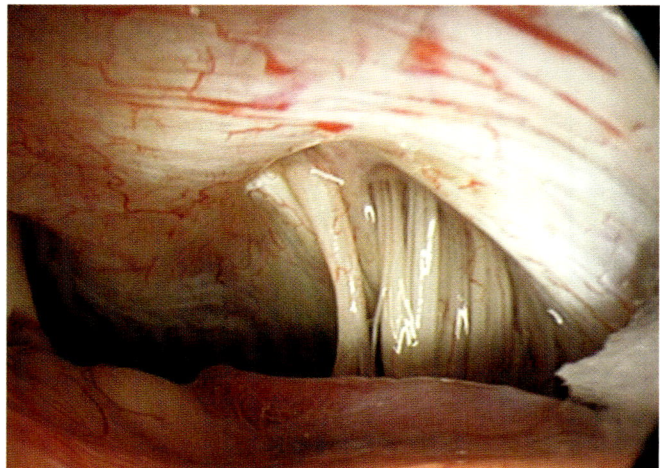

Fig. 5.3: Endoscopic picture showing the cochlear nerve is inferior (caudal) and close to the lower cranial nerves

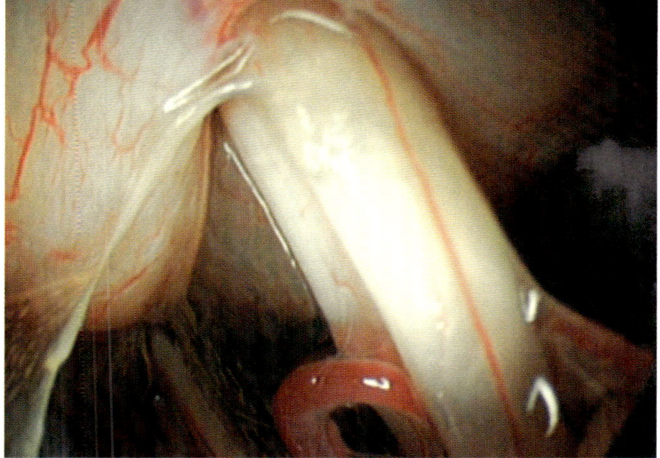

Fig. 5.4: Endoscopic picture showing that the facial nerve is closer to vestibulocochlear nerve along its cisternal course to lie in anterosuperior quadrant at porus

nerve appears grayish as compared with the cochlear nerve. The key point of the procedure is to know that there is always an intervestibulocochlear cleavage plane in its cisternal course to the porus and is often marked by a small blood vessel running over this cleavage plane. Although the vestibular and cochlear nerves fuse within the internal auditory meatus (IAM), the intervestibulocochlear cleavage plane is apparent both by gross examination and on histological study. When the arachnoid wrapping is dissected away from the nerve bundle, a groove along the vestibulocochlear nerve is visible and well marked near the porus (Figs 5.2 and 5.3). This cleavage plane divides the vestibulocochlear nerve into two parts. The origin of the facial nerve is located anteroinferior to the vestibulocochlear nerve and thus it remains ventrally (anteriorly) positioned being hidden from the view in the cerebellopontine angle (CPA) and comes closer to the vestibulocochlear nerve along its cisternal course to lie in the anterosuperior quadrant at porus (Figs 5.4 and 5.5). The anterior inferior cerebellar artery (AICA) is often closely related to the vestibulocochlear and facial nerves (Figs 5.2 and 5.4), running either caudal, cephalad or occasionally between them. The position of the facial nerve and AICA can be confirmed with endoscope, if required (Figs 5.2 to 5.5).

Once the vestibulocochlear nerve is well identified and the cleavage plane between them delineated (Figs 5.6 and 5.7), the superiorly lying vestibular nerve is transected at the medial part of its course in CPA near the brainstem. As discussed earlier, specially adapted micro-instrumentation set with bayonet handle facilitates visualization with the keyhole approach. Conventional otologic instruments are too short and the usual neurosurgical instruments are too bulky. A small dissector inserted into this partition line divides the acoustic nerve into its two parts (Fig. 5.8). Vestibular neurotomy is performed initially with long microsurgical scissors (Sterker's scissors) transecting the majority of the superiorly lying vestibular nerve (Figs 5.9 to 5.12), but leaving the terminal fibers with close relation to the inferiorly lying cochlear nerve. The final fibers of

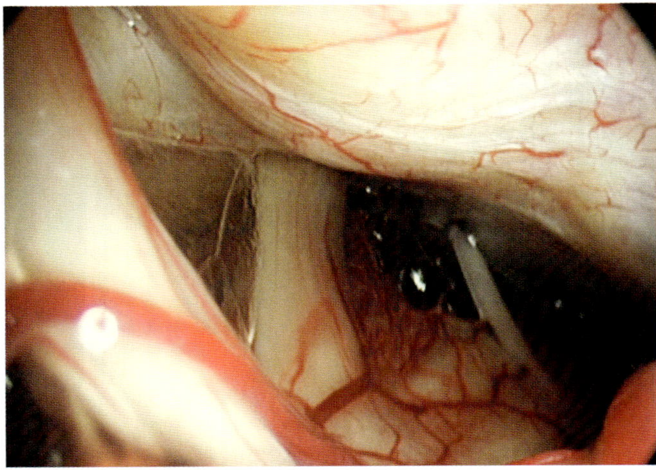

Fig. 5.5: The origin of the facial nerve at lateral pontomedullary junction is located anteroinferior to the vestibulocochlear nerve and thus it remains ventrally (anteriorly) positioned being hidden from the view in CPA

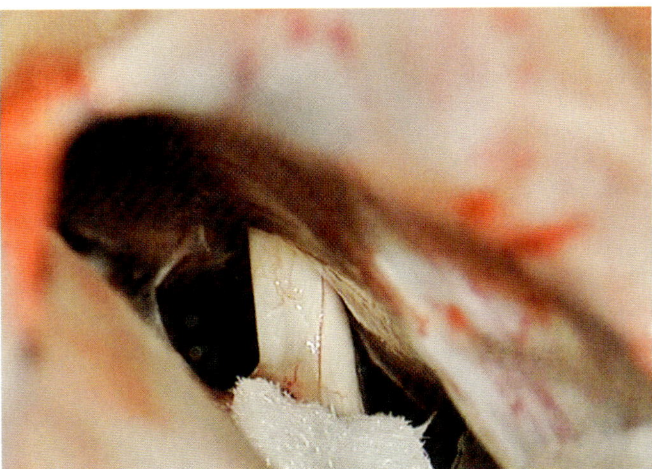

Fig. 5.6: Microscopic picture showing the vestibulocochlear nerve after the arachnoid surrounding the acousticofacial nerve bundle is dissected completely

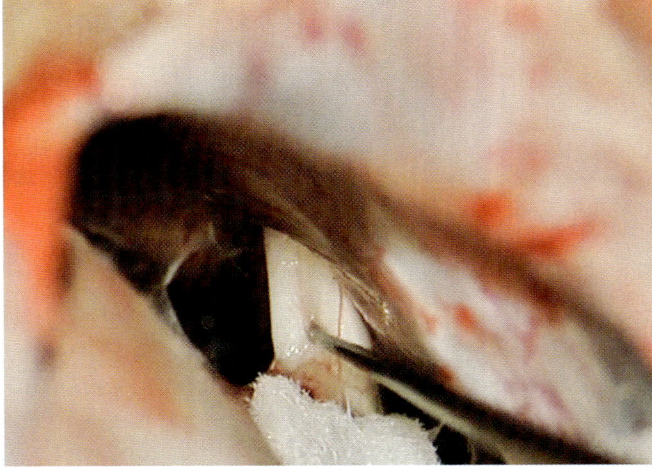

Fig. 5.7: The intervestibulocochlear groove separates the vestibulocochlear nerve. A blunt probe marks the intervestibulocochlear cleavage plane and isolates the vestibular (that lies superiorly) from the inferiorly positioned cochlear nerve

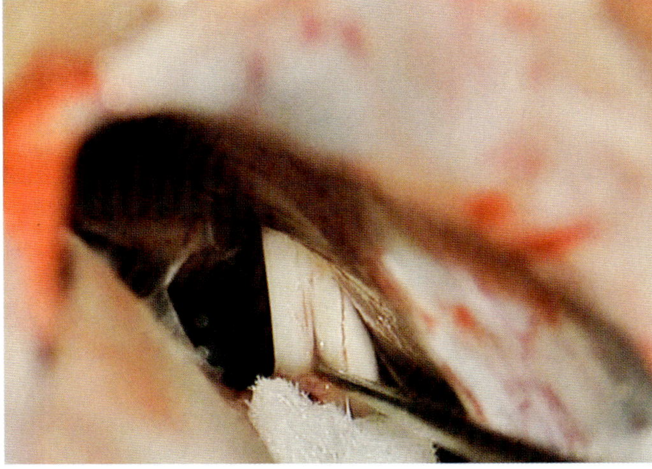

Fig. 5.8: Under microscopic view, a small dissector is inserted in the intervestibulocochlear cleavage plane and isolates the vestibular from the cochlear nerve

the vestibular nerve are transected by blunt hook/probe till the nervus intermedius fibers are seen (Figs 5.13 and 5.14). After complete neurotomy, the ends of the nerve retract spontaneously (Fig. 5.15), so that the surgeon need not perform the resection of a segment of nerve (neurectomy). The facial nerve, which runs anteroinferior, is widely separated at the medial end of the CPA and is usually safe from injury. One should always visualize the course of AICA before transecting the vestibular nerve. The position of the facial nerve and AICA can be asserted during surgery by gentle retraction of the cisternal course of the vestibulocochlear nerve (Figs 5.16 and 5.17). The nervus intermedius is formed by the various connecting nerve fibers between the vestibulocochlear and facial nerves, which enter the former at the cleavage plane anteriorly and forms a good landmark for completion of the vestibular nerve section (Fig. 5.17). We do not use the endoscope routinely in vestibular neurotomy, but it gives an excellent orientation of the neighboring AICA and facial nerve (Figs 5.18 and 5.19).

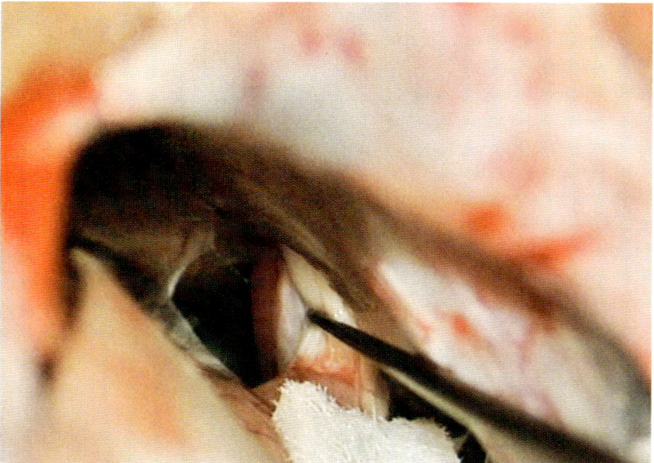

Fig. 5.9: The facial nerve is closer to vestibulocochlear nerve along its cisternal course to lie in anterosuperior quadrant at porus. The position of the facial nerve and AICA is reconfirmed under microscopic view by retracting the vestibulocochlear nerve before dividing the vestibular division

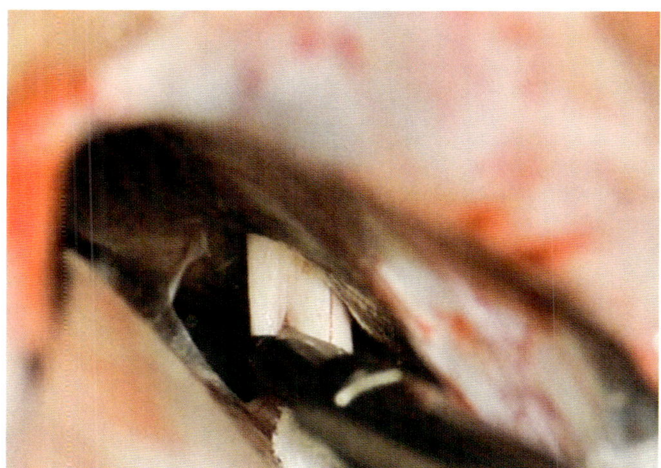

Fig. 5.10: Vestibular neurotomy is performed with microscissors

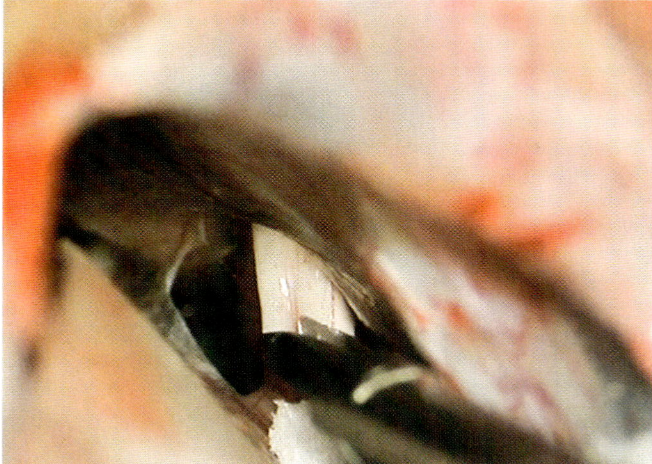

Fig. 5.11: Vestibular neurotomy is performed by microscissors with one flange in the intervestibulocochlear cleavage plane and another superior to the vestibular nerve

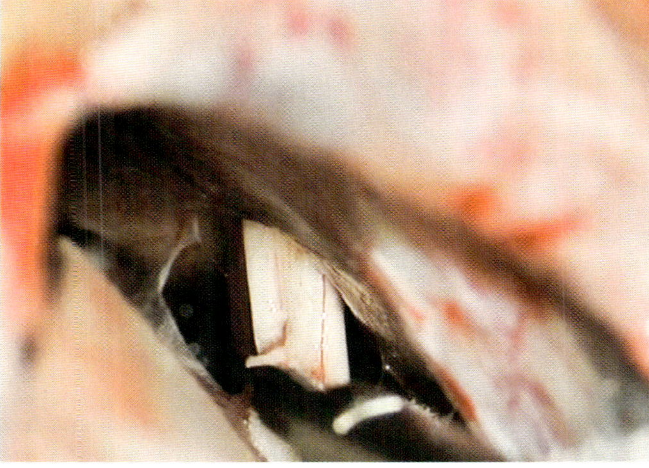

Fig. 5.12: Vestibular neurotomy is performed with microscissors. A few fibers of vestibular nerve are still attached to the cochlear nerve

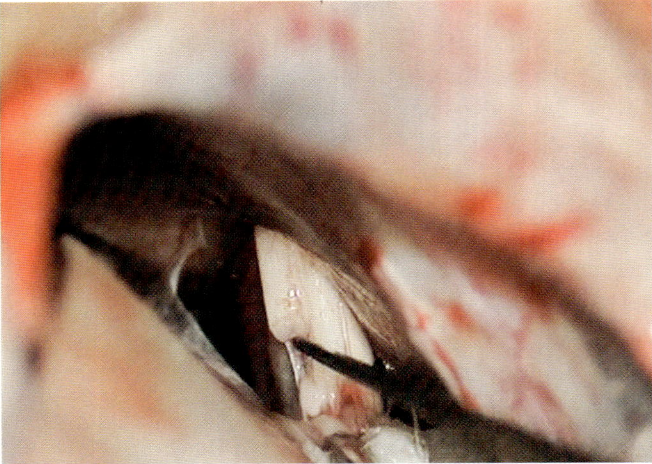

Fig. 5.13: The last few fibers of vestibular nerve are still attached to the cochlear nerve and are transected by blunt hook/probe with blunt dissection (microscopic view)

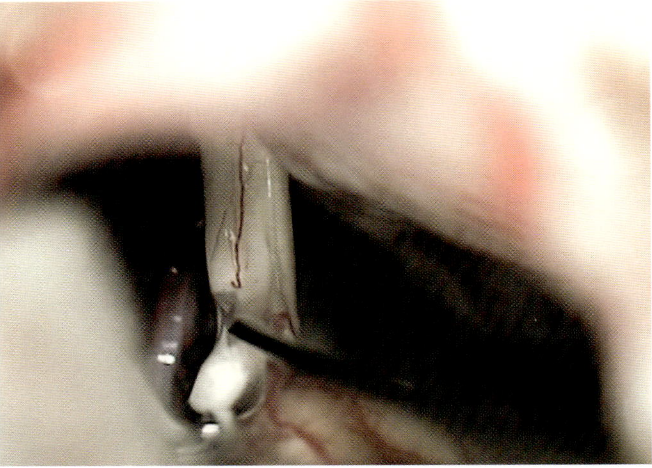

Fig. 5.14: A few fibers of vestibular nerve still attached to the cochlear nerve are resected with blunt dissection (endoscopic view)

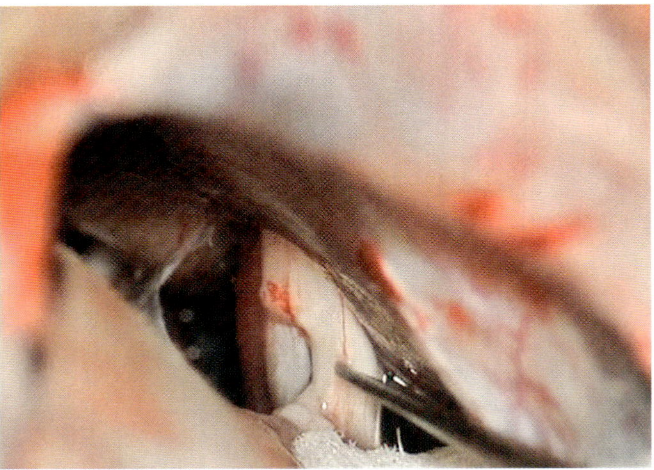

Fig. 5.15: Vestibular neurotomy completed

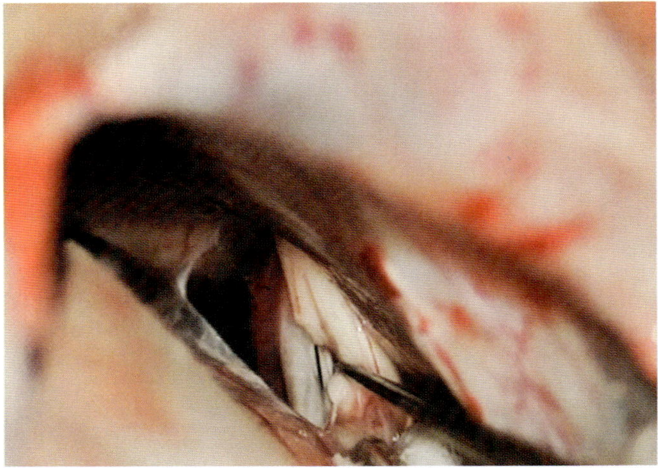

Fig. 5.16: Nervus intermedius is an important landmark suggesting complete vestibular nerve section as it is located at the junction of the vestibular and facial nerve

Care is taken to avoid unnecessary stretching or injury to the internal auditory (labyrinthine) artery. Using this technique, there is virtually no injury to the cochlear nerve fibers and its blood supply, and gives good postoperative hearing results. In fact, the main risk of vestibular neurotomy is a partial section of the vestibular component that should be suspected postoperatively in a patient with a delayed and unsatisfactory rehabilitation concomitant to an absence of complete areflexia. The use of intraoperative cochlear monitoring and vestibulocochlear mapping solves this possibility of partial resection.

COCHLEAR NERVE MONITORING AND MAPPING FOR VESTIBULAR NEUROTOMY

The major indication for the vestibular neurotomy is the disappearance of attacks of vertigo without any change in the function of the cochlear and facial nerve due to surgery. Cochlear and facial nerve monitoring and mapping help in achieving this target. It is relatively easier to set the dorsal cochlear nucleus action potential (DNAP) and facial nerve

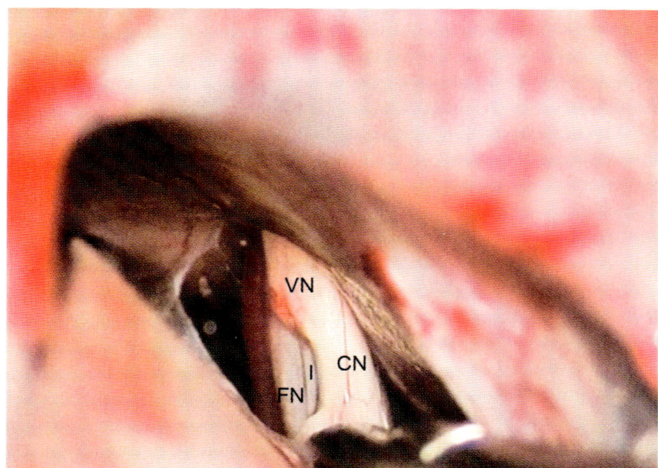

Fig. 5.17: Final microscopic picture at the end of vestibular neurotomy showing resected vestibular nerve, cochlear nerve, AICA, facial nerve and nervus intermedius

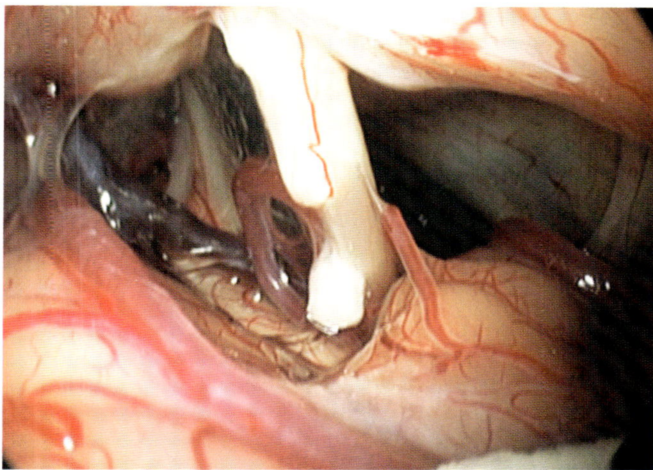

Fig. 5.18: Final endoscopic picture at the end of vestibular neurotomy showing resected vestibular nerve, cochlear nerve, AICA and facial nerve. After sectioning, the ends of the vestibular nerve retract spontaneously. Flocculus covers the medial 3–5 mm of the vestibulocochlear nerve

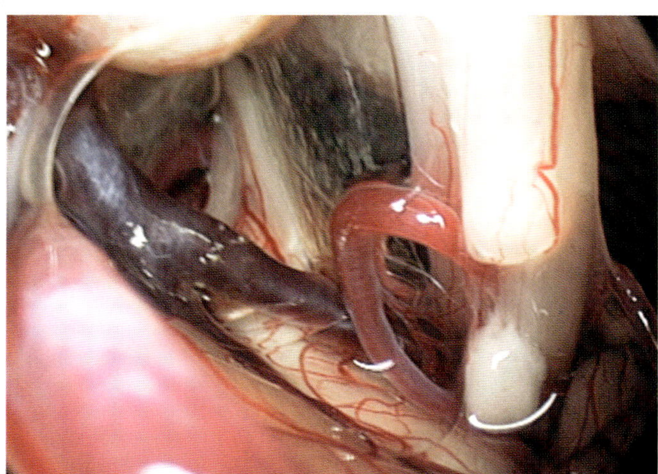

Fig. 5.19: Final endoscopic picture at the end of vestibular neurotomy showing resected vestibular nerve, cochlear nerve, AICA and facial nerve

root evoked muscle action potential (FREMAP) electrodes in comparison to acoustic tumor surgery.

After setting the DNAP and FREMAP electrodes, cochlear nerve mapping is performed. Through the stimulation on the cochleovestibular nerve with an electrical current of 0.1 or 0.2 mA, the electrophysiological cleavage line of the cochlear nerve and vestibular nerve are identified (Figs 5.20 and 5.21). After the vestibular neurotomy, cochlear nerve mapping is performed on the cross section of the incised vestibular nerve and also remnant cochlear nerve fibers (Fig. 5.22) that are anatomically indistinguishable from the vestibular nerve to confirm the complete section of the vestibular nerve. Variations in distribution pattern of the cochlear and vestibular nerve are known within the eighth cranial nerve at the CPA and it is sometimes difficult to identify the cleavage line on the microscopic view. Insufficient section of the vestibular nerve will give an insufficient result[39] and the purpose of the surgery is not fulfilled. To make a safe and perfect section of the vestibular nerve, this electrophysiological mapping technology is extremely effective.

At the end, the dura and soft tissue are closed as discussed in Chapter 4. The average time for this procedure is one and a half hours. The patient returns to the ward on the same day postoperatively, and is usually discharged after 1 week. Vestibular suppressants are given for initial 2 days to avoid severe vertigo and vegetative symptoms. The patient is encouraged early mobilization, initially with support and later independently to augment vestibular compensation. Patients are taught vestibular rehabilitation exercises before discharge from the hospital by the physiotherapist specially trained in vestibular rehabilitation. The most common side-effect of the procedure is the CSF leak in 3% of cases. A postoperative chronic headache is unusual in our patients after keyhole retrosigmoid approach. Some patients complain of pain in the field of Arnold's nerve owing to both the perioperative positioning of the head and the postoperative tension of the neck muscles, which can be solved using local treatment. Neither postoperative facial paralysis, nor total hearing loss has occurred in any patient in our series. The postoperative asymmetric pattern toward the operated size improves

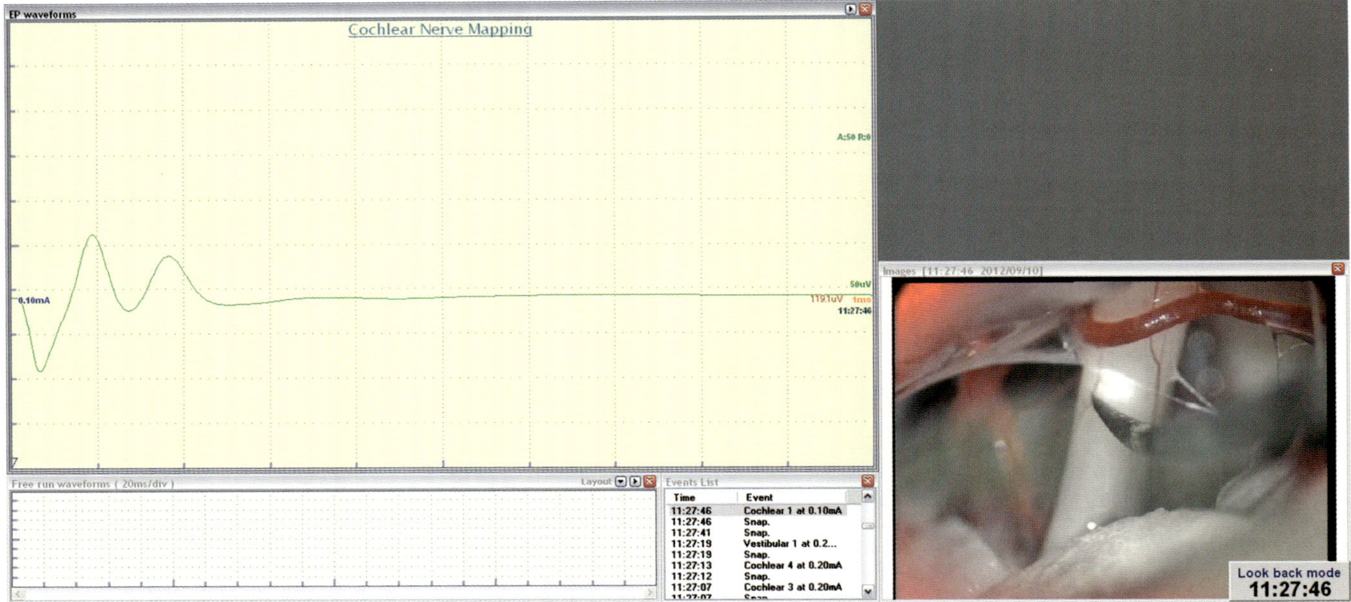

Fig. 5.20: Cochlear nerve mapping by 0.1 mA stimulation and recording DNAP. Cochlear nerve fibers can be identified due to two peaks at 1 and 2 ms

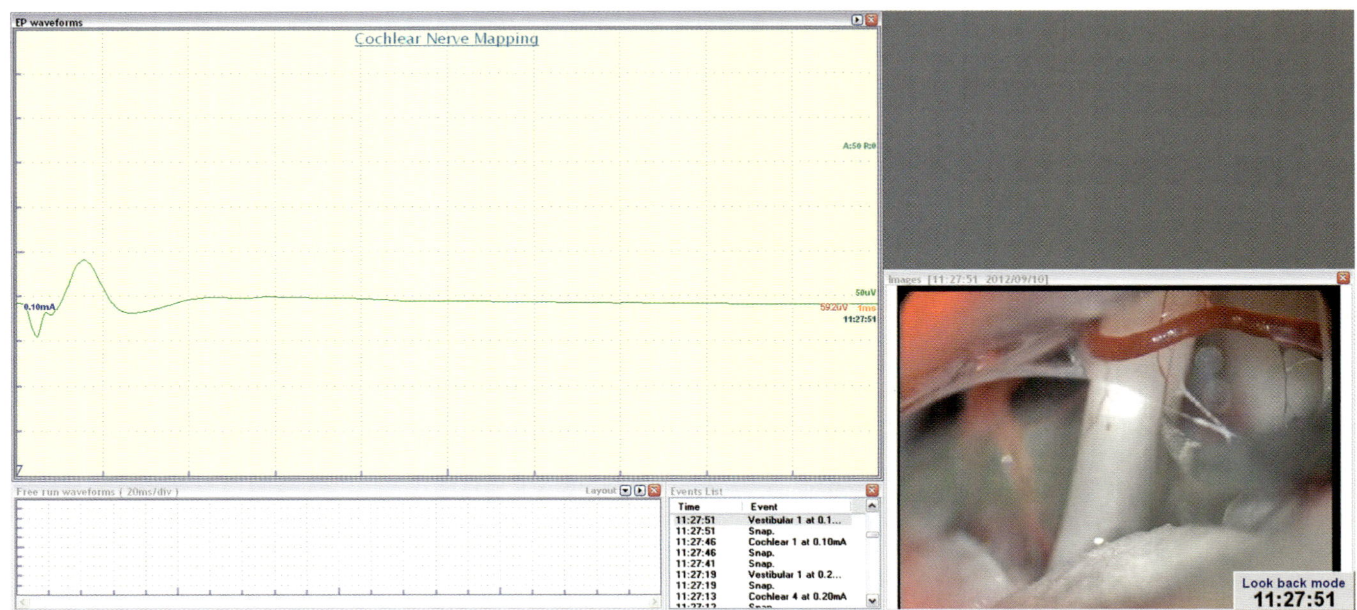

Fig. 5.21: Cochlear nerve mapping by 0.1 mA stimulation and recording DNAP. Stimulating probe identifies the vestibular nerve as there is no peak at 2 ms

progressively in 1 month for the head and the step, in 3 months for the walking performances. Cyclotorsion and vertical perception takes longer to recover.

RESULTS

During the 25-year period from 1974 to 2008, we performed 509 vestibular neurotomies in Menière's disease patients. None of our patients of vestibular neurotomy till date had any anacusis or immediate complete facial palsy. We presented our results from 1974 to 1998 of 283 cases of retrosigmoid vestibular neurotomy.[3] There were 54% males and 46% females. The mean age was 49 years (range, 17–79 years). Each patient underwent a thorough neurological investigation prior to therapy. All patients

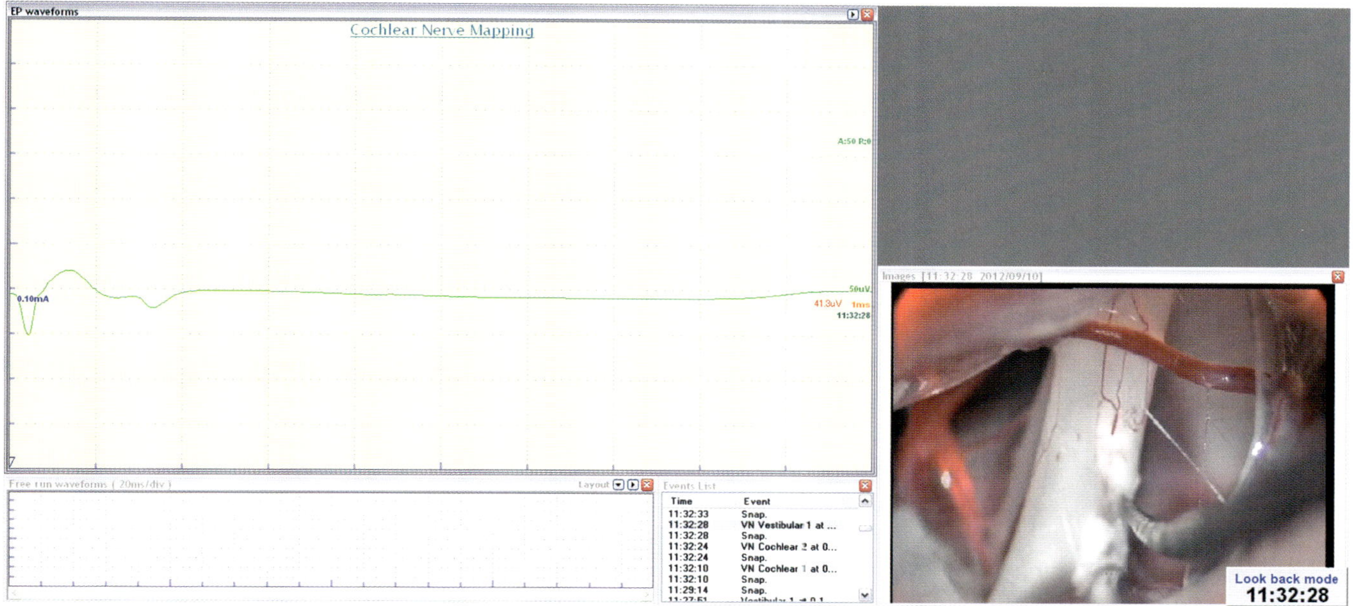

Fig. 5.22: Conducting a cochlear nerve mapping on the remaining nerve fibers after section of the vestibular nerve. It could be identified as the fiber of vestibular nerve as there is no peak at 2 ms

were medical failures (mean duration between onset of disease and surgical treatment of 6 years), and 38 had experienced previous endolymphatic decompression. When seen initially, 274 patients had unilateral classic Menière's disease and nine bilateral diseases. Finally, the decision is made to proceed with surgery by the patients themselves, based on impairment of hearing in the affected ear and on the other side, their professional status and most importantly when their vertigo produced sufficient disability in their lifestyle to outweigh the surgical reluctances.

Vertigo

The severity of the disability caused by vertigo can be judged by the changes in their employment activity and their daily routine. About 18% lost their original job, 39% stopped working, 28% reduced their employment activities and 15% could not find any job because of their disability. The severity before surgery was estimated by the frequency of attacks of acute vertigo. Prior to surgery, 38% of patients complained of daily crisis, 44% of cases complained of weekly crisis, and 18% of cases, of monthly crisis. Of 283 patients, 270 were relieved of their vertigo (95.5%). In the remaining 13 cases, recurrent rotatory vertigo occurred in six cases (five cases of bilateral disease, and one relapse following incomplete vestibular section), and seven cases mentioned severe imbalance. Ice water caloric stimulation revealed no response in all cases but one. Some patients continued to mention an occasional brief feeling of unsteadiness, but were able to carry on with normal activities. The assessment of "patient's point of view" was stressed by Reid et al.[6] by sending out a questionnaire. Patient satisfaction with unilateral retrosigmoid vestibular neurotomy was recorded as follows. Vertigo cured and patient back to normal activities in 62% of cases (165 patients), vertigo cured and imbalance only in specific circumstances, as in the dark or with fast movement of the head in 21.5% of cases (61 patients), vertigo cured but significant walking unsteadiness in 9.5% of cases (36 cases), vertigo cured but dissatisfaction in eight patients (2.5% of cases) for various reasons and further vertigo in 4.5% of cases (13 cases). None of the patients had vertigo worse than that before surgery. Lastly, 83% of patients expressed a high level of satisfaction. The 36 cases with a chronic feeling of being off balance were interpreted as having incomplete vestibular compensation, and required complementary vestibular rehabilitation. Eight patients expressed their dissatisfaction in spite of the fact that their vertigo had been cured, due to persistent aural fullness (four cases), visual problems (two cases) and incapacitating tinnitus (two cases).

Hearing

Most of the patients undergoing vestibular neurotomy had serviceable hearing in the involved ear at the time of surgery. Of the 283 patients, 23 had a pure tone audimetry (PTA) of between 0 and 20 dB, 49 of them, between 21 and 40 dB, 140 of them between 41 and 60 dB, 55 of them between 61 and 80 dB and 16 had total or near total preoperative hearing loss. The preoperative mean hearing level was 49 dB.

Immediate Follow-up

Audiological assessment was routinely performed in each patient during the postoperative period before leaving the unit and 1 month later. No patient suffered total postoperative hearing loss. According to the AAO guidelines,[40] hearing was improved in 21%, unchanged in 66% and decreased in 13%. But the variance of the PTA scores in patients with hearing improvement and in those with worsened hearing shows a similar average for the pre- and postoperative hearing thresholds. Furthermore, the 13% with worsened hearing correspond to the poorest hearing level obtained by the patient before surgery. In other words, these data do not mean worsening due to surgery, but only the inability of the surgical procedure to retain the fluctuating hearing of the patient at the best level.

One-Year Follow-up

Two hundred and thirty-seven (237) patients were available for postoperative PTA at 1 year after the operation. The PTA had improved postoperatively by over 15 dB in 59 patients (25%), had remained unchanged in 155 patients (66.5%), and had declined by over 15 dB in 23 patients (8.5%). When the preoperative and postoperative PTA variance was reduced to 10 dB, hearing had improved in 40%, and had worsened in 29%. Therefore, after 1 year, the average hearing threshold was slightly better than 46 dB.

Five-Year Follow-up

Only 93 patients were available for PTA at 5 years after vestibular neurotomy. Of these, 5 had a PTA between 0 and 20 dB, 18, between 21 and 40 dB, 46, between 41 and 60 dB and 24, between 61 and 80 dB. Patients with a preoperative hearing loss of more than 80 dB were excluded from this long-term follow-up. The average hearing threshold had decreased by 4 dB compared to the preoperative hearing threshold and by 7 dB compared to the 1-year postoperative threshold, reaching 53 dB. However, it was the same case in the other ear.

There was particular interest in studying the outcome of patients with good preoperative hearing (between 10 and 20 dB). Fifteen patients were selected according to this criterion. At one month postoperatively, hearing was unchanged in 13 patients and decreased by less than 20 dB in two patients. At one year postoperatively, hearing was unchanged in 12 patients, and had decreased by more than 20 dB in one patient and by less than 20 dB in two patients. Only nine patients were followed for more than 5 years postoperatively. Hearing was stable in five of these patients and had decreased in four (one by more than 20 dB and three by less than 20 db).

Using class A, B, C and D definitions for the control of vertigo and stabilization of hearing after 1 year postoperatively, 25% of patients were class A, 66.5%, class B and 8.5%, class C. After 5 years postoperatively, 9% of patients were class A, 75%, class B, and 15%, class C. In several long-term follow-up studies of successful hearing preservation cases, deterioration over time has been demonstrated.[7,8] Our experience leads to less negative conclusions. We found that hearing was stable over the long term in 70% of patients operated on for Menière's disease. Rosenberg et al.[4] and Goksu et al.,[5] respectively, reported no change or better hearing in 66 and 89% of their patients after a 2-year period. This data is of particular interest for patients with good or serviceable hearing, and suggest that surgery should be performed at an early stage of Menière's disease, to preserve the hearing in the affected ear.

Tinnitus

The subjective evaluation of tinnitus depends on the versatile behavior of the patients. Immediately after surgery the trend was toward disappearance or reduction. Tinnitus usually only stabilizes after several months, and 55% of patients graded their tinnitus at the same level as prior to the surgery, while 22% of patients were free of this symptom.

Aural Fullness

Aural fullness improved or resolved in the majority of cases except four patients who experienced worsened aural fullness.

CONCLUSION

The infrequency of complications and the efficiency of the vestibular compensation allows considering retrosigmoid vestibular neurotomy as the safest procedure of choice for incapacitating Menière's disease when residual hearing still exists (particularly to arrest further hearing loss), until we find the etiopathogenic and medical treatment of such a disease.

REFERENCES

1. Silverstein H, Smouha E, Jones R. Natural history vs surgery for Menière's disease. Otolaryngol Head Neck Surg. 1989;100:6.
2. Magnan J, Bremond G, Chays A, Gignac D, Florence A. Vestibular neurotomy by retrosigmoid approach: technique, indications and results. Am J Otol. 1991:12; 101–4.
3. Magnan J. Vestibular neurotomy by retrosigmoid approach for Menière's disease 1999. Update. In: Sterkers O, et al. (Eds.). The Hague: Kugler Publications; 2000: 65–9.
4. Rosenberg S, Silverstein H, Hoffer M, Thaler E. Hearing results after posterior fossa vestibular neurectomy. Otolaryngol Head Neck Surg. 1996;114:32–7.
5. Goksu N, Bayazit Y, Beder L. Posterior fossa vestibular nerve section for the management of peripheral vertigo. Eur Arch Otorinolaryngol. 1999;256:230–2.
6. Reid C, Eisenberg R, Halmagyi M, Fagan P. The outcome of vestibular nerve section for intractable vertigo: the patient's point of view. Laryngoscope 1996;106:1553–1556.
7. Papas D, Pappas D. Vestibular nerve section: long-term follow up. Laryngoscope. 1997;107:1203–9.
8. Wazen J, Spitzer J, Kasper C, Anderson B. Long-term hearing results following vestibular surgery in Menière's disease. Laryngoscope. 1998;108:1470–3.
9. Hirsch B. Kammerer D. Intratympanic gentamicin therapy for Menière's disease. Am J Otol. 1997;18:44–51.
10. Driscoll C, Kasperbauer J, Facer G, Harner S, Beatty C. Low-dose gentamicin and the treatment of Menière's disease: preliminary results. Laryngoscope. 1997;107:83–9.
11. Abou-Halawa A, Poe D. Efficacy of increased gentamicin concentration for intratympanic injection therapy in Menière's disease. Otol Neurotol. 2002;23:494–502.
12. Kaplan D, Nedzelski J, Chen J, Shipp D. Intratympanic gentamicin for the treatment of unilateral Menière's disease. Laryngoscope. 2000;110:1298–1305.
13. Rauch S, Oas J. Intratympanic gentamicin for treatment of intractable Menière's disease: a preliminary report. Laryngoscope. 1997;107:83–9.
14. Minor L. Intratympanic gentamicin for control of vertigo in Menière's disease: vestibular signs that specify completion of therapy. Am J Otol. 1999;20:209–19.
15. McFeely W, Singleton G, Rodriguez F, Antonelli P. Intratympanic gentamicin treatment for Menière's disease. Otolaryngol Head Neck Surg. 1998;118:589–96.
16. Nedzelski J, Schessel D, Bryce G, et al. Chemical labyrinthectomy: local application of gentamicin for the treatment of unilateral Menière's disease. Am J Otol. 1992;13:8.
17. Toth A, Parnes L. Intratympanic gentamicin therapy for Menière's disease: preliminary comparison of two regimens. J Otolaryngol. 1995;24:340.
18. Zakir M, Dickman J. Regeneration of vestibular otolith afferents after ototoxic damage. J Neurosci. 2006;26(11): 2881–93.
19. Schmerber S, Dumas G, Morel N, Chahine K, Karkas A. Vestibular neurectomy vs. chemical labyrinthectomy in the treatment of disabling Menière's disease: a long-term comparative study. Auris Nasus Larynx. 2009;36:400–5.
20. Colletti V, Carner M, Colletti L. Auditory results after vestibular nerve section and intratympanic gentamicin for Menière's disease. Otol Neurotol. 2007;28(2):145–51.
21. Hillman T, Chen D, Arriaga M. Vestibular nerve section versus intratympanic gentamicin for Menière's disease. Laryngoscope. 2004;114:216–22.
22. Sajjadi H, Paparella MM. Menière's disease. Lancet. 2008;372(9636):406–14.
23. Leveque M, Seidermann L, Tran H, Langagne T, Ulmer E, Chays A. Vestibular function outcomes after vestibular neurectomy in Menière's disease: can vestibular neurectomy provide complete vestibular deafferentation? Auris Nasus Larynx. 2010;37:308–13.
24. Haberkamp T, Silverstein H. Vestibular neurectomy from posterior fossa approaches: a summary of the the techniques. Oper Tech Otolaryngol-Head Neck Surg. 2001;12(3):116–21.
25. Fisch U. Vestibular nerve section for Meniers's disease. Am J Otol. 1984;5:543–5.
26. Garcia-Ibanez E, Garcia-Ibanez L. Middle fossa vestibular neurectomy: a report of 373 cases. Otolaryngol head Neck Surg. 1980;88:486–90.
27. Dandy W. Menière's disease: diagnosis and treatment of thirty cases. Am J Surg. 1933;20:693–8.
28. Green R, Douglas C. Intracranial division of the eighth nerve for Menière's disease: a follow-up study of patients operated on by Dr Walter Dandy. Ann Otol Rhinol Laryngol. 1951;60:610–21.
29. Aubry M, Ombredanne M. Deux cas de section partielle du nerf auditif avec guérison des vertiges et conservation de l'audition. Ann Otolaryngol. 1935;52:535–9.
30. House W. Surgical exposure of the internal auditory canal and its contents through the middle cranial fossa. Laryngoscope. 1961;71:1363–5.
31. Fluur E, Tovi D. Microscopic intracranial section of vestibular nerve. Acta Otolaryngol (Stokh). 1965;59:604–6.
32. Bremond G, Garcin M, Magnan J, Bonnaud G. L'abord à minima de l'angle ponto-cérébelleux. Cah ORL 1974:9: 443–60.
33. Bremond G, Garcin M. Microsurgical approach to the cerebellopontine angle. J Laryngol Otol. 1975;89:237–48.
34. Millen S, Meyer G. Retrosigmoid intracanicular vestibular nerve section: an alternative surgical approach for Menière's disease. Am J Otol. 1986;7:330–2.
35. Silverstein H, Haberkamp T. A comparison of retrosigmoid IAC, retrolabyrinthine, and middle fossa vestibular neurectomy for treatment of vertigo. Laryngoscope. 1987;97:165–73.

36. Silverstein H, Wanamaker H, Flanzer J, Rosenbergs. Vestibular neurectomy in the United States 1990. Am J Otol. 1992;13:23–30.
37. Jackler R, Whinney D. A century of eight nerve surgery. Otol Neurotol. 2001;23;401–16.
38. Perez R, Chen J, Nedzelski J. The status of the contralateral ear in established unilateral Menière's disease. Laryngoscope. 2004;114:1373.
39. Leveque M, Seidermann L, Tran H, Lanqaqne T, Chays A. Vestibular function outcomes after vestibular neurectomy in Menière's disease: can vestibular neurectomy provide complete vestibular differentiation? Auris Nasus Larynx. 2010;37(3):308–13.
40. Monsell E, Balkany T, Gates G, et al. Committee on hearing and equilibrium guidelines for the diagnosis and evaluation of therapy in Menière's disease. AAOHNS. Otolaryngol Head Neck Surg. 1995;113:181–5.

Vascular Compression Syndromes

6

INTRODUCTION

The vascular compression syndromes of cranial nerves include a number of entities that share similarities among them like the anatomical site [the cerebellopontine angle (CPA)], the pathophysiology, the radiological investigation by magnetic resonance imaging (MRI) and the surgical treatment wherein the therapeutic principle is to "decompress" the related cranial nerve by isolating the "offensive" vessel. The common basic finding in all the so-called "vascular compression syndromes" is the contact between the offending blood vessel (usually artery) and the related cranial nerve and undisputable resolution of the patients' symptoms by eliminating this contact by "microvascular decompression (MVD)." So, it was logical to search for these vascular contacts and to treat the cause for these pathologies. Usually in any disease, the study of etiopathology explains all the clinical features and points to the way of therapy. These vascular compression syndromes are different from other diseases because we have various other ways for transitory successful treatment (especially for trigeminal neuralgia) and some are not yet sure of the pathophysiology of the disease and how the surgery for vascular decompression works.

Though the pathophysiology is likely to be similar for all the vascular compression syndromes, clinical presentation is obviously quite different depending on the cranial nerve involved. That leads us to the following neurovascular syndromes which need to be presented separately.

- Trigeminal neuralgia for trigeminal nerve
- Hemifacial spasm for facial nerve
- Glossopharyngeal neuralgia for glossopharyngeal nerve
- Certain unilateral tinnitus and disabling positional vertigo for vestibulocochlear nerve.

PATHOPHYSIOLOGY

A cranial nerve is composed of a central nervous system (CNS) segment and a peripheral nervous system (PNS) segment separated by the transitional zone. The PNS and CNS segments of cranial nerves are histologically distinct entities that are separated by a transitional zone or the Obersteiner-Redlich zone. In the CNS segment, the oligodendroglia are responsible for axonal isolation, and in PNS segment outside brainstem this function is of Schwann cells. Thus at this point, there is a transition from oligodendrocytes myelin to Schwann cell myelin. In this area, a number of axons have a marginal or no isolation at all.

A number of properties of the PNS segment make it more resistant to compression than the CNS segment. The PNS segment consists of undulating nerve fibers, and it is thus protected from traction by its elasticity. The nerve fibers in the PNS segment are organized in fasciculi (funiculi). Each nerve fiber is supported by a layer of endoneurium, and each funiculus is surrounded by thin perineurium. The sheath around the entire nerve (epineurium) is present in the peripheral segment and is replaced by pia mater near the entry/exit of the cranial nerve from the brainstem. Conversely, the CNS segment has a structure similar to that of white matter of the CNS, consisting of parallel traveling nerve fibers, and it lacks funicular structure. Nerve fibers are embedded in supporting tissue, but specific endo, peri- and epineurium are absent. A layer of pia mater surrounds the CNS segment. This CNS segment is also less vascularized than the PNS segment. The myelination of the CNS and PNS segments also differs in structure and is not as well organized in the CNS segment as compared with the PNS segment. Therefore, the central portion of the cranial nerves is much more vulnerable than its peripheral portion. The transition zone or Obersteiner-Redlich zone is the interpenetration of a few millimeters, of the central (glial) into the peripheral (Schwann) type of cells. Although vascular compression can occur at any point along the cranial nerve, it has been generally assumed that only vascular contact at the root entry/exit zone (REZ) of the affected cranial nerve can cause symptoms. It was at this point of fragility, "Achilles heel" of the nerve, that the vascular loops may cause disruptive irritation. Its location varies depending on the considered cranial nerve[1] and defines the so-called REZ. For the trigeminal nerve, the REZ is variable in the cisternal course of the nerve and extends 7–8 mm, occasionally up to the entrance of Meckel's cave. In the facial nerve, the REZ extends only 1–3 mm after its emergence from pontomedullary junction. For the vestibulocochlear nerve, the REZ may reach 9–11 mm and may be located up to the porus. A correlation exists between the length of the central nervous system segment of the root outside the brainstem and the incidence of the corresponding compression syndrome.[1] The incidence of microvascular compression syndromes differs. Trigeminal neuralgia[2] has a higher incidence than hemifacial spasm,[3] which has a higher incidence than glossopharyngeal neuralgia or cochlear component of vestibulocochlear cranial nerve compression.[4]

Several hypotheses regarding the development of cranial nerve compression syndromes have been published.[1] Jannetta[5] suggested that vascular compression develops when blood vessels elongate, leading to formation of vascular loops and an increased risk for vascular compression of one or more cranial nerves. He postulated that the mechanical effect of a pulsating blood vessel was the cause of the disease. He further hypothesized that the compression must be at the root entry zone of the cranial nerve to cause symptoms.[5] Leclercq et al.,[6] Ryu et al.[7] and Møller[8] suggested that the compression can occur at any point along the cranial nerve, especially at the CNS segment, and not only at the root entry zone. In addition, there is considerable evidence that any vascular contact (not only artery but even vein) can cause symptoms[8] and pulsations from the artery is not always found. The compression of the associated cranial nerve by an artery or vein results in a focal demyelination at the compression site.

Initially it was hypothesized that the abnormal neural stimulation of the cranial nerves was caused by the compression of blood vessels only. There were many theories proposed to explain the abnormal neural activity, the principle among them to get maximum acceptance was the "ephaptic transmission theory." The ephaptic transmission theory was described by Nielsen et al.[9] for hemifacial spasm and was based on the finding of demyelination of the facial nerve at the root entry zone. According to this theory,[9] mechanical stress caused by a vascular loop in this demyelinated area would slow the conduction velocity in nervous fibers. This would trigger formation of false synapse or ephapse between axons of facial nerve fibers at the site of compression. "Ephapsis" is the ability of nerve impulse to pass from original nerve fiber to multiple surrounding nerve fibers. Demyelinated conflict site becomes a great potential discharge, which means that its firing rate is likely to increase. So after the initial discharge, the mechanism is self-maintained and the genesis of new influx could in turn reinitiate the system. In short, a kind of "short-circuit" allows nerve impulse to choose an unnatural path out of the axon which it originally conveyed to the place of the short-circuit. The events once initiated follow and assemble in a "cascade effect." Demyelinated nerve fiber discharges and produces an impulse that initiates a muscle response in the corresponding motor unit and, second, enables adjacent fibers in a state of hyperexcitability. Thus at the site of conflict, ephaptic transmission occurs that allow primary impulses to diffuse to adjacent nerve fibers. In short, the vessel in contact with the nerve induces a chronic compression that leads to focal demyelination through which ephaptic transmissions can occur.

In a healthy subject, the stimulation of a branch of the facial nerve only induces contractions of motor fibers innerved by this branch, whereas in patients suffering from hemifacial spasm, the same stimulation would induce contractions in expected muscles and also in other territories. This phenomenon can be recorded on electromyograph (EMG) from facial muscles innervated by different branches of facial nerve in patients of hemifacial spasm and is known as "lateral spread" or abnormal muscle response (AMR)[11] and explains the synkinesis observed. The AMR can be elicited in every patient with HFS by EMG preoperatively and intraoperatively (Fig. 6.1). The electrophysiological hallmarks on EMG of HFS consist of spontaneous, high-frequency (as many as 150 impulses per second), synchronized firing and an AMR elicited clinically in preoperative period with the trigeminofacial or "blink" reflex. Blink reflex is used in the clinic by tapping on the supraorbital area and recording the EMG from orbicularis oculi and mentalis muscles. AMR is elicited intraoperatively by recording of muscle action potentials from orbicularis oculi on stimulating the marginal mandibular branch of facial by insert electrodes and vice versa from mentalis by stimulating zygomatic branch of facial nerve (Fig. 6.1). Ephaptic transmission is judged to be eliminated once the "lateral spread" of impulses from one motor branch of the facial nerve to the muscles innervated by other motor branch is eliminated despite intraoperative facial nerve branch stimulation. Since the AMR often disappears when the offending vessel is lifted off the facial nerve in MVD, its use has been suggested as an intraoperative guide to success (Figs 6.2 and 6.3).

The other hypothesis supports the role of hyperactivity of the associated cranial nerve nucleus in causing the signs and symptoms of hemifacial spasm (HFS) and trigeminal neuralgia (TN).[8,12,13] This was based on the intraoperative electromyographic data from patients of hemifacial spasm.[14] The abnormal spread of contraction to other facial territories called "lateral spread" of motor responses was calculated from nerve conduction studies to originate in the facial motor nucleus and not from facial nerve. It suggests that the symptom is caused by reduced segmental inhibition of respective central nucleus along with excitatory input from abnormal nerve. It suggests that ephaptic transmission at demyelinated nerve does not cause the "cross transmission" but it occurs at the level of facial/trigeminal nerve nucleus.

Both the peripheral "ephaptic" and central "nucleus" theories are not mutually exclusive and the subsequent data suggested a combination theory that postulates "a peripheral etiology and a central pathogenesis." The combined hypothesis suggests that the hyperactivity of the respective nucleus is caused by the irritation of the respective nerve.[8,10,12] That means the central and peripheral hypotheses are not mutually exclusive. Though the initiation of the pathology is at the REZ of the nerve, the signs and symptoms are caused due to central nucleus. The vascular contact along with the probable "second cause" like nerve injury causes the irritation of the nerve, which is then conveyed to the central nucleus causing "kindling effect" on the nucleus[11] that results in seizure-like discharges from the nucleus. Fromm[13] proposed that the nuclear hyperactivity causing the pain of trigeminal neuralgia results from impaired segmental inhibition, which is caused by irritation of the trigeminal nerve root in combination of increased activity in afferent fibers of

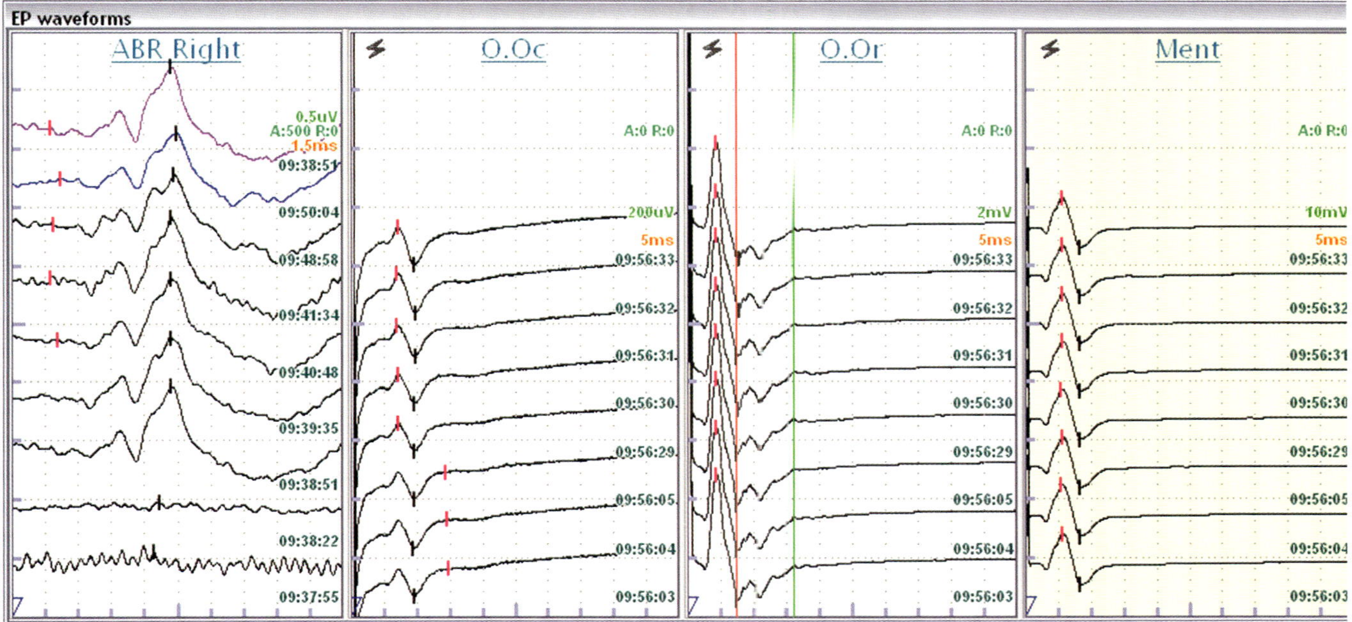

Fig. 6.1: Intraoperative electromyograph (EMG) of facial muscles to demonstrate abnormal muscle response (AMR). In a healthy subject, the stimulation of a branch of the facial nerve only induces contractions of motor fibers innerved by this branch, where in this patient with hemifacial spasm, the same stimulation would induce contractions in expected muscles and also in other territories. In this case, AMR is elicited by recording of muscle action potentials from orbicularis oris on stimulating the marginal mandibular branch of facial nerve by insert electrodes. Abnormal muscle response at orbicularis oris is observed between red and green line when the mentalis muscle is electrically stimulated prior to microvascular decompression

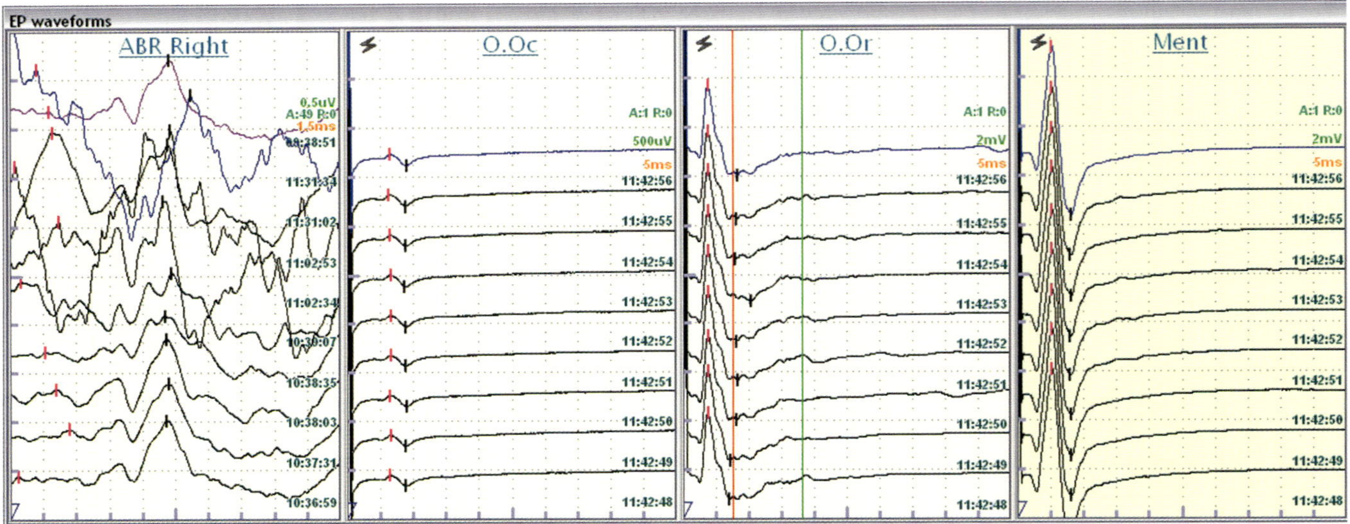

Fig. 6.2: The abnormal muscle response (AMR) often disappears when the offending vessel is lifted off the facial nerve in microvascular decompression (MVD). Ephaptic transmission is judged to be eliminated once the "lateral spread" of impulses from one motor branch of the facial nerve to the muscles innervated by other motor branch is eliminated despite intraoperative facial nerve branch stimulation. No AMR is observed at orbicularis oris muscle when the mentalis muscle is electrically stimulated after the MVD

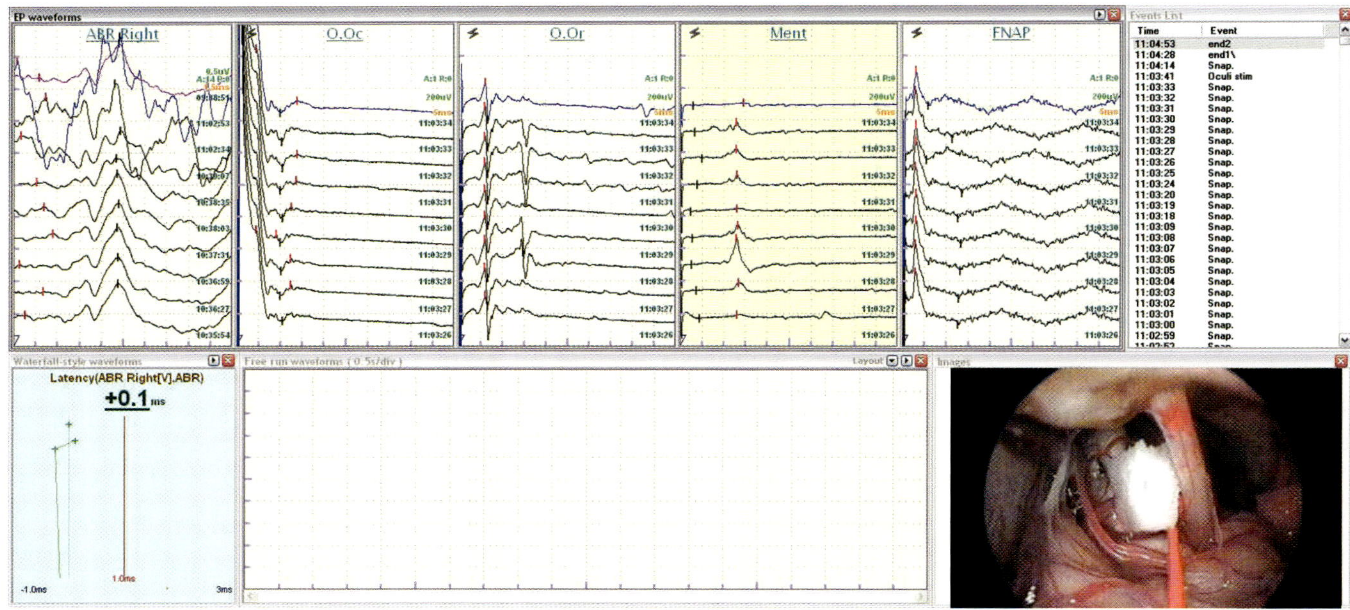

Fig. 6.3: Endoscope image and electrophysiological tests after successful microvascular decompression (MVD) for hemifacial spasm. Facial nerve root exit zone evoked muscle action potential electrode set as a stimulant electrode is on top of the facial nerve. Teflon is sandwiched in between and REZ of the facial nerve

the nerve due to spikes and possibly crosstalk (ephaptic transmission) between injured fibers. The reduction in segmental inhibition could be caused by chronic irritation of the trigeminal nerve by a blood vessel. The results of animal studies have supported the hypothesis that hyperactivity of cranial nerve nucleus is caused by irritation from the respective nerve. Thus, repeated electrical stimulation to the injured facial nerve can cause hyperexcitability of the facial motor nucleus. This "central switch down" causing reduced central inhibition of related nucleus due to repeated irritative stimulus from the injured peripheral part of cranial nerve is described as the "Kindling effect." "Kindling theory" suggests that the culprit conflicting vessel on the nerve root causes ectopic excitation, which induces chronic stimulation and impulses are conveyed to the periphery as well as to the nucleus. The abnormal vessel contact with the related cranial nerve at the REZ results in ectopic excitation of the nerve with antidromic impulses traveling back to nucleus and reorganization within nucleus results in increased discharge. This hyperactivity travels orthodromically down the respective nerve. This hyperexcitable and hyperactivated nucleus triggers an abnormally high burst of action potentials producing the pain or spasm. Thus trigeminal neuralgia begins with chronic vascular compression of the trigeminal nerve that causes focal demyelination. This leads to local dysfunction of inter-inhibitory neurons and also to the development of ectopic neuronal foci. The combination of increased input by afferent ectopic foci and the failure of the intersegmental inhibitory neurons lead to hyperactivity of the core of the trigeminal nucleus. This result in attacks of severe pain along areas innervated by trigeminal nerve after stimulation of its afferent fibers by activities such as brushing of teeth, eating or even by touching the face.

The universally good and rapid result of the MVD surgery is due to removal of the peripheral irritative contact of the artery/vein from the nerve. It prevents the abnormal transmission to the nucleus by allowing the separation of the demyelinated axons and reducing the spontaneous generation of the impulses. It also reverses compression-induced conduction block.[10]

However, this theory of vascular compression causing these disorders was soon disputed,[15] with the valid arguments that vascular contacts are common in CPA and that other treatments are also effective in trigeminal neuralgia. Vascular contact with a cranial nerve is common; however, symptoms of vascular compression are rare. The question that remains unanswered is that why not all the patients with vascular contacts develop these disorders. The exact association between vascular contact and related disorder is still not completely understood. There is a hypothesis that perhaps there are multiple other factors (unknown at present) required to cause the hyperexcitability of the nucleus[11] or it is necessary to have prior injury to the associated nerve[15] (in form of either viral neuritis or trauma as happens to trigeminal nerve occasionally after dental extraction) and the patients with this predisposition are susceptible to the associated vascular compression syndrome. This means that perhaps another factor such as a previous minor injury is necessary for creating symptoms such as hemifacial spasm, trigeminal neuralgia and glossopharyngeal neuralgia in persons who has neurovascular conflict. With MVD surgery, the surgeon attempts to remove one of the precipitating factors and hope for the resolution of the hyperexcitability of the cranial nerve nucleus. This explains the excellent results after the MVD surgery and occasional delayed benefit after the surgery. This also explains that there may be more ways than one to cure these disorders. However, the most logical and reliable decision to definitively cure such neurovascular compression syndrome is without any doubt the surgical procedure of neurovascular decompression.

IMAGING OF NEUROVASCULAR CONFLICTS OF CPA

The common basic etiology in the vascular compression syndromes is the contact between the offending artery and the nerve in CPA. MRI is an essential element in the work-up of these pathologies. MRI is able to reproduce the anatomy of the CPA and to demonstrate the presence of a neurovascular conflict.[16-22] It also eliminates other potential causes such as a tumoral process or multiple sclerosis. The typical radiological images of the MRI assessment correlate with the surgical intraoperative findings in such neurovascular pathologies in the CPA. The MRI of the CPA in three-dimensional high-resolution acquisition has been the principle examination of all syndromes or suspected vascular compression syndrome of the cranial nerves. MRI makes the diagnosis, accurately assesses the responsible vessels and finally dictates the indication for surgery.[17]

Magnetic resonance imaging in both T1 and T2 three-dimensional Fourier transform (3DFT) sequences is the most effective method of delineating both the cranial nerves and the surrounding vascular structures in the CPA. The protocol for imaging that we follow includes beginning with whole-brain T2 or FLAIR sequence to exclude multiple sclerosis, followed with axial and coronal T1 imaging of brainstem and CPA cistern (preferably with contrast) to look for venous cause, cranial neuritis, perineural tumor and cisternal tumor. High-resolution thin-section T2 imaging of brainstem and CPA cistern is performed next and is the best sequence to look for offending artery. The T2 is carried out using 3D CISS (constructive interference in steady state by Siemens) or 3D FIESTA (fast imaging employing steady-state acquisition by GE healthcare) sequences. Imaging of the CPA is done with serial thin slices preferably of 0.4–0.7 mm thickness. The axial plane offers the most comprehensive and demonstrative images. 3D CISS/FIESTA imaging offers high spatial resolution and excellent contrast resolution and depicts both the artery and the vein responsible for the neurovascular conflict.

To confirm the diagnosis, the single presence of a neurovascular contact is not sufficient. Several radiological criteria are required, with some variability depending on the involved cranial nerves. The common criteria include a perpendicular contact between the vascular loop and the cranial nerve at its root exit zone (REZ), visualized along two different perpendicular planes, and a distortion of the nerve or other neural structures. For the trigeminal nerve, the reduction in its diameter is an additional criterion (Figs 6.4 and 6.5). The most common offending vessel is the superior cerebellar artery (SCA), but in 20% of cases, a venous structure (aberrant trigeminal vein) might be the cause of the conflict, and it is visible only on T1 with gadolinium. For the facial nerve, the location of the conflict at the REZ of the nerve and the distortion of the brainstem at this level are additional criteria (Fig. 6.6). The most common offending vessels are the PICA and a dolicho vertebral artery. For the auditory nerve, we expect to see displacement of the nerve with a certain distance between the facial and cochlear nerves, with an imprint on the nerve and reduction in its diameter (Fig. 6.7), and with brainstem distortion caused by the vascular structure at the level of the REZ of the facial nerve.

Magnetic resonance imaging findings correlate very reliably with the surgical findings, and give a rather precise idea of the neurovascular conflict that is expected to be encountered during surgery. We have followed a classification to denote the offending vessel. The classification SAPV Ve is described below:

- Type S is a conflict caused by Superior cerebellar artery (SCA)
- Type A is a conflict caused by Anterior inferior cerebellar artery (AICA)
- Type P is a conflict caused by Posterior inferior cerebellar artery (PICA)
- Type V is a conflict caused by Vertebral artery (VA)
- Type Ve corresponds to a conflict caused by a cerebellar vein.

The capital letter is used when the radiological criteria of conflict are met. The lowercase is reserved if there is just a contact between neurovascular structures without fulfilling the radiological criteria. This classification is used in all types of neurovascular conflicts, regardless of the number of blood vessels in question. For example, in the hemifacial spasm, a conflict of type V + P is a conflict between the facial nerve and the vertebral and posterior inferior cerebellar artery. In case of conflict between the trigeminal nerve and SCA and a vein, it will be a Type S + Ve. This classification thus has a predictive nature of the difficulty or simplicity of the surgical decompression and therefore a prognostic value on the cure rate. Finally, it allows better analysis and comparisons of the MVD procedures.

Five examples of analysis by MRI and its correlation with intraoperative findings are shown below.

- *Case 1*: Correlation between MRI and intraoperative findings in a patient with right trigeminal neuralgia due to SCA (Figs 6.8–6.11).

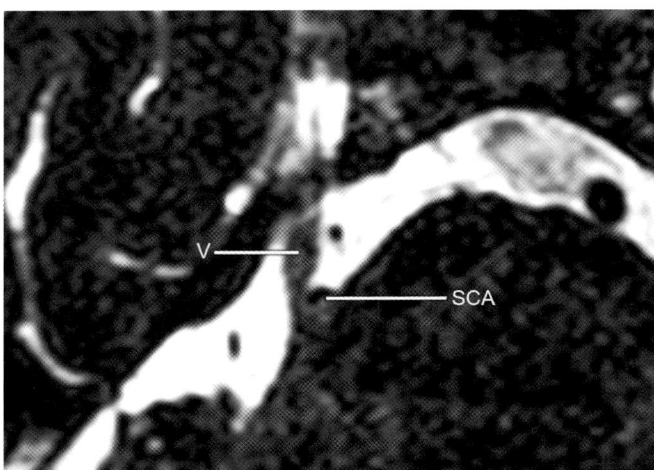

Fig. 6.4: Axial MRI of CPA in CISS sequence in a patient with right trigeminal neuralgia showing perpendicular contact between SCA and V at REZ causing distortion and reduction in V diameter

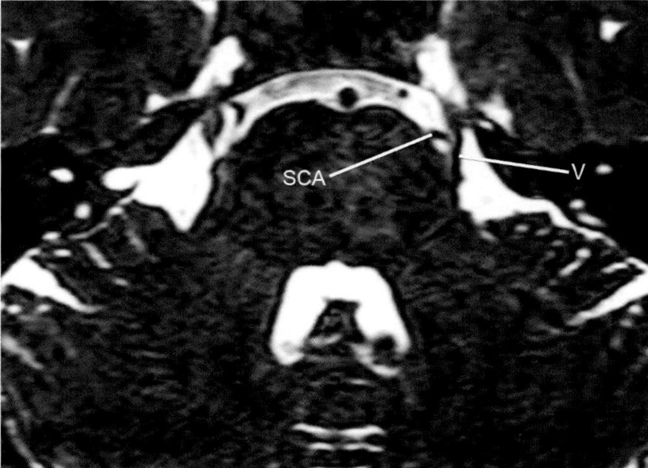

Fig. 6.5: Axial MRI of CPA in CISS sequence in a patient with left trigeminal neuralgia showing SCA having perpendicular contact with V and causing distortion of V at more lateral cisternal part and not at REZ

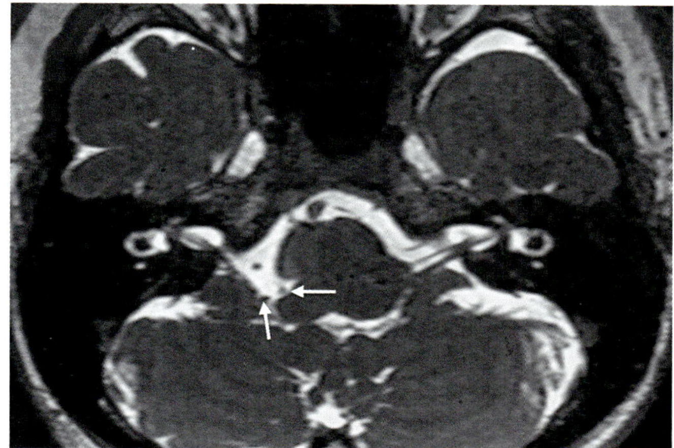

Fig. 6.6: Axial MRI of CPA in CISS sequence in a patient with right hemifacial spasm showing PICA having perpendicular contact with VII at REZ with distortion of the brainstem at this level

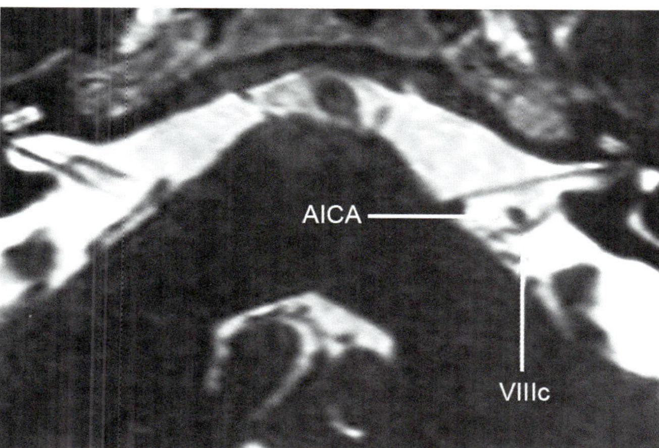

Fig. 6.7: Axial MRI of CPA in CISS sequence in a patient with left tinnitus showing displacement of the cochlear nerve from the facial nerve, with an imprint on the nerve and reduction in its diameter

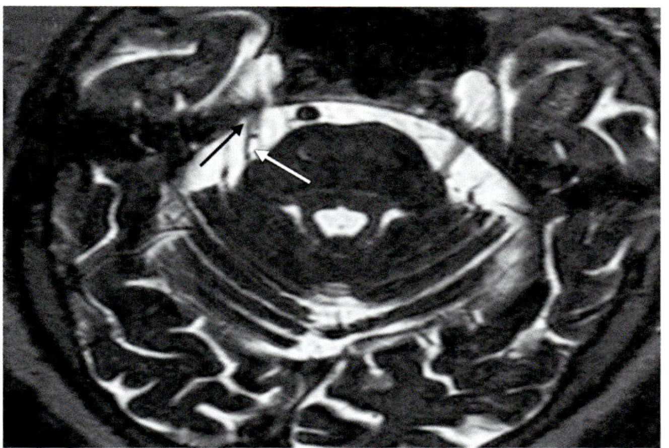

Fig. 6.8: Case 1: Axial MRI showing right trigeminal neuralgia due to SCA

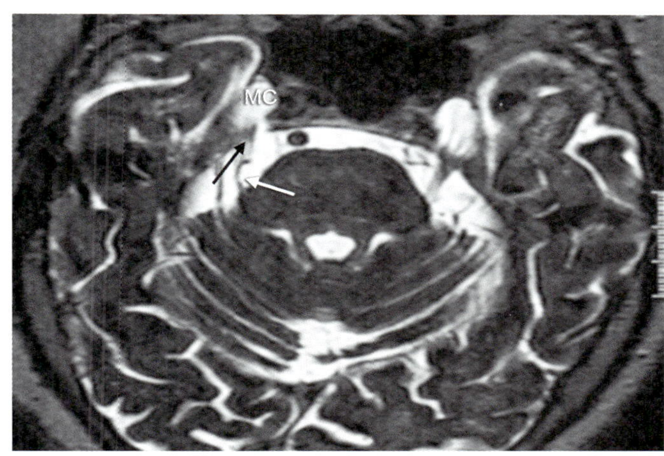

Fig. 6.9: Case 1: Axial MRI showing right trigeminal neuralgia due to SCA

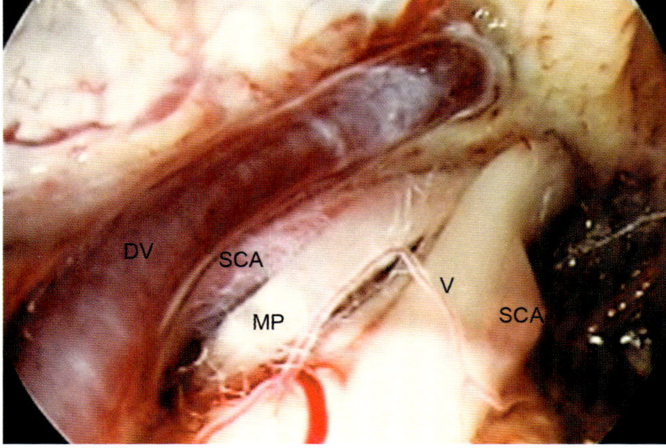

Fig. 6.10: Case 1: Intraoperative endoscopic picture showing right trigeminal neuralgia due to SCA impinging into the V at REZ

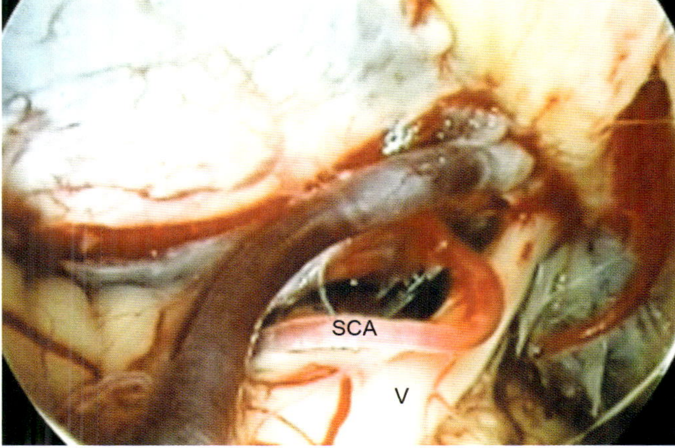

Fig. 6.11: Case 1: Intraoperative endoscopic picture after "decompression" of V from the distortion caused by SCA

- *Case 2*: Correlation between MRI and intraoperative findings in a patient with right trigeminal neuralgia due to SCA and a vein (Figs 6.12–6.14).
- *Case 3*: Correlation between MRI and intraoperative findings in a patient with right hemifacial spasm due to PICA (Figs 6.15–6.17).
- *Case 4*: Correlation between MRI and intraoperative findings in another patient with right hemifacial spasm due to PICA (Figs 6.18–6.21).
- *Case 5*: Correlation between MRI and intraoperative findings in a patient with right hemifacial spasm due to VA (Figs 6.22 and 6.23).

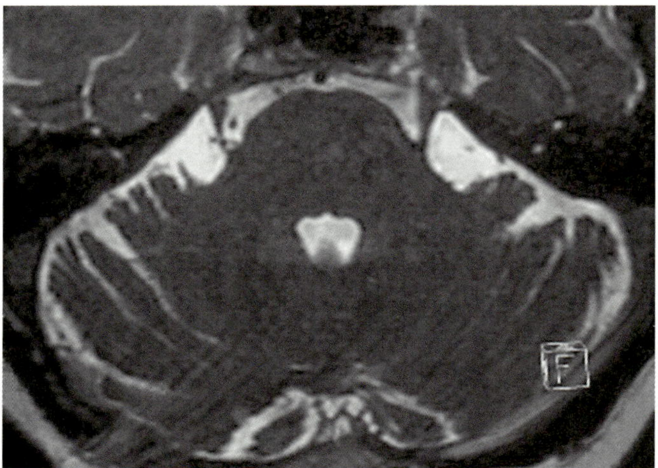

Fig. 6.12: Case 2: Axial MRI showing right trigeminal neuralgia due to SCA and a vein showing perpendicular contact between SCA and V at REZ medially and vein laterally causing distortion and reduction in V diameter

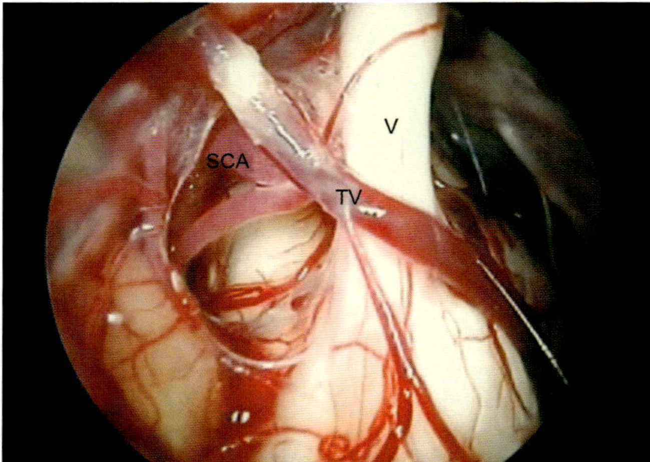

Fig. 6.13: Case 2: Intraoperative endoscopic picture showing right trigeminal neuralgia due to SCA medially and vein laterally impinging into the V

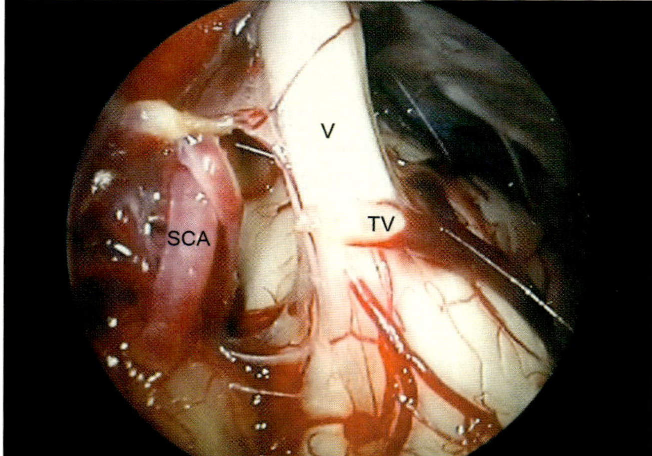

Fig. 6.14: Case 2: Intraoperative endoscopic picture after "decompression" of V by mobilizing the SCA and coagulation of vein

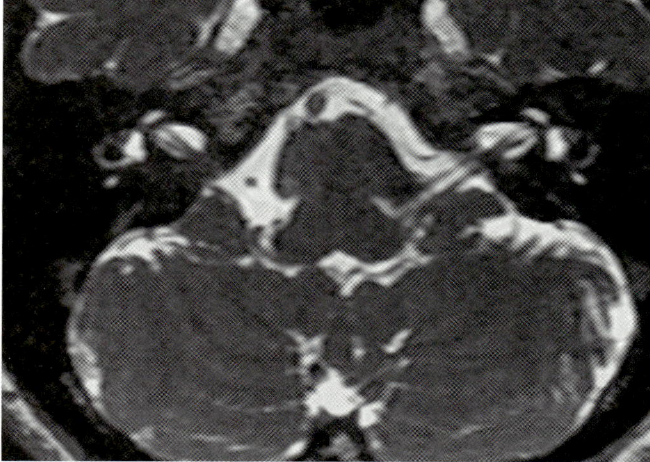

Fig. 6.15: Case 3: Axial MRI in a patient with right hemifacial spasm showing PICA having perpendicular contact with VII at REZ with distortion of the brainstem at this level

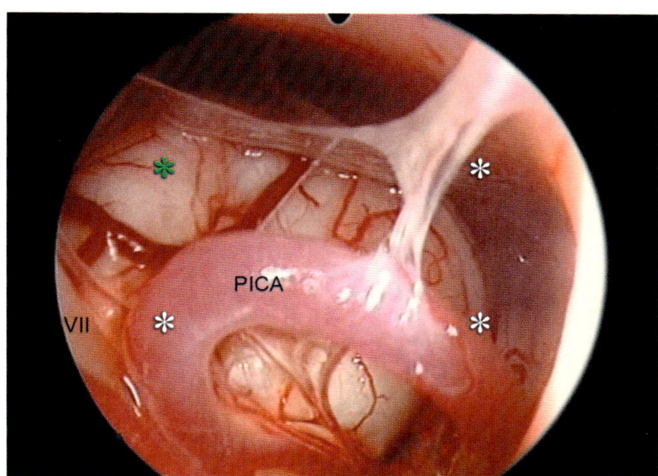

Fig. 6.16: Case 3: Intraoperative endoscopic picture in a patient with right hemifacial spasm showing PICA having perpendicular contact with VII at REZ

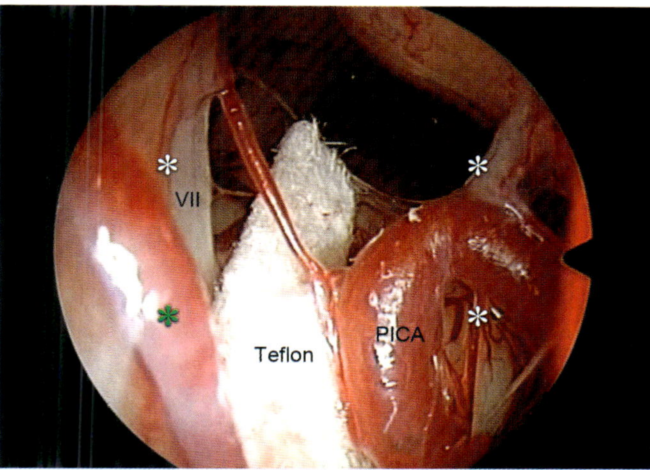

Fig. 6.17: Case 3: Intraoperative endoscopic picture in a patient w th right hemifacial spasm after "decompression" of VII at REZ by mobilizing PICA and interposition of Teflon insulation

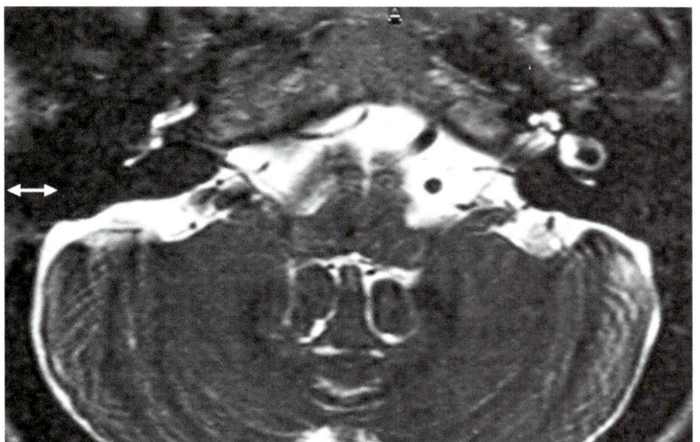

Fig. 6.18: Case 4: Axial MRI in a patient with left hemifacial spasm showing PICA arising from VA and having perpendicular contact with VII at REZ with distortion of the brainstem at this level

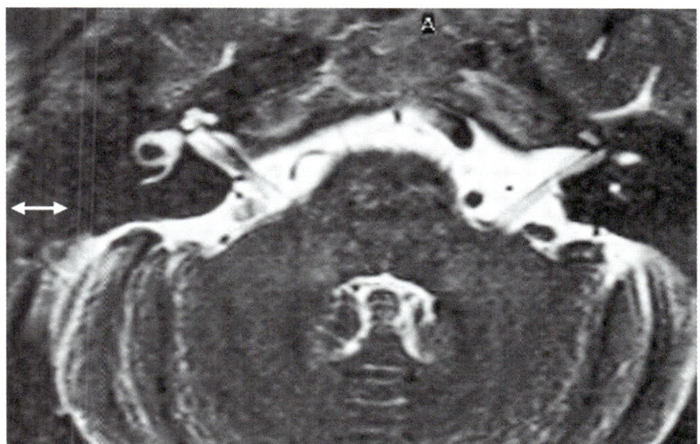

Fig. 6.19: Case 4: Axial MRI in a patient with left hemifacial spasm showing PICA arising from VA and having perpendicular contact with VII at REZ with distortion of the brainstem at this level

VASCULAR COMPRESSION SYNDROMES

Trigeminal neuralgia, hemifacial spasm, intractable vertigo, tinnitus and glossopharyngeal neuralgia are disabling functional cranial nerve disorders that can impair severely the quality of life of the patients. The efficacy of conservative management usually is limited over time, and patients ultimately seek a definitive surgical solution to their problem. Although MVD is gratifying for the patient and the surgeon, it is the surgeon's duty to prevent any devastating complications in these functional disorders. To achieve cure without complications necessitates a perfect knowledge of the anatomy of the area as well as mastering every step of the surgical technique. The following neurovascular syndromes are associated with their respective cranial nerves and will be presented separately to have better understanding of their diagnosis and management:

- Trigeminal neuralgia for trigeminal nerve
- Hemifacial spasm for facial nerve
- Glossopharyngeal neuralgia for glossopharyngeal nerve
- Certain unilateral tinnitus and disabling positional vertigo for vestibulocochlear nerve.

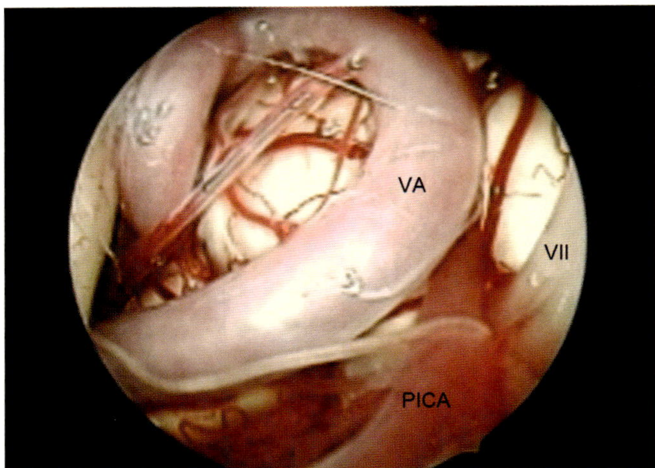

Fig. 6.20: Case 4: Intraoperative endoscopic picture in above case showing PICA arising from VA and having perpendicular contact with VII at REZ

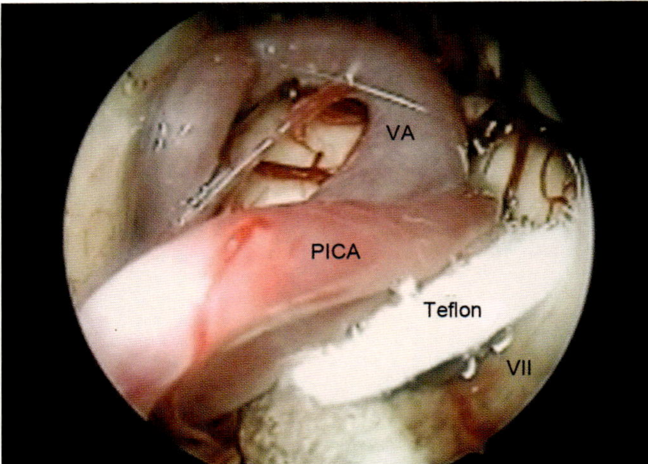

Fig. 6.21: Case 4: Intraoperative endoscopic picture in above case after "decompression" of VII at REZ by mobilizing PICA and interposition of Teflon insulation

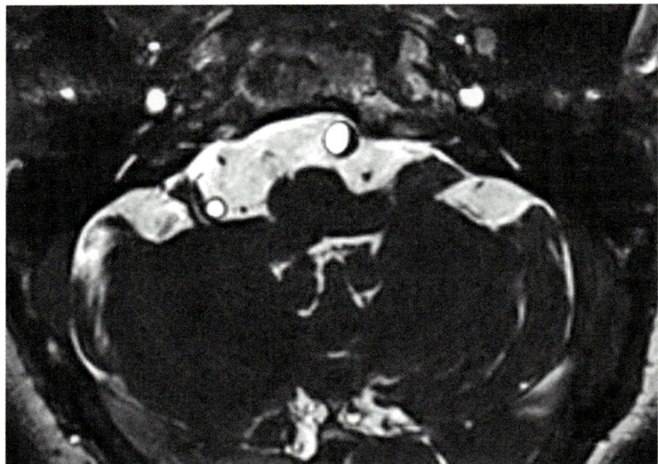

Fig. 6.22: Case 5: MRI in a patient with right hemifacial spasm due to dolichovertebral artery having perpendicular contact with VII at REZ

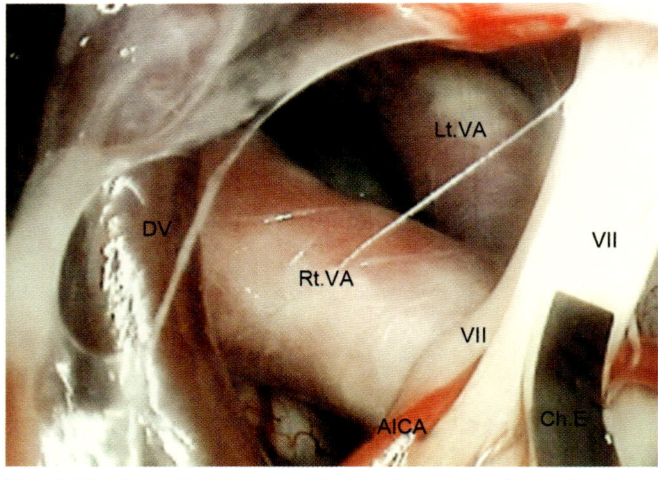

Fig. 6.23: Case 5: Intraoperative endoscopic picture in above case showing dolichovertebral artery having perpendicular contact with VII at REZ. Contralateral vertebral artery is also seen

Trigeminal Neuralgia: Vascular Compression Syndrome of Trigeminal Nerve

The trigeminal neuralgia was first described by Dandy[23] in 1935, as compression syndrome of the trigeminal nerve, from his operative findings made on 215 patients who underwent surgery in the CPA for trigeminal neuralgia and he described the presence of the SCA in contact with the trigeminal nerve in 45% of his cases and hypothesized that the vascular compression may be responsible for the painful phenomenon. The MVD surgery for trigeminal neuralgia was performed for the first time in 1959 by Gardner,[24,25] but it was popularized by Jannetta[26-28] after late 1960s, who is now considered the father of "MVD surgery."

Clinical Features

The clinical syndrome of trigeminal neuralgia was a well-defined entity and the term "tic douloureux" was used by Nicolas Andre in 1756.[29] Its incidence is four cases per 100,000 inhabitants,[30] with more prevalence in woman (61%) (1.5 times that in males). Involvement is unilateral, predominantly right (55%). Bilaterality was reported in around 2% of cases by Barker (19 of 1185 cases)[31] and Fukushima (38 of 1866).[32] Trigeminal neuralgia is a disease of midlife. Three out of four times the pain is felt after 50 years, with an average of 55 years and range of 18–83 years.

The pain of trigeminal neuralgia is paroxysmal, severe type often compared to electric shock. Though it can affect any territory of the face innervated by trigeminal nerve, it is most often in the territory of the second (V2) and/or third (V3) division of trigeminal nerve. It lasts for a few seconds to a minute or two. Between bouts of crisis, there is no pain, but the patient has anxiety for the next episode. The pain is aggravated by speech, chewing, brushing teeth, wind or by the contact at the "trigger zone" of skin (unilateral cheek and/or nose). In most of the cases, the phenomenon disappears at night, during sleep. The evolution of trigeminal neuralgia is almost never continuous, with painful periods separated by remissions. Trigeminal neuralgia usually begins as a relapsing disease with pain-free intervals that may last months or years. These intervals, however, typically grow shorter and eventually disappear. As the disease progresses, patients can have difficulty talking, eating and washing face out of fear of triggering the pain. There is no sensory deficit, no decrease in corneal reflex and no symptom in the other cranial nerve territories. Atypical trigeminal neuralgia has similar pain but with a constant background burning or aching pain and may be associated with sensory loss. Secondary trigeminal neuralgia represents 2% of cases and is due to tumors or vascular lesions compressing the trigeminal nerve or due to multiple sclerosis.

It is essential to distinguish typical trigeminal neuralgia from atypical trigeminal neuralgia, as the underlying etiopathology and the prognosis for treatment differs in both. The typical trigeminal neuralgia includes "lancinating" pain in one or more of the branches of the trigeminal nerve, a typical course in time, and one or more typical pain triggers are essential for diagnosing typical trigeminal neuralgia. In typical trigeminal neuralgia, on examination no neurological deficit is found in trigeminal nerve distribution. Atypical trigeminal neuralgia is described as a burning and continuous pain (neuropathy). In a longer existing trigeminal neuralgia a continuous underlying pain with a more continuous nature may exist between the attacks.

MRI Findings

Magnetic resonance imaging allows eliminating the causes such as tumor, multiple sclerosis or aneurysm/AV malformation. Besides the study of cisternal course of nerve in MRI, we must also take note of the nerve at the Meckel's cave and the position of the internal carotid artery. The precise imaging for the culprit vessel identifies, in order of frequency, the SCA (79%), trigeminal vein (20%), AICA (5%) and ectasia of the vertebrobasilar artery (3%) as the cause for conflict. It locates the exact site of the conflict on the trigeminal nerve, at REZ in 48% of cases, at the cisternal course of the nerve in 40% of cases and at the exit of the nerve at the entrance of Meckel's cave in 25% of cases.[16]

Therapeutic Options for Trigeminal Neuralgia

Typical trigeminal neuralgia usually responds very well to medical treatment trial with carbamazepine, at least initially and is pathognomonic of diagnosis. Carbamazepine is started in doses of 100 mg bid and increased as per requirement up to 800–1000 mg per day based on the tolerance of the patient. As the time passes, however, in many of these patients drug become ineffective or the patient develops adverse effects to the drug. Surgery is indicated after failure of medical treatment by anticonvulsants. When drug therapy fails or the patient wants a more permanent solution, a choice must be made from the other options: a percutaneous ablative technique or surgical treatment such as the MVD. The patients are educated regarding factors concerning the method itself, known results regarding effectiveness, side effects and risks and factors regarding the patient's general health and age. We personally believe the MVD surgery should precede other ablative techniques, such as radio-frequency thermocoagulation, glycerol rhizotomy or balloon compression. MVD may be considered a treatment of choice, as this modality is safe, provides the only curative solution, is not associated with any sensory loss as a result of surgery, has high long-term success rate, and is associated with the lowest rate of pain recurrence.[31–35]

Hemifacial Spasm: Vascular Compression Syndrome of Facial Nerve

The clinical syndrome of hemifacial spasm was first described by Gowers,[36] in 1888, distinguishing it from other motor abnormalities of the face. As early as 1909, Hunt[37] explained the hemifacial spasm by a "reflex" theory where the trigeminal nerve acted as an activating factor. In 1912, Sicard and Bollack[38] proposed a supranuclear origin. In 1952, Wartenberg[39] proposed hyperactivity at the nuclear level. Alajouanine and Thurel[40] proposed the presence of a lesion along the nerve itself whether in the CPA or in the intrapetrous segment. Gardner[41] in 1960 published the presence of a vascular loop as a cause of surgically reversible hemifacial spasm. Jannetta[42,43] confirmed and developed in the 1970s the concept of neurovascular conflict as a cause for hemifacial spasm.

Clinical Features

The hemifacial spasm is an involuntary contraction of the muscles of the face, is an isolated event with sudden onset and disease-free intervals in between the episodes. The incidence of idiopathic hemifacial spasm was evaluated by Auger to 0.8 per 100,000 population and a prevalence of 7.4 per 100,000 in men and 14.5 per 100,000 in women.[44] This disease has a female predominance (65%) of 2:1. The average age of onset of HS is 48 years with a range from 18 to 81 years. The mean time from onset of symptoms and surgery in our study[45] was 8 years ranging from 1 to 30 years. The hemifacial spasm, as the name suggests, is unilateral with predominance on the left (59%). This contraction usually begins in unilateral orbicularis oculi (blepharospasm occurring in both orbicularis oculi is concerned a different entity) and gradually spread to involve muscles of lower face in several months or years. The typical spasm, the most frequent condition, starts with involuntary twitching of the orbicularis muscles, gradually involving all the muscles on the same side, and finally the platysma or frontalis muscle or both. These contractions are synchronous in the involved muscles. After this initial period of clonic movements, a tonic phase usually supervenes, producing a grinning expression of face called risus sardonicus. This phase produces a forced ipsilateral eye closure interfering with binocular vision. This results in asymmetric faces that have nothing in common with the voluntary mimicry. Emotional or physical stress and voluntary contraction of any facial muscles make it worse. This contracture is isolated without pain or paralysis or hearing impairment. Unilateral tinnitus is found in 5% of cases. Patients with HFS often suffer from social embarrassment and depressive symptoms as their main handicap. These problems may lead to low self-esteem, social isolation, depression; consequently reduced life quality.

Differential Diagnosis

In 1–2% of symptomatic hemifacial spasms, other definitive cause for spasm are found like arachnoid cysts, vascular lesions (Arnold Chiari malformation, vertebrobasilar aneurysms, ischemia of the pons), tumors (brainstem or CPA tumors), Paget's disease and multiple sclerosis. Post-paralytic spasms are one of the differential diagnoses. Here, a period of facial palsy is found in the patient's past history and spasm is characterized by contracture at rest, clonical contractions at blinking, abnormal voluntary movements with loss of functional synergy and above all some residual facial weakness. Neuromuscular dystonia are characterized by their central origin and affect both sides of the face. Idiopathic blepharospasm leads to complete or partial closure of both the eyes. Oromandibular dystonia or Meige's syndrome corresponds to bilateral blepharospasm associated with periodic contraction of muscles from the lowest part of the face. Cervical dystonia or spasmodic stiff neck affects shoulder and neck muscles. Convulsive tics occur in children and they disappear during sleep or with voluntary control. Myokimia are most of the time very localized, especially on the orbicularis oris or orbicularis oculi, which tremble. They can be found in anxious patients and physicians must look for a metabolic disorder or multiple sclerosis as an underlying cause.

MRI Findings

Radiological exploration of the CPA in hemifacial spasm is always based on MRI. Its objectives are to confirm clinical diagnosis by showing a neurovascular conflict, to eliminate differential diagnosis and to realize a precise preoperative vascular mapping. Magnetic resonance imaging eliminates an intrinsic tumor or extrinsic compression from surrounding CPA pathology. It starts by a gadolinium enhanced T1 MRI, to eliminate differential diagnosis and followed by the axial and coronal T2 CISS 3DFT sequences to allow an analysis of the path of facial and vestibulocochlear nerves, seeking for a vascular loop and evaluate the deformation of the lateral recess of the pons and medulla. There are three radiological signs of neurovascular compression in hemifacial spasm: a neurovascular contact must be seen at the REZ, the vessel should be perpendicular to the facial nerve and a deformity of the nerve or the pons is observed.[16] MRI cannot be interpreted without any data concerning the patients' clinical background, as up to 3% of asymptomatic patients have a neurovascular contact on the MRI, and 0.5% of asymptomatic patients present a neural deformity. The culprit vessel with deformation induced in neural structures (facial nerve and/or lateral pons) was detected in 73% of our cases.[16] Nociceptive contact is at the REZ of the facial nerve in 95% of cases and at the porus in 5%. The combination of posterior inferior cerebellar artery and vertebral artery is responsible for 32% and the posterior inferior cerebellar artery alone in only 37%. Arterial multiple conflicts are frequent (40%). A vein is solely responsible for this in 1% of our cases[45,46] and in 2.9% of cases in study published by Jannetta team.[47] In the patients younger than 18 years with hemifacial spasm, vein or a small artery is involved with a plexiform aspect of the REZ in 67% of case.[46]

Therapeutic Options for Hemifacial Spasm

Many patients undergo various medical treatments such as antidepressants, anxiolytics, neuroleptics, etc., but none is efficient on the spasm itself. Two main definitive treatments are proposed for control of spasmodic episodes. Botulinum toxin injected at neuromuscular endings of facial muscles locks neuromuscular transmission of the nervous signal and therefore prevents facial contractions. The effects of the toxin may be very satisfying initially. They are nevertheless transitory, lasting for 2–4 months depending on the type and the amount of toxin injected.[48–51] It is not a curative treatment of hemifacial spasm, and it controls its symptoms for a short period only.

The most successful form of treatment to date has been MVD of the facial nerve at the brainstem.[52–56] The procedure has been improved in the 1990s by Magnan[46,57,58] with the complementary help of endoscope and the development of minimally invasive retrosigmoid approach. Surgical treatment is preferred in case of persistent and severe hemifacial spasm, immediately or after botulinum toxin injections, which do not modify surgical prognosis and results. Surgical treatment based on neurovascular decompression combining the use of both microscope and preoperative endoscope is the only curative treatment. It is efficient and has a very low morbidity rate. The good results obtained are long lasting and patients rapidly go back to their social and professional lives that they expected.[52–56]

Disabling Tinnitus: Vascular Compression Syndrome of Cochlear Nerve

There are several etiologies for tinnitus. Among these, cochlear nerve compression by an arterial loop or a vein in the CPA represents a very small percentage which is difficult to quantify. Therefore, the vascular compression theory of the auditory cranial nerve has remained still questionable, and has not yet gained the large acceptance that the trigeminal and facial nerve decompression received for trigeminal neuralgia and hemifacial spasm, respectively.

The specification of tinnitus as due to a neurovascular conflict is difficult. The decision to perform a MVD is not made unless a full work-up has been done. Patients with tinnitus are quite demanding of a radical solution, and thus, decision making should be very careful, and the patients must have specific clinical and test battery criteria before being advised surgery.

Most important is the unilaterality of the tinnitus whatever its characteristics. In addition to the audiogram and auditory evoked responses, we also order a MRI to search for any associated pathology along the path of the auditory pathways, and in particular at the level of the CPA.[59]

SELECTION CRITERIA FOR OPERATIVE TREATMENT

Clinical Criteria

Tinnitus has to be: unilateral, severe (following Reed's classification[60]: affecting significantly the quality of life and considered as a handicap for the patient), present since several months and persistent despite trials of therapy with the available medical treatments.

Though patients in general present with persistent continuous tinnitus, nonpulsatile and of high frequency. The pulsatile nature and the tonality of the tinnitus are not decision-influencing criteria. In addition, tinnitus associated with a low-frequency fluctuating hearing loss as in Ménière's disease or with progressive hearing loss was for us an exclusion criterion for MVD.

Radiological Criteria

As discussed earlier, MRI is able to reproduce the anatomy of the CPA and to demonstrate the presence of a neurovascular conflict. It also eliminates other potential causes of unilateral tinnitus such as an acoustic neuroma. It helps in delineating both the acoustic-facial nerves and the surrounding vascular structures in the CPA and the IAC. The image assessment includes all the CPA with serial thin slices of 0.4 mm thickness. The vascular compression is at the transition zone of the eighth nerve, which varies in its location along the course of nerve. Consequently, the sites of the vascular conflicts can occur anywhere along the nerve from the brainstem to the internal auditory canal.[61] To confirm the diagnosis, the single presence of a neurovascular contact is not sufficient. Other radiological criteria required are perpendicular contact between the vascular loop and the nerve along two different perpendicular planes, displacement of the cochlear nerve (with a certain distance between the facial and cochlear nerves) and imprint on the cochlear nerve and reduction in its diameter. Brainstem distortion caused by the vascular structure at the level of the root entry zone of the cochlear nerve, if present further strengthens the suspicion. The presence of an arterial loop in the internal auditory canal (IAC) may be responsible for tinnitus, but is not a sufficient criterion by itself. MRI for search of neurovascular conflict according to radiological criteria, usually found the anterior inferior cerebellar artery (77% in study by Moller et al.,[61] 60% in our study[59]) as the culprit artery.

Electrophysiological Criteria

Pure tone audiometry: Pure tone audiometry can identify a unilateral sensorineural hearing loss, on the same side as the tinnitus, in general of moderate severity over all the frequencies tested (250 to 8 kHz), but predominantly at the higher frequencies. This hearing loss is of statistical significance when we compare it to the contralateral ear ($p < 0.05$) and is a proof that the nerve is in a pathological state.

Auditory brainstem response (ABR): ABR in the case of a retrocochlear lesion will reveal a prolongation of the latencies or a desynchronization. We use Moller's criteria[61] to identify pathological ABRs with a prolonged interwave latency of peaks I–III of more than 0.2 ms or loss of synchronization of wave V.

Videonystagmography (VNG): Vestibular tests allow searching for an ipsilateral vestibular deficit on the same side as the tinnitus, even though it may be a subclinical deficit. The vascular compression might be responsible for a vestibular deficit following the same mechanism as that of tinnitus.

In summary, the diagnosis of a neurovascular conflict with the cochlear nerve requires the combination of a clinically incapacitating unilateral tinnitus, radiological presence of a vascular compression and electrophysiological alteration of ABR with increased latencies or desynchronization of waves.[59]

These criteria should convince the surgeon of the involvement of the CPA vessel in the etiology of tinnitus and the possible benefit of the decompression. We noted that it was not uncommon that making the diagnosis of a vascular compression on the cochlear nerve as a cause of tinnitus reassured the patient, rendered the tinnitus more tolerable, and consequently did not require operative treatment in many patients.

Disabling Positional Vertigo: Vascular Compression Syndrome of Vestibular Nerve

The term disabling positional vertigo (DPV) was first described by Jannetta in 1975.[62] The symptoms include severe motion-induced dizziness, continuous disequilibrium and unsteadiness while patient is in motion, visually induced nausea and instability.[63–66] The DPV is relieved by standing still, sitting or lying down. Symptoms do not come in attacks and are not fatigable and are not relieved by vestibular rehabilitation or medical treatment.[67] DPV is usually not accompanied by other aural symptoms, although tinnitus, hearing loss, fullness, ear pain can be present in various degree. The vascular compressive neuropathy should induce vestibular nerve irritation that results to hyperactivity and hyperexcitability of the nuclei and central nuclear dysfunction.

On audiometric examination, a unilateral high or middle frequency loss is found in more than 70% of the cases and 22% have middle frequency loss.[66]

The validity of the diagnosis of DPV was questioned by Bergsneider and Becker.[68] "It would appear that the syndrome of DPV might encompass a broad spectrum of other vertigo syndromes, predominantly what would be considered variants or atypical symptoms of classic syndromes."

Abnormal auditory brainstem response (ABR) is found in up to 40% of cases.[69] The pressure on the VIIIth cranial nerve by an offending vessel would result in a delay of wave II or an increase in the latency between peaks I and II which corresponds to the distal auditory nerve. The most relevant Moller's criteria for ABR abnormalities are wave I–III interval difference > 0.2 ms, wave I–III interval difference > 0.16 ms if low or absent wave II, wave II amplitude 33% to contralateral side, ipsilateral wave I–III absolute interval > 2.3 ms.

Imaging: Magnetic resonance imaging (MRI) is the key of assessment of neurovascular conflicts. It must include the whole course of vestibulocochlear nerve in CPA. The variability of the vascular anatomy of the CPA and the frequency of the presence of a vascular loop having contact with the vestibulocochlear nerve in many asymptomatic subjects results in the skepticism regarding the likelihood of pathology arising from cross compression.[70,71] Reliable radiologic diagnostic criteria of neurovascular conflict are required before claiming a cross compression of the vestibulocochlear nerve secondary to a vascular loop.[16] There are two criteria, the presence of orthogonal contact between the nerve and the vessel; and the presence of neural structure distortion by the offending vessel. In cases of DPV, an abnormal ABR associated with a MRI showing a vascular conflict with the eighth nerve are sufficient indications for surgical decompression of the nerve.[66]

Jannetta and Moller[63,64] reported the results of three series of DPV patients who underwent MVD. Without going into details, out of 71 patients, the result was considered as "excellent" in 76% or "significantly improved" in terms of vertigo symptoms or quality of life. McCabe and Gantz,[65] out of 29 patients, published 23 cases of relief of vertigo and motion intolerance. Sakaki et al.,[72] out of 18 patients, vertigo disappeared in 11, and improved markedly in 2. The House clinic experience,[67] based on 20 patients, reports 85% improvement of their overall disabling rating. In our experience, out of 25 patients who underwent MVD, the procedure was successful in 14 cases (56%) with complete disappearance of the complaint. One case showed a sudden sensorineural hearing loss (20 dB), 1 month post-operatively. ABR returned to normal in 5 cases. In the remaining 11 cases (44%) the decompression procedure was ineffective.

So far, Schwaber's conclusions[69] still summarize the efficiency of "this controversial treatment for a controversial illness." MVD of the vestibular nerve eliminates the disequilibrium in approximately half of the cases, improves the symptoms in one-fourth of cases and fails to control the symptoms in an another one-fourth of cases.

Glossopharyngeal Neuralgia: Vascular Compression Syndrome of IX, X Nerves

Harris first introduced the term glossopharyngeal neuralgia[73] describing two idiopathic cases that he considered to be caused by a disease of the glossopharyngeal nerve. The term vagoglossopharyngeal neuralgia was proposed later by White and Sweet.[74] The glossopharyngeal neuralgia is rare, its incidence 0.3–0.5% of the number of cases of trigeminal neuralgia.[75] It is characterized by paroxysmal electric-shock-like pain in the innervation territory of the glossopharyngeal nerve and pharyngeal branches of the vagus nerve with unilateral severe, stabbing pain for a few seconds to 2 min at the base of the tongue, pharynx, tonsillar region or sometimes ear, caused by swallowing. It is essential to rule out multiple primary causes like pharyngeal cancer, temporo-maxillary joint dysfuction CPA tumors and AV malformations. Some patients with glossopharyngeal neuralgia experience sudden excessive vagal outflow during an attack that can result in arrhythmia, hypotension and syncope. Neuralgic pain gives rise to a massive volley of afferent impulses that reach the motor nucleus of the vagus nerve causing excessive parasympathetic outflow. Ephaptic transmission through artificial synapses between cranial nerves IX and X at the level of their respective ganglia and presence of collaterals between the nucleus of tractus solitarius and dorsal motor nuclei of the vagus nerve have been proposed.

A useful way for confirming the glossopharyngeal neuralgia is to spray the pharynx and the supraglottic area with 5% xylocaine spray during the attack and if the pain disappears it is highly likely to be neuralgic pain from IX or X cranial nerve. The other way to suggest the diagnosis is the relatively good response to carbamazepine. Surgical intervention is indicated if medical treatment fails despite the use of the highest tolerated dosage of medication. Similar to trigeminal neuralgia, many surgical procedures for glossopharyngeal neuralgia have been described. It includes extracranial or intracranial nerve section or MVD of glossopharyngeal nerve.

The PICA alone or with vertebral artery is the commonest cause for compression. Among these, dolichoectasia of the vertebral artery makes it difficult to maintain the decompressed glossopharyngeal and vagal rootlets to remain distinct from the artery. Section of the glossopharyngeal nerve has been then recommended, and not random decompression of it, because keeping the vertebral artery away without distortion of the glossopharyngeal nerve may be uncertain. However, a loop of the posterior inferior cerebellar artery is amenable to a vascular decompression surgery with good results.[75-78]

MICROVASCULAR DECOMPRESSION SURGERY

The technique of MVD was first proposed in 1960 by Gardner,[24,25] but was subsequently made popular by Peter Jannetta[26,27] who was the first to use the operating microscope for this surgery. This surgery, also known as "Jannetta technique," is performed on a patient in lateral decubitus position, by suboccipital approach, with the help of technical monitoring of the facial nerve and the cochlear nerve. The surgical approach that we follow is keyhole minimally invasive retrosigmoid approach in supine position and has been discussed in detail in Chapter 4.

Indications

- Trigeminal neuralgia
- Hemifacial spasm

- Selected cases of tinnitus
- Glossopharyngeal neuralgia.

Vascular Decompression Technique

Identification of Neurovascular Conflict by Endoscopy

The operating microscope in spite of its qualities of brightness, magnification and depth of field provides only axial view to the operator. Yet, the site of the conflict is to be found most often against the brainstem at the emergence of cranial nerves, which then requires a mechanical retraction of cerebellum and other neural structures. According to the landmark paper of Janetta group,[79] the pioneer and stalwart in the field of MVD "Turning the corner is the most dangerous stage of the operation and must be executed with patience and the utmost care," and that most complications can be attributed to cerebellar retraction. The intraoperative endoscopy, thanks to its panoramic vision and angulated view, allows a complete exploration of the CPA without retraction of the cerebellum or brainstem and leaves no hidden areas to be missed.[57,58] It is therefore the procedure of choice to locate the site of conflict without significant cerebellar retraction, positively identify the vessels responsible as well as their path, and define the best maneuver to decompress the artery. Hopkins autoclavable rigid 30° angled endoscope (22 cm long, 4 mm in diameter) with attached video monitor is necessary for such endeavor. Once the endoscope is placed into the cranial opening, it should be moved either in a straight in-and-out direction along the axis of the shaft or rotated about the axis of the shaft. It should not be moved in a side-to-side direction. To change its trajectory, the tip should be withdrawn. The direction is then changed, and the endoscope is reintroduced in a straight line. Swinging motions of the tip, which put the cranial nerves and vascular structures at the greatest risk, should be limited as much as possible. Cranial nerves are much more prone to damage by retraction and surgical manipulation because they lack supporting and protective epineurium in their cisternal course. The endoscope should not be kept more than a minute in the same place or in contact with neural structures, as the heat produced at its hot tip can damage these structures. The site for compression/s by one or more artery or vein is identified. Compression is defined as a grossly appreciable change in appearance of the nerve in the area of contact with a vessel, including indentation, discoloration, or evidence of trauma to the nerve.

Vascular Decompression Using the Operating Microscope

Whatever the site of neurovascular conflict, the principle of vascular decompression surgery is to mobilize the offending vessel from the affected cranial nerve, then maintain its new position away from the cranial nerve affected. Once the site for neurovascular conflict is identified by the endoscope, we shift to microscope for separation of the conflicting vessel from the nerve. Under the vision of operating microscope, the loop responsible for pressure is cautiously and gradually mobilized using bayonet shaped curved elevators. This displacement of the vessel is relatively easy in cases where the vertebral artery is the offending vessel and more delicate and difficult in other vessels like the posterior inferior cerebellar artery (due to its internal and inferior situation), the SCA (due to the presence of perforating arteries) and the anterior inferior cerebellar artery (due to the presence of a labyrinthine artery and its location between facial and vestibulocochlear nerves).

The artery is maintained in this new remote place by interposition between the artery and nerve of inert synthetic insulating material (like pledgets of Teflon, Gelfoam, Dacron or silastic) and/or by fixation of the artery to the adjacent dura mater with suture or glue. We prefer pledgets of Teflon felt to insulate the compression site over the cranial nerve from the artery and occasionally use fibrin glue to fix artery in its new position. When a vein is responsible, it is coagulated and sectioned, after ensuring thorough surgical exploration of the CPA that it is not the only route of venous drainage. There are two important considerations that we follow: any contact of the artery with the affected hyperexcitable nerve must be isolated and secured and even asymptomatic vascular conflict on a nerve in the neighborhood should be treated.

Confirmation of Microvascular Decompression by Endoscopy and Nerve Monitoring

Because of the narrow and deep operative field, the view for placement of Teflon pledgets is partially obstructed. Therefore after decompression of the conflict under microscopic guidance, we use the endoscope to check the right place of the Teflon pledget and the absence of any residual neurovascular contact, without changing the position of the existing structures. Intraoperative electrophysiological tests must recover their normality, but this is inconsistent in various disorders and will be discussed individually.

In MVD operation, similar to other functional disorders of CPA, functions of the cochlear and facial nerves should not be altered after the surgery. For that purpose, we are conducting the intraoperative monitoring by auditory brainstem responses (ABR), dorsal cochlear nucleus action potential (DNAP) and facial nerve root exit zone evoked muscle action potential (FREMAP) for the hemifacial spasm surgery. In this surgery, it is rare to conduct cochlear nerve and facial nerve mappings, but measurement of an AMR (also called lateral spread response; LSR) which is widely prevalent as an indicator of pressure removal is conducted by using a FREMAP electrode (Figs 6.1 to 6.3). Besides these, measurement of blink reflex and various other electrophysiological tests using facial nerve stimulation probe are possible. It could be mentioned that in case of a trigeminal neuralgia surgery, routine intraoperative monitoring may be avoided as there would be no effect on the acoustico-facial bundle if excessive retraction of the cerebellum could be avoided.

VARIATIONS IN SURGICAL TECHNIQUE IN DIFFERENT VASCULAR SYNDROMES

Microvascular Decompression for Trigeminal Neuralgia

Vascular decompression of trigeminal nerve is done in a particularly deep and medial location (Fig. 6.24) but fortunately we have a comparatively wide and strong cranial nerve. The endoscope is used to visualize the entire path of the trigeminal nerve up to its entrance into the Meckel's cave (Figs 6.25 and 6.26). Regions of the nerve that are not clearly visualized under the microscope (Fig. 6.27) are carefully examined for evidence of additional nerve–vessel conflicts. These areas include the medial and inferior faces of the nerve root entry zone; the superior, inferior and medial aspects of the cisternal portion of the nerve; and the site of entry of the nerve into Meckel's cave. Proximal and distal mapping of all offending vascular structures is conducted under the endoscope. Microsurgical access to the nerve can be obstructed either by the petrosal vein of Dandy or by a bulging posterior wall of the petrous apex (Fig. 6.24). If the petrosal vein (Dandy's vein) obstructs progress, it usually can be sacrificed without complications. If it is particularly large and thought to constitute a substantial portion of the drainage of the cerebellum, it should be dissected out as much as possible and work should be performed around it. The endoscope must pass the vein on the way to the trigeminal cistern without placing traction on it, thus avoiding the danger of rupturing it. The trigeminal nerve is resistant to surgical trauma, but it is particularly sensitive to contact and deformation. This represents a risk factor for recurrence by postoperative fibrosis that may change the relationships between neurovascular structures after the surgery despite it being initially effective. It is therefore essential to place the SCA against tentorium (and preferably glue the artery to tentorial dura with fibrin glue), without even indirect support of the trigeminal nerve, and ensuring that its loop will not secondarily extend toward the nerve. Since there is no need for retractors to maintain the view (due to surgical position and the use of endoscope), there is little chances for stretching of the facial and vestibulocochlear nerve and thus leading to the facial weakness and hearing loss. If a lateral decubitus approach (park bench position) is used instead, the facial–vestibulocochlear nerve complex encountered before the trigeminal nerve are at increased risk of stretch injury and great care is required to avoid retracting these nerves laterally to prevent damage from retraction. However, care should be taken while inserting and using endoscope to avoid traction or thermal injury to the cranial nerves by being too close to the nerves for longer duration.

In the case of a conflicting artery, the vessel is detached from the nerve and pons by dissecting the pia-arachnoidal filaments that maintain the artery adherent to the neighboring nervous structures, with microscissors (Fig. 6.28). The artery is transposed away from the

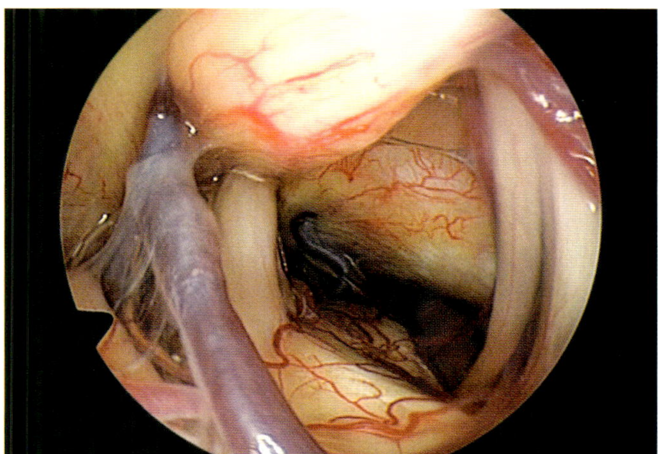

Fig. 6.24: Endoscopic picture showing trigeminal nerve and its vascular conflict with SCA. The SCA is the most commonly conflicting vessel. Also seen proximally is Dandy's vein entering superior petrosal sinus and acoustico-facial bundle entering IAC. Ipsilateral vertebral artery continuing as basilar artery is seen inferiorly

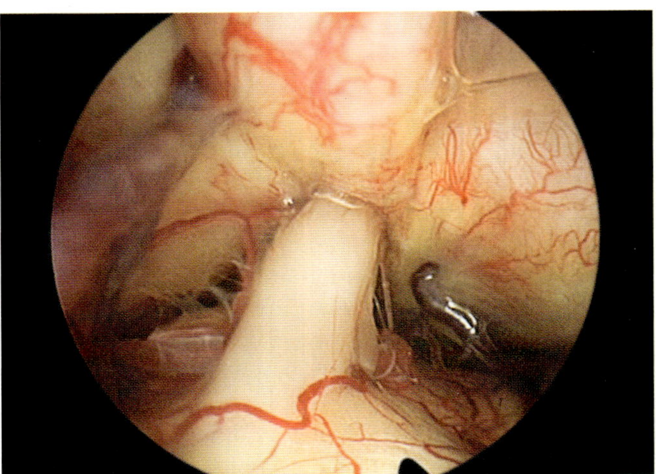

Fig. 6.25: Closer endoscopic view showing main trunk of SCA impinging into REZ of V

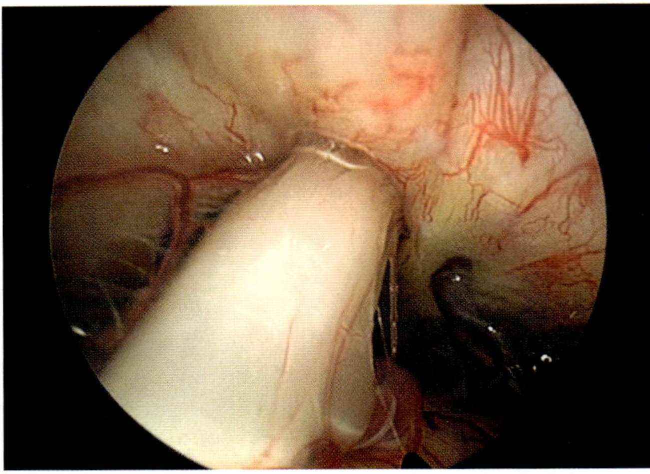

Fig. 6.26: Further closer endoscopic view showing main trunk of SCA impinging into REZ of V. The cisternal course of V and its entry into Meckel's cave is free of any vascular conflicts

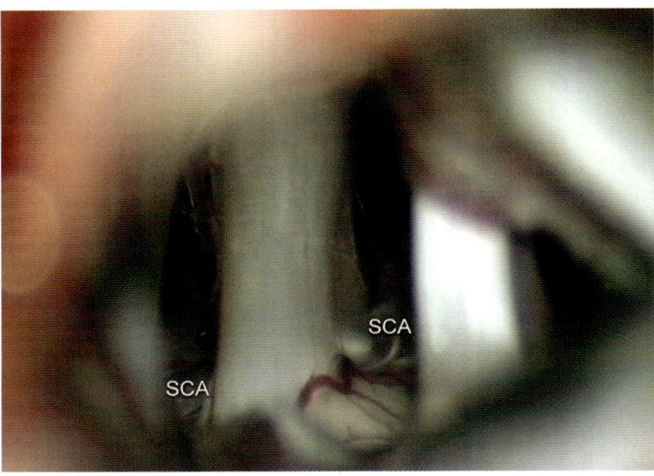

Fig. 6.27: Microscopic view showing main trunk of SCA impinging into REZ of V

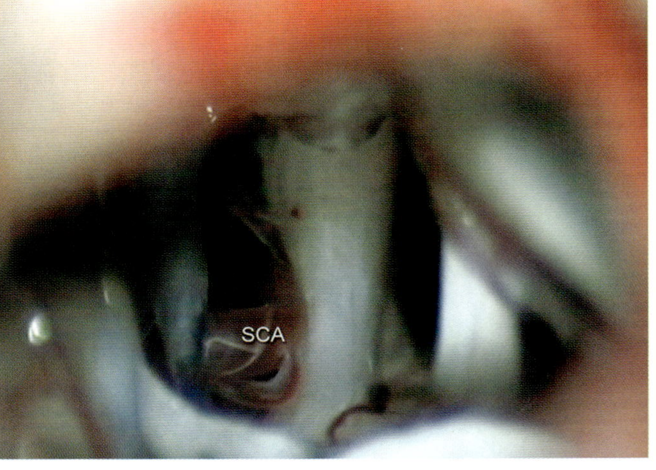

Fig. 6.28: Microscopic view showing main trunk of SCA after displacing its position from conflict site at REZ of V

trigeminal root toward the tentorium (Figs 6.29 and 6.30) and adhered to later using fibrin glue. The conflicting artery is further kept apart from the trigeminal nerve in a horizontal position toward the tentorium by means of one or several pieces of Teflon pledgets (Figs 6.31 to 6.35). Throughout the vascular manipulations, one should always notice for any spasms in the related artery and if noticed, apply a Gelfoam soaked in papaverin to avoid mechanical vasospastic reactions in the arteries.

Different Types of Conflicts Observed in MVD for Trigeminal Neuralgia

The SCA is the commonest source for neurovascular conflict in trigeminal neuralgia (Figs 6.24 to 6.35), either its main trunk or its branches. Its normal anatomic situation corresponds to a course from anterior to posterior around the pons, with a bifurcation into rostral and caudal branches at a certain distance superior to the REZ of trigeminal nerve, before distributing to the medial and lateral superior cerebellar surface and the dorsolateral aspect of the peduncle. When responsible for a neurovascular conflict, the SCA is elongated and of one of the following two types: anteromedially positioned or superiorly positioned.

In the neurovascular conflict by the SCA (Figs 6.36 to 6.38), the vessel is transposed upward under the tentorium and parallel to it (Fig. 6.39). Care is taken to avoid kinking of the elongated artery and tearing or avulsion (or

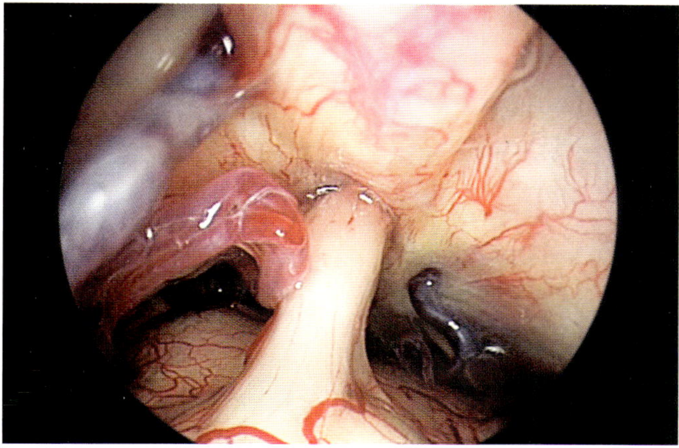

Fig. 6.29: Endoscopic picture showing main trunk of SCA along with its cephalic and caudal branches after displacing its position from conflict site at REZ of V

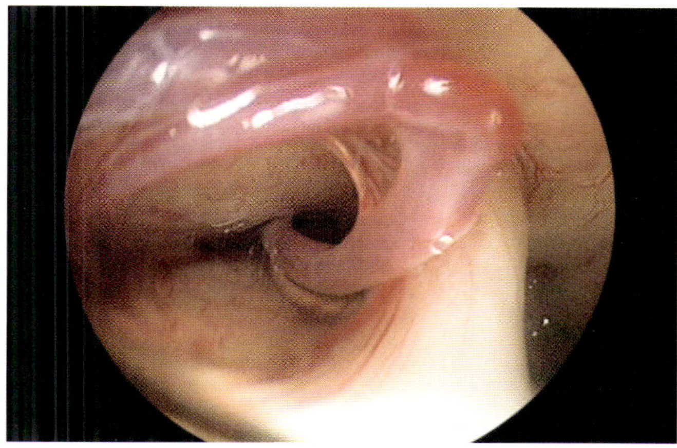

Fig. 6.30: Endoscopic picture showing main trunk of SCA along with its cephalic and caudal branches are displaced superiorly toward tentorium

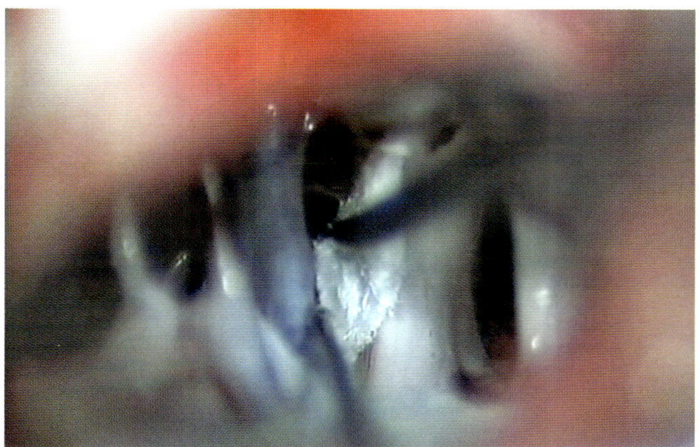

Fig. 6.31: Microscopic picture showing placement of Teflon pledget in between the V and SCA

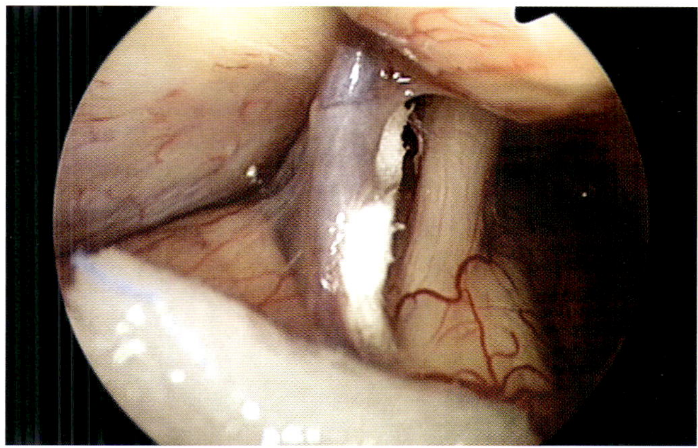

Fig. 6.32: Endoscopic picture showing new position of SCA secured in between the tentorium and cerebellum by Teflon pledgets and fibrin glue

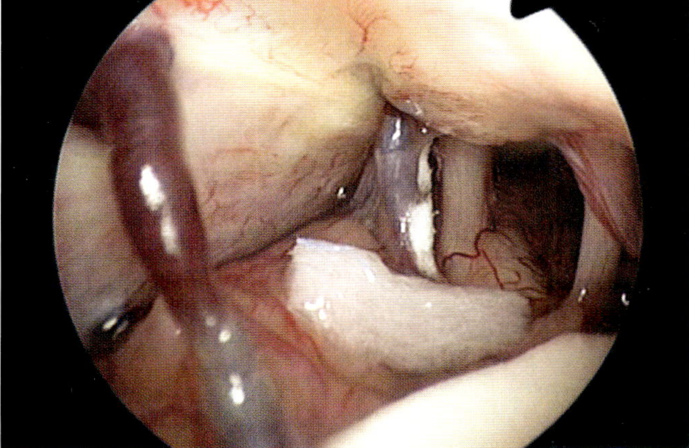

Fig. 6.33: Endoscopic picture showing new position of SCA secured in between the tentorium and cerebellum by Teflon pledgets and fibrin glue

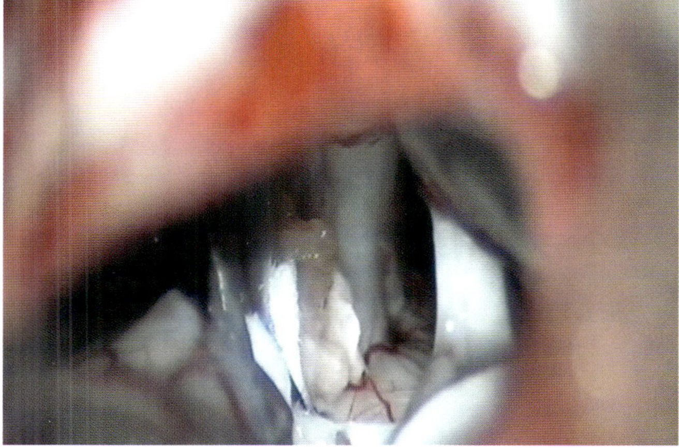

Fig. 6.34: Microscopic picture showing stabilization of Teflon pledgets and prevention of its displacement into the V course by free fat tissue

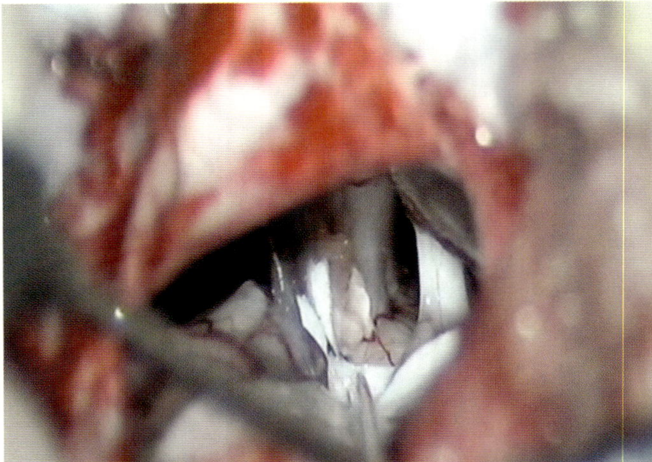

Fig. 6.35: Final picture showing the decompression of trigeminal nerve for trigeminal neuralgia by MIRA. Note the size of craniotomy, relations with adjoining structures like Dandy's vein and acoustico-facial bundle

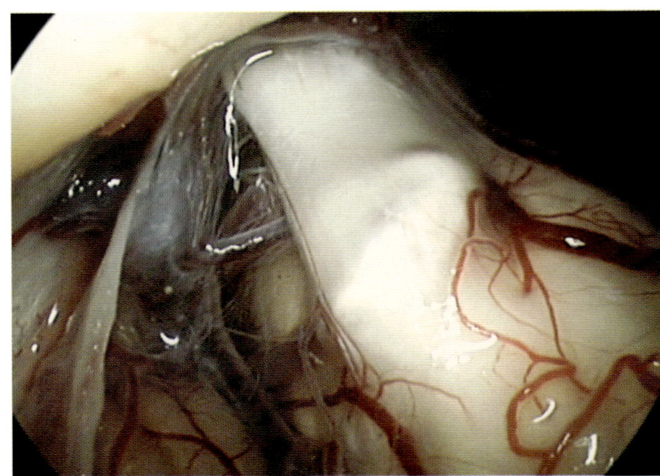

Fig. 6.36: Another case of trigeminal neuralgia due to vascular conflict by SCA at REZ of V

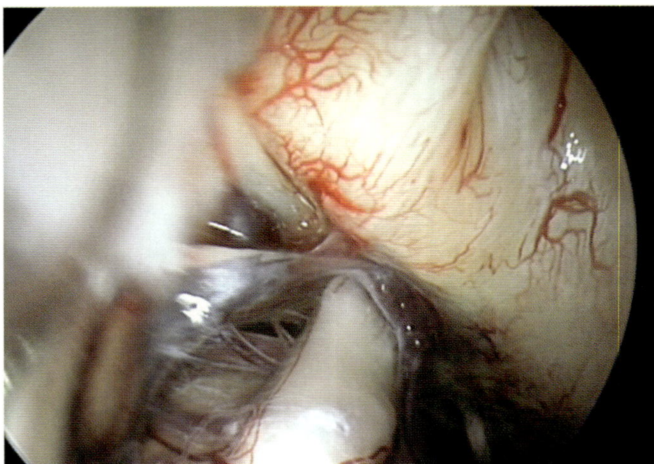

Fig. 6.37: Apart from obvious conflict by SCA, note the presence of vein running perpendicular to the V at Meckel's cave

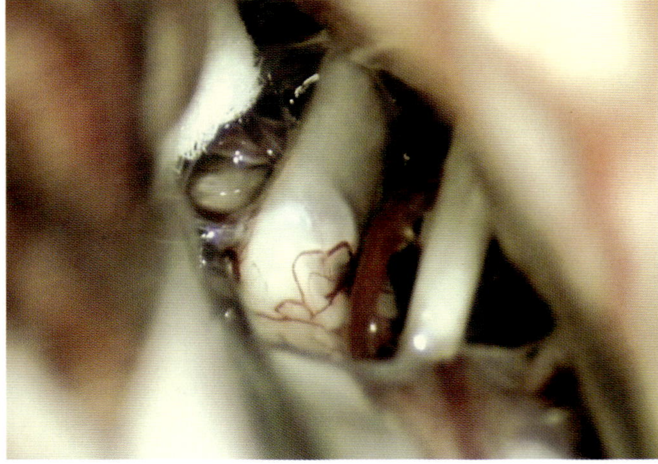

Fig. 6.38: Microscopic picture showing vascular conflict by SCA at REZ of V

both) of the tiny collateral branches circumferential to the brainstem. Because these collaterals are generally long vessels, transposition of the SCA is relatively easy. SCA is placed against tentorium and preferably glued to the tentorial dura with fibrin glue (Fig. 6.40) and prevents its loop to extend toward the nerve. The conflicting artery is further kept apart from the trigeminal nerve in a horizontal position by means of one or several pieces of Teflon pledgets (Fig. 6.41). The SCA and its branches are blocked toward the midline generally by squeezing it between the superior surface of the cerebellum and the inferior aspect of the tentorium (Fig. 6.40), if necessary with additional packing of Teflon (Fig. 6.41). Care must be taken to avoid rupturing of any infratentorial bridging vein. To prevent displacement of the repositioned artery, a square piece of Teflon felt is placed on the superior petrosal vein to hold the artery in place.

Initially, we used Telfon felt directly over the trigeminal nerve. But after a couple of incidences of Teflon migration into Meckel's cave, Teflon granuloma and deep invagination of Teflon felt into the trigeminal nerve trunk on revision surgeries, we now routinely interpose a small fibrofatty tissue between the nerve alone (Figs 6.42 to 6.46) or with the Teflon felt to prevent aforementioned

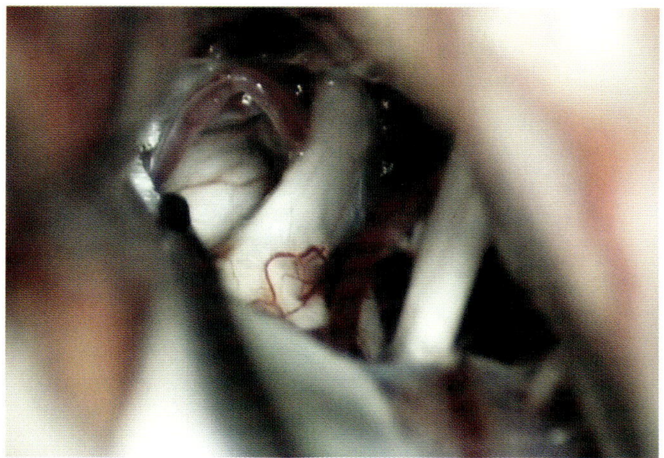

Fig. 6.39: Microscopic picture showing displacement of SCA superiorly after carefully disentangling the loop from REZ of V

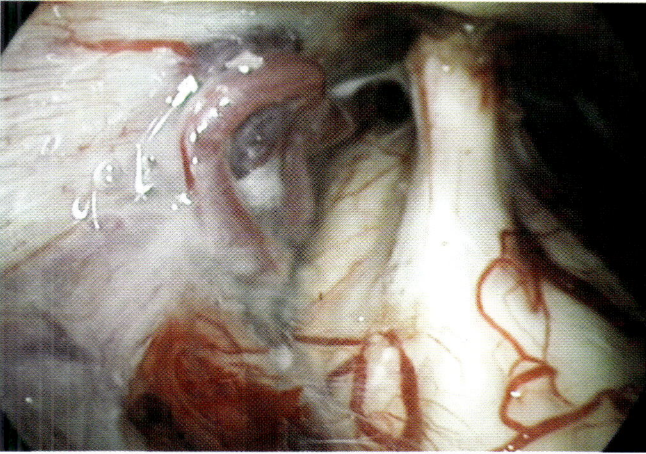

Fig. 6.40: Endoscopic picture showing new position of SCA secured to the tentorial dura by fibrin glue

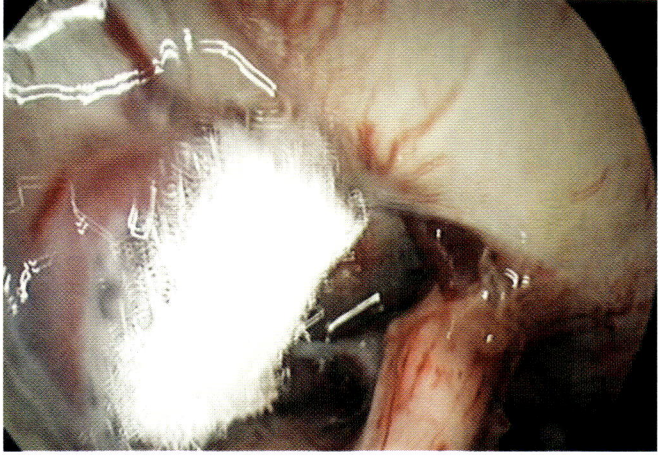

Fig. 6.41: Endoscopic picture showing new position of SCA secured to the tentorial dura by Teflon pledget and fibrin glue. Also note that the vein running perpendicular to the V at Meckel's cave has been cauterized and cut

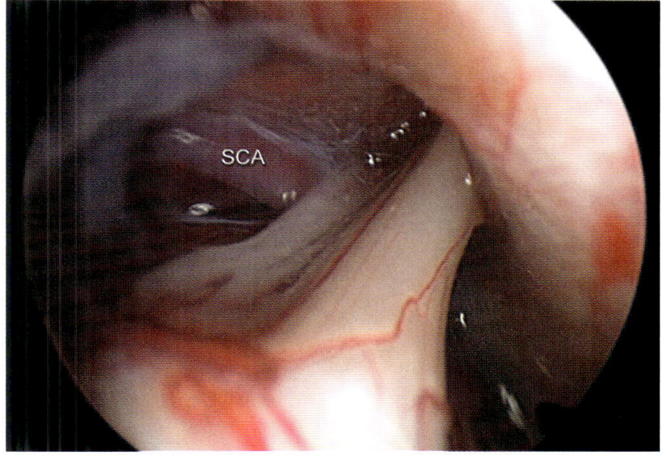

Fig. 6.42: Another case of trigeminal neuralgia due to vascular conflict by SCA with V at its cisternal course and close to Meckel's cave

complications (Figs 6.34 and 6.35). The Teflon piece is passed between the conflicting artery and nerve.

Apart from the SCA as the sole conflicting artery, its association with the AICA or one of several satellite veins is the next common cause for neurovascular conflict in trigeminal neuralgia. AICA can be the sole conflicting artery or can be an additional conflict along with the SCA (inducing a vascular "forceps" compression) (Fig. 6.47). For the AICA conflict, nerve compression generally is exerted by an upward loop of AICA, which indents the caudal surface of the REZ (Figs 6.47 to 6.64). When the AICA is implicated, the cross compression is therefore almost always is located on the inferior (or the posteroinferior) aspect of the pars major (Figs 6.50, 6.51, 6.54, 6.55), usually at the REZ. Because of the frequent presence of short collaterals that correspond to important perforators for the adjacent brainstem and, sometimes, because of a labyrinthine artery arising from the loop itself, transposition of the AICA away from the nerve should be performed very carefully. In most cases, the loop can be pulled away and maintained apart from the trigeminal nerve by Teflon pledget as with the SCA (Figs 6.52 and 6.64).

For veins, it is often difficult to be certain of their involvement except when they create a marked segmental groove in the root. When veins are concerned, the site of

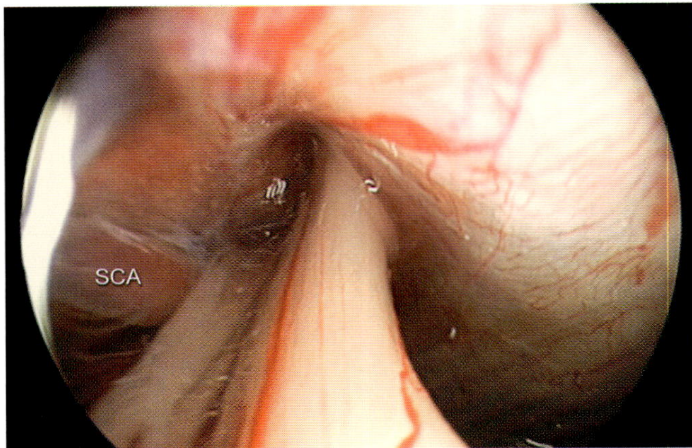

Fig. 6.43: Endoscopic picture showing vascular conflict by SCA with V close to Meckel's cave

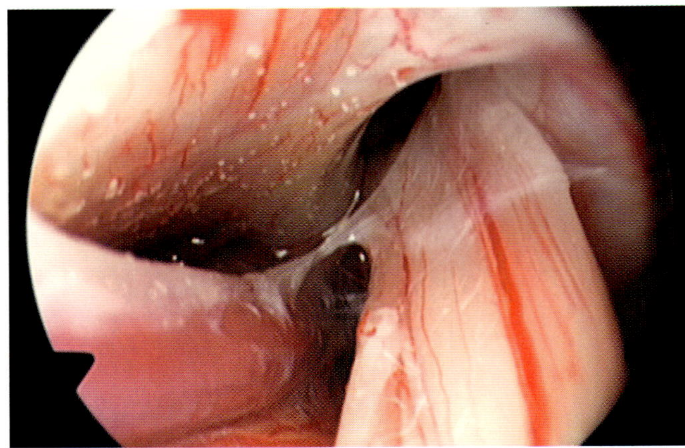

Fig. 6.44: Endoscopic picture showing vascular conflict by SCA with V close to Meckel's cave has been displaced superiorly

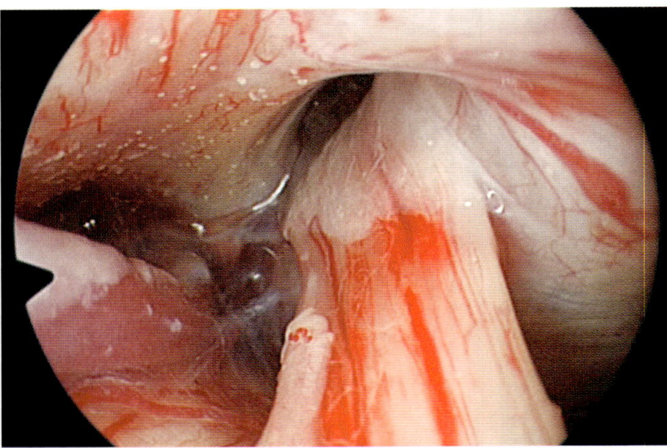

Fig. 6.45: Endoscopic picture showing dissection of all arachnoid adhesions between SCA and V. Also note the distortion of the V by the vascular conflict

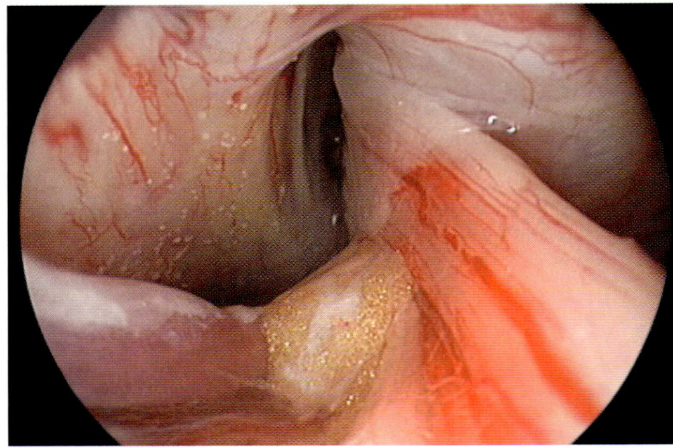

Fig. 6.46: Endoscopic picture showing placement of free fatty tissue to maintain the new position of SCA

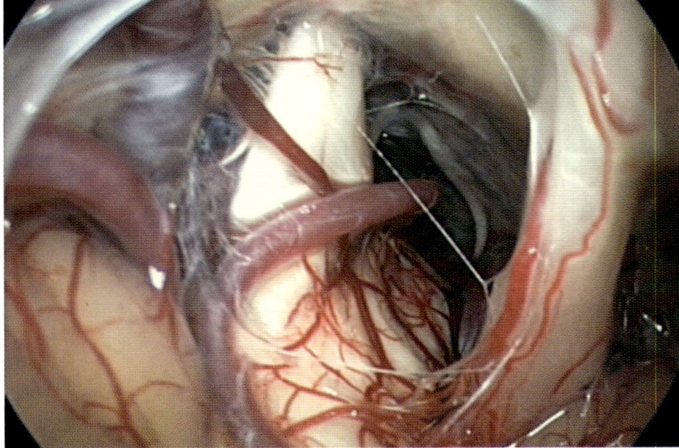

Fig. 6.47: Endoscopic picture in another case of right trigeminal neuralgia showing vascular conflict by SCA superomedially and AICA inferolaterally. Also present is the vein between V and AICA conflict site

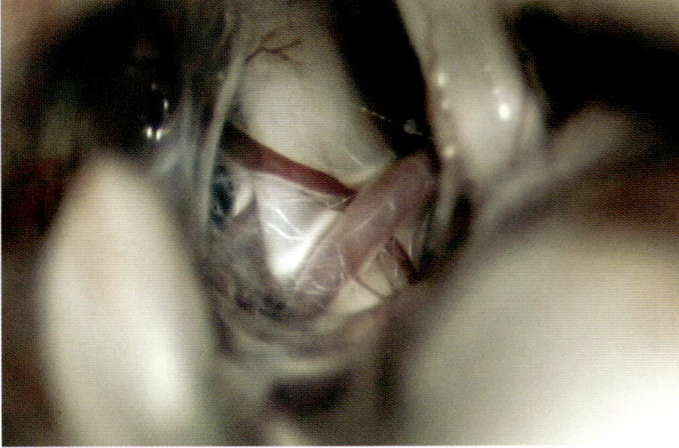

Fig. 6.48: Microscopic picture showing vascular conflict by SCA superomedially, AICA inferolaterally and vein over the lateral surface of V

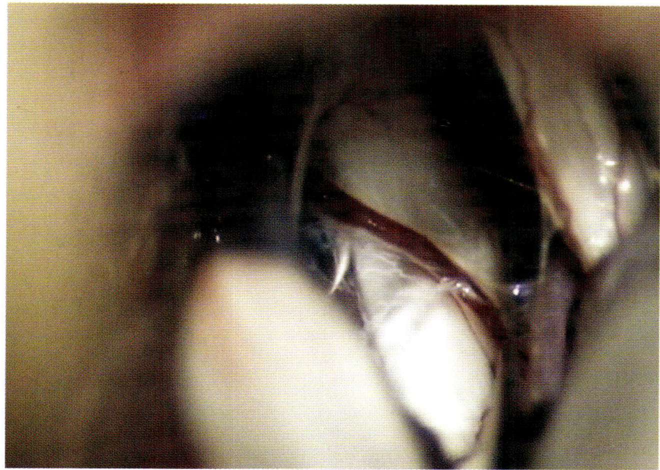

Fig. 6.49: Dissection of AICA from V by dividing the arachnoid adhesions

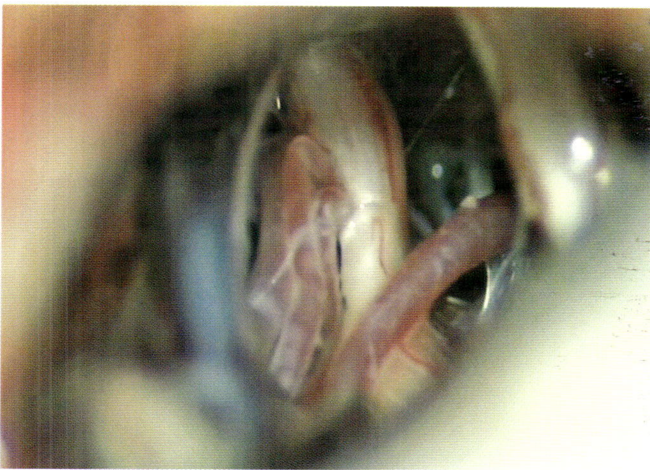

Fig. 6.50: Microscopic picture showing dissection of AICA and SCA with its branches from V. Note the vein between V and AICA has been cauterized and cut

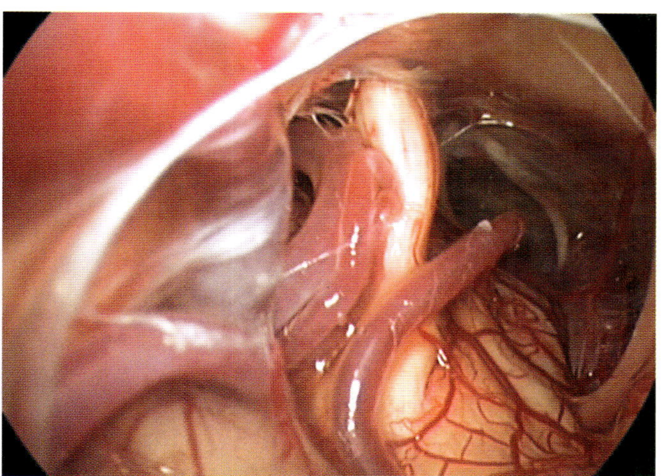

Fig. 6.51: Endoscopic picture showing dissection of AICA and SCA with its branches from V. The V appears to be distorted at the site of conflict

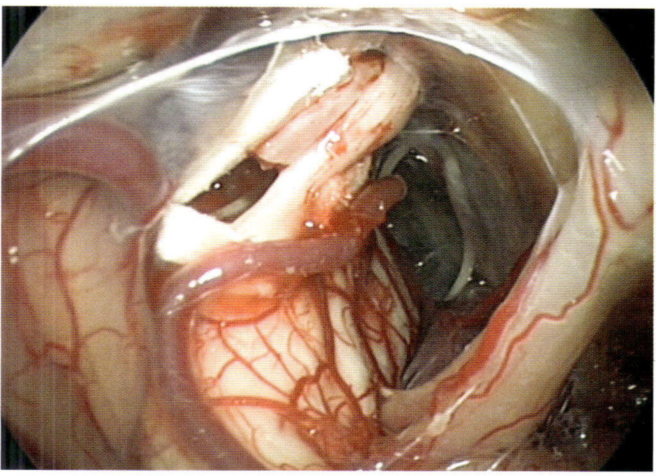

Fig. 6.52: Endoscopic picture showing "decompression" of V from SCA and AICA by Teflon pledgets and free fat tissue

the compression is most often on the lateral part of the pars major owing to a pontine tributary of the superior petrosal venous sinus (Figs 6.65 to 6.67). In the case of a cross-compressing vein making groove in the REZ laterally or inferiorly over the pars major, most of the time it is difficult if not impossible to transpose the vein away from the nerve. It is preferable to coagulate the vein using a fine bipolar forceps, divide it and recoagulate both the ends (Fig. 6.68). When there is a large vein coursing parallel to the nerve and adjacent to it (usually a satellite vein originating from the pons and running near the undersurface of trigeminal nerve, before entering the Meckel's cave), it is difficult to be certain of its pathologic role. If there is no obvious responsible offending artery, however, this vein may be considered as playing a role and has to be isolated by Teflon pledgets (Figs 6.68 and 6.69). More common is an additional vein around the nerve at the entrance of Meckel's cave inferiorly and posteriorly. Such venous structure must be coagulated and divided (Fig. 6.68).

In our cases of MVD for trigeminal neuralgia,[81,82] a vascular decompression procedure was performed on SCA in 76%, on a venous structure in 29% and on other artery in 17%. Dolicovertebral artery is an uncommon cause for trigeminal neuralgia (Figs 6.70 to 6.75).

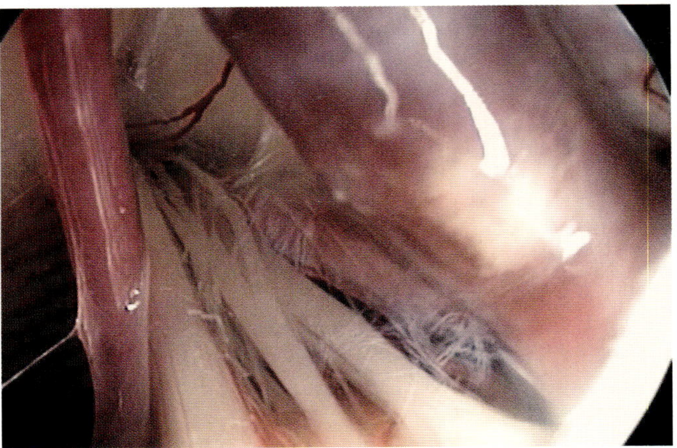

Fig. 6.53: Endoscopic picture in another case of left trigeminal neuralgia showing vascular conflict by SCA superomedially and AICA inferolaterally

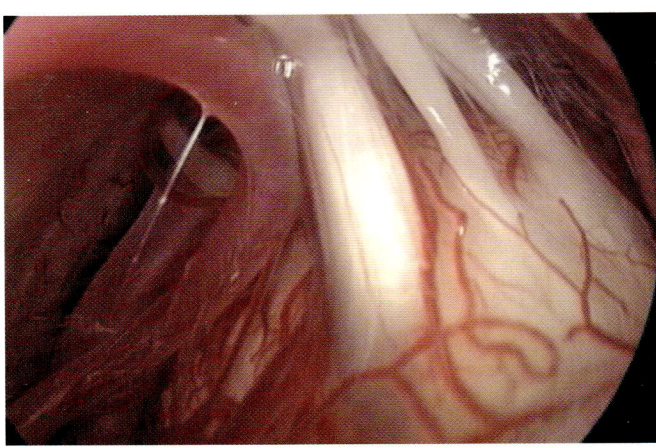

Fig. 6.54: Endoscopic picture showing vascular conflict by AICA inferolaterally

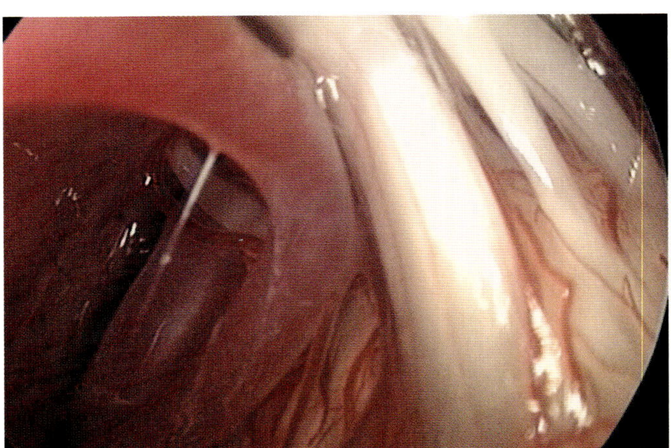

Fig. 6.55: Closer endoscopic picture showing vascular conflict by AICA inferolaterally

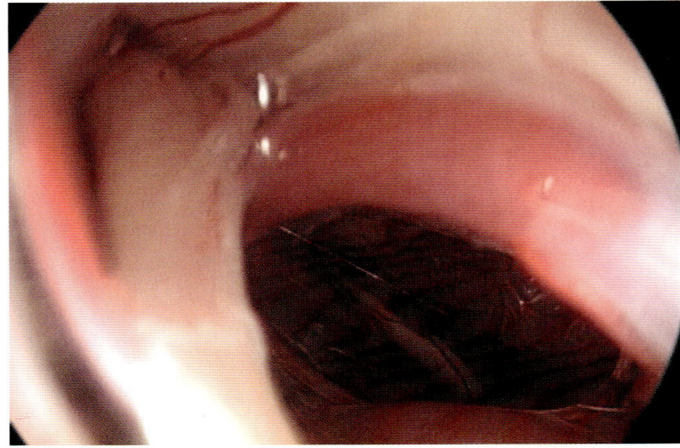

Fig. 6.56: Endoscopic picture showing vascular conflict by SCA superomedially

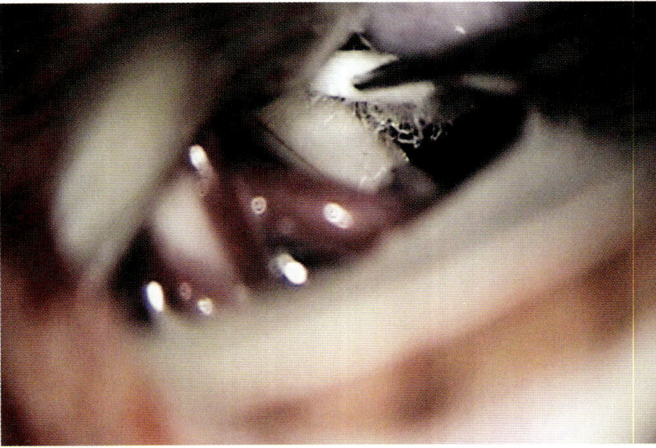

Fig. 6.57: Microscopic picture showing placement of Teflon pledget between V and SCA

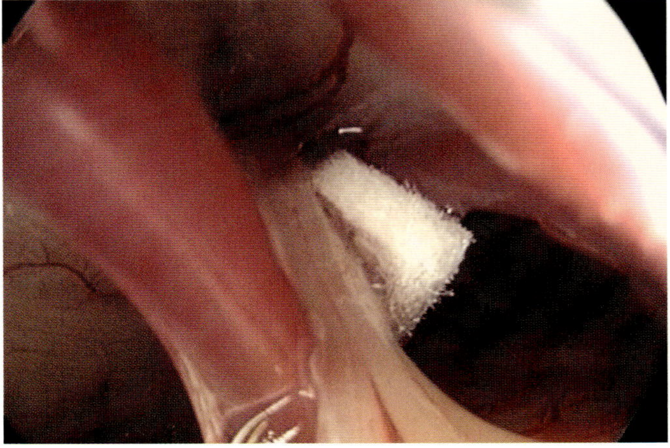

Fig. 6.58: Endoscopic picture showing Teflon pledget between V and SCA

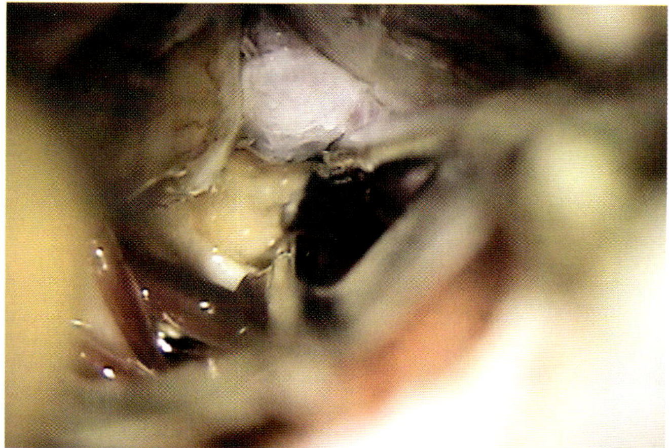

Fig. 6.59: Microscopic picture showing placement of free fat tissue between V and Teflon pledget to prevent displacement of later

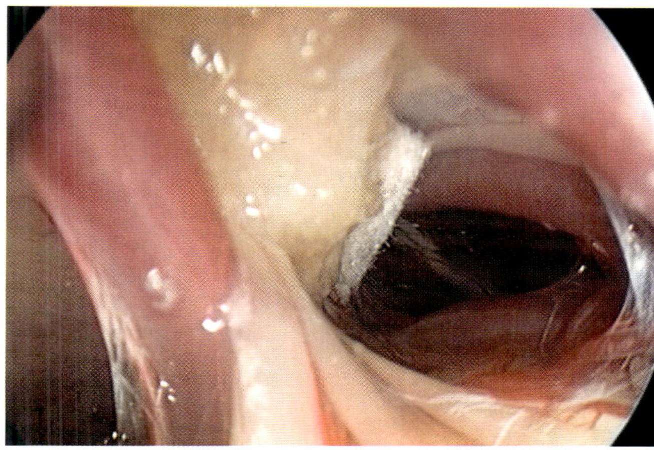

Fig. 6.60: Endoscopic picture showing placement of placement of free fat tissue between V and Teflon pledget to prevent displacement of later

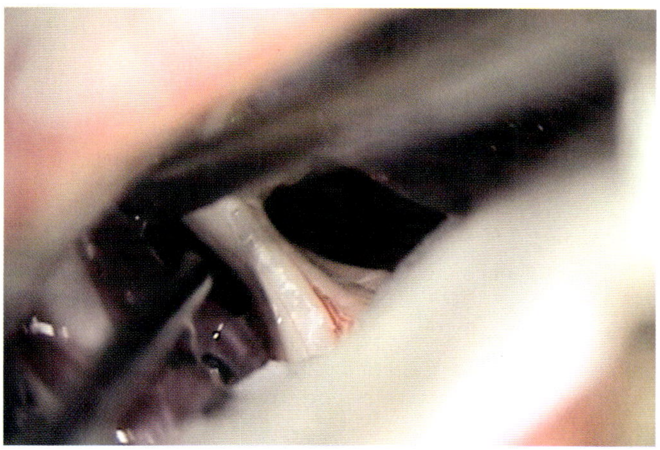

Fig. 6.61: Microscopic picture showing displacement of AICA from V

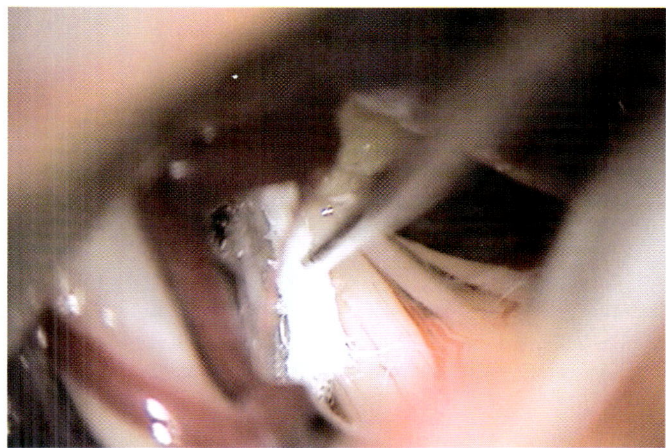

Fig. 6.62: Microscopic picture showing placement of Teflon pledget between V and AICA

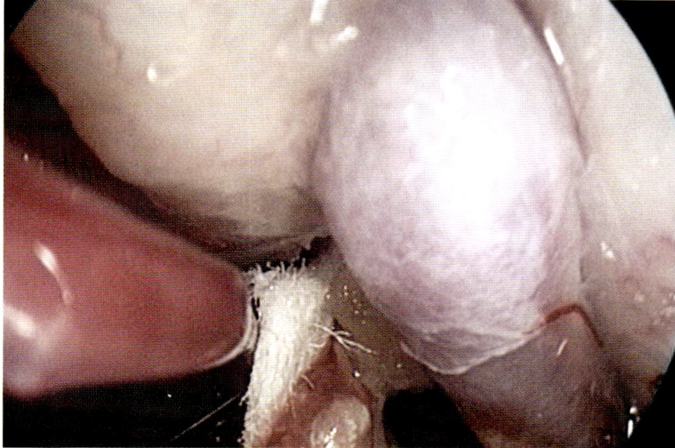

Fig. 6.63: Endoscopic picture showing Teflon pledget between V and AICA

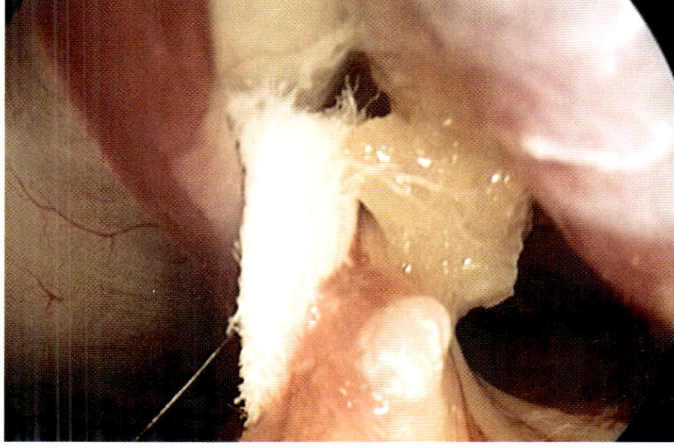

Fig. 6.64: Endoscopic picture showing Teflon pledget between V and AICA

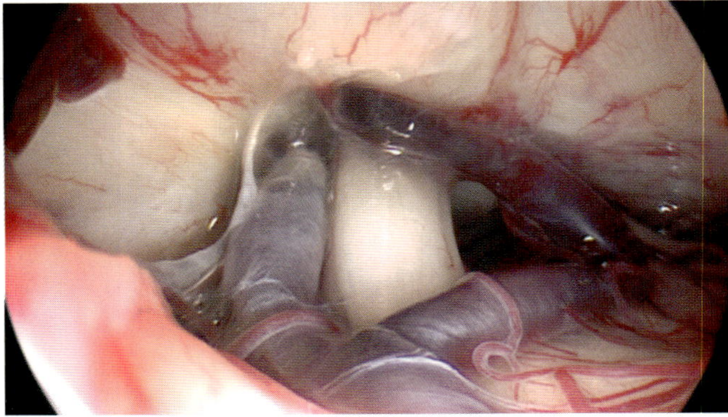

Fig. 6.65: Endoscopic picture in another case of right trigeminal neuralgia showing multiple large veins in contact with lateral surface of V. No obvious arterial conflict was found

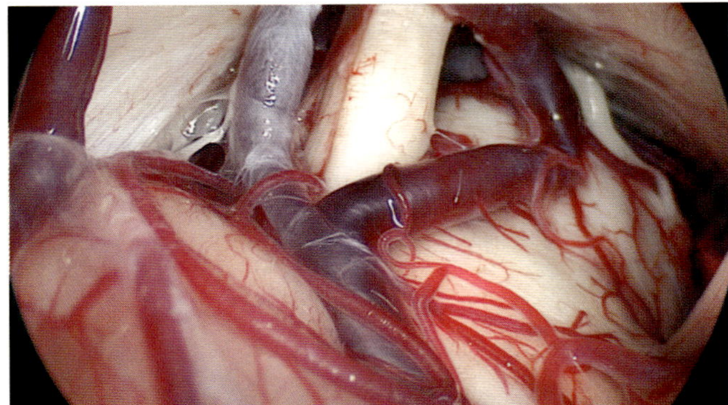

Fig. 6.66: Endoscopic view of REZ of V having close contact with trigeminal vein

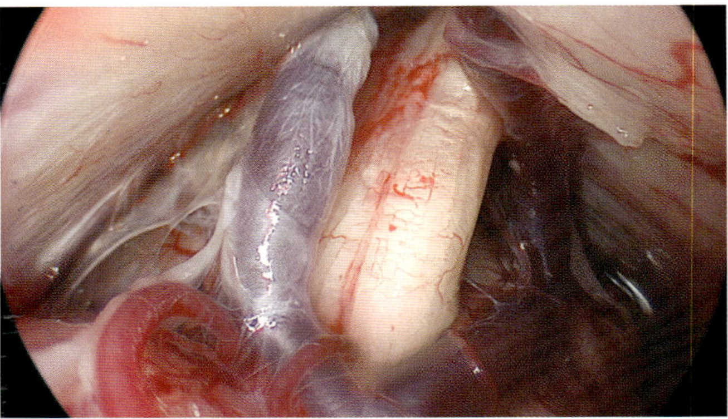

Fig. 6.67: Endoscopic view of Meckel's cave of V having close contact with another draining trigeminal vein

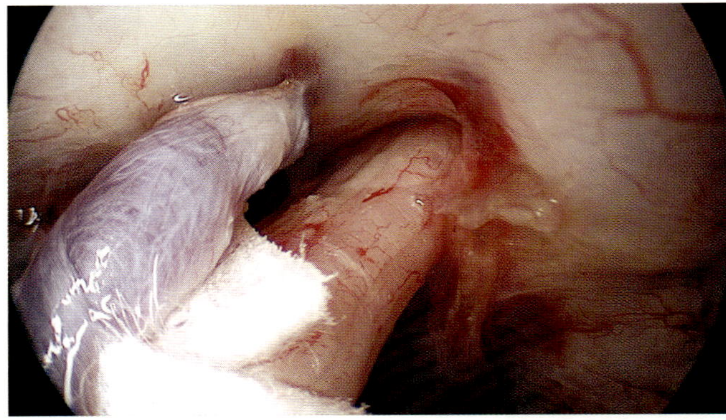

Fig. 6.68: Endoscopic view of Meckel's cave of V showing the cauterized vein. Cisternal part of V is isolated from large trigeminal vein by multiple pledgets of Teflon

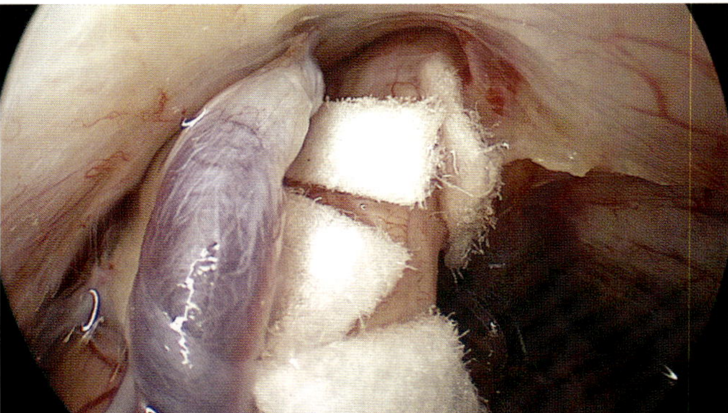

Fig. 6.69: Endoscopic view of cisternal part of V showing its isolation from large trigeminal vein by multiple pledgets of Teflon

Prevention of Recurrences

The most common cause of immediate failure is an incomplete dissection of the SCA with a persistent contact with the trigeminal nerve. It can be due to one of the two branches of the SCA hidden behind the medial side of the REZ between it and the pons or the trunk of the SCA still in contact with the anterior border of the trigeminal nerve close to the Meckel's cave. Occurrence of more than one vessel is high (25% in our experience), but to miss a vessel especially with the complementary help of endoscopy is exceptional. The surgeon should search carefully for an additional several conflicting vessels after successfully removing one conflicting artery. In some cases it is difficult to be certain of the involvement of a vein if it does not create groove in the root significantly and when the course of the vein goes inside the Meckel's cave. Even if it is rare, the surgeon has to be aware that the slipping of the insulating material in Meckel'cave is responsible for immediate failure with increase in pain in the immediate postoperative period, thus requiring immediate revision.

The most common reason for recurrence could be recompression of the affected nerve due to same vessel

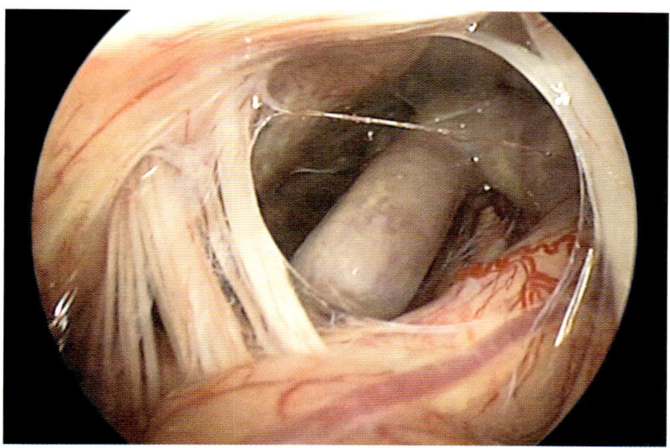

Fig. 6.70: Endoscopic picture in another case of left trigeminal neuralgia showing severely dolichovertebral artery

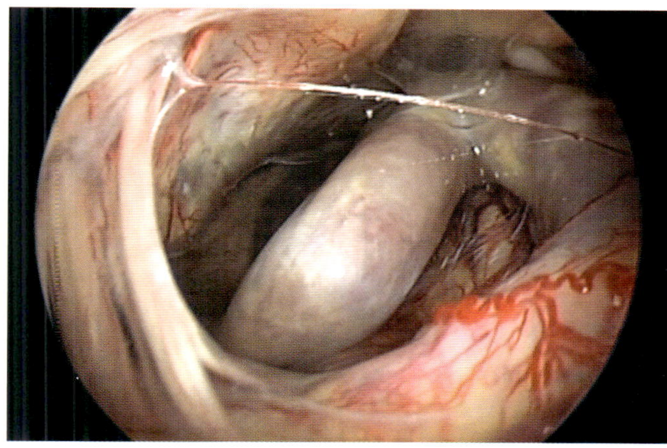

Fig. 6.71: Endoscopic picture showing dolichovertebral artery causing severe displacement of V

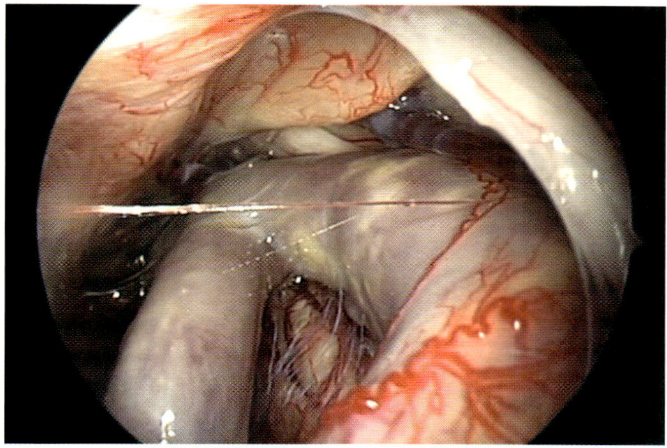

Fig. 6.72: Closer endoscopic picture showing dolichovertebral artery causing severe displacement of V

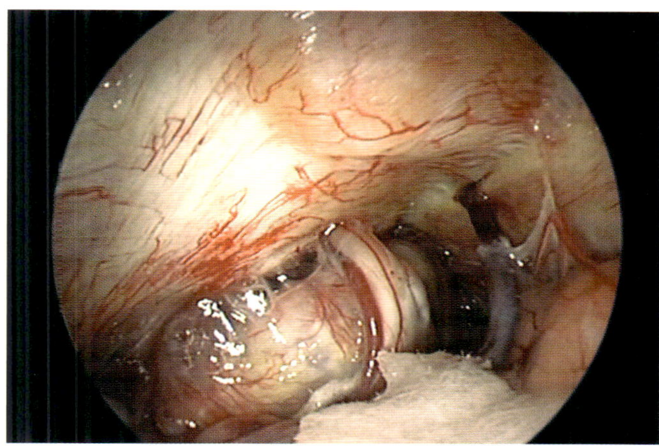

Fig. 6.73: Endoscopic picture showing dolichovertebral artery causing severe displacement of acoustico-facial bundle as well as V

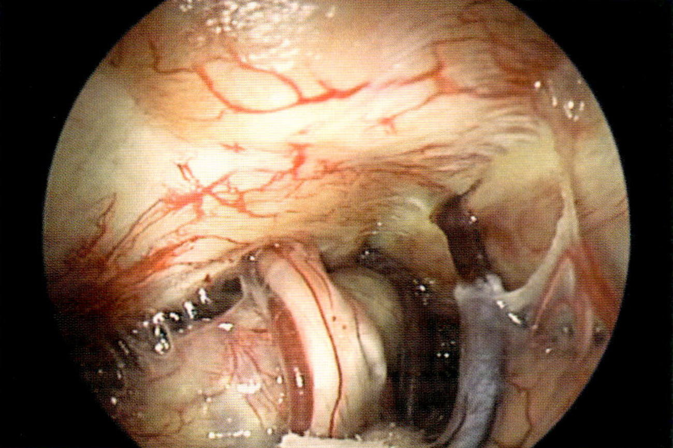

Fig. 6.74: Closer endoscopic showing dolichovertebral artery causing severe displacement of acoustico-facial bundle as well as V

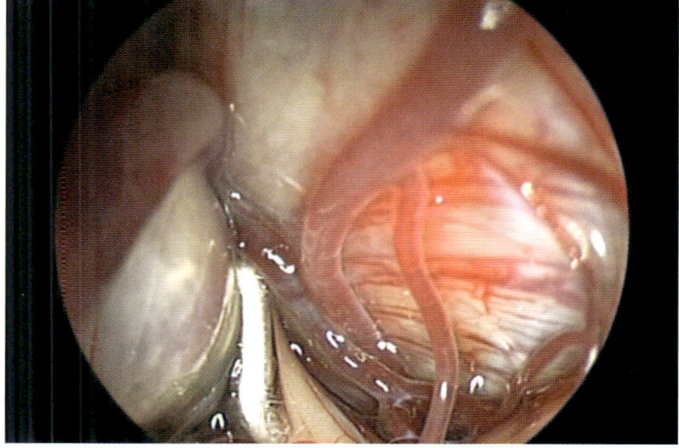

Fig. 6.75: Endoscopic picture showing placement of Teflon pledget between V and dolichovertebral artery. Also seen is SCA in contact with V superiorly

or due to a new conflict due to scar tissue and the timing is usually between 6 months and 1 year (67% of the recurrences). The use of absorbable material like Gelfoam to keep the offending artery apart gets resorbed and there is recompression. The spontaneous resorption of the fat or other soft tissue interposed between the nerve and the artery may lead to a new offending effect of the vessel. Possible materials are autologous muscle, fascia, subcutaneous fat tissue (all harvested from the operative wound) and fibrin glue. Occasionally the flattening and hardening of Teflon pledgets over the time itself transmit the pulsations of the adjacent artery due to loss of its insulating character or due to direct compression. Neocompression can be due to slipping or migration of the Teflon prosthesis, if insufficiently secured at the time of surgery. After several years, recurrence can occur due to subsequent fibrosis or Teflon granuloma leading to scarring around the nerve and causing irritation of the nerve.

The ideal method for achieving a real pure decompression when an elongated artery is the conflicting vessel would be to transpose the vessel away from the root and to maintain it apart without implantation of material of any kind. If implants are inserted between the root and artery, this might lead to neocompression. However, in most cases, implantation is necessary to secure transposition and in certain situations it is impossible to immobilize the conflict artery due to anatomical constraints. In such cases, it is better to avoid interposition of Teflon pledget at the REZ such that it itself causes the compression of the root (to achieve real decompression) and perform atraumatic dissection of the artery and the root by minimal manipulation in this area. Secure transposition of the artery to the tentorium with fibrin glue or a small piece of fibrofatty tissue around the artery (provided the artery is mobilized away from the nerve). Preserve the veins because, in addition to the fact that this would prevent venous congestion and hemorrhagic infarction, the veins are sometimes useful for holding the Teflon pledgets, so that they do not touch the root or migrate.

MICROVASCULAR DECOMPRESSION OF HEMIFACIAL SPASM

We follow the same approach and incisions in all types of vascular compression syndromes (Figs 6.76 to 6.81 right side) as well as other retrosigmoid surgeries like vestibular neurotomy and acoustic neuroma surgery. The patient position and the sites for craniotomy do not differ in trigeminal neuralgia, hemifacial spasm or glossopharyngeal neuralgia. In hemifacial spasm surgery, before evaluating the REZ of facial nerve for neurovascular conflict, it is necessary to dissect the arachnoid covering the lower cranial nerves, facial and vestibulocochlear nerves and the flocculus (Figs 6.81 and 6.82). Deep and anterior (anteromedially) to the flocculus, the choroid plexus of the foramen of Luschka is seen (Fig. 6.82). Approximately 5 mm rostral to the origin of glossopharyngeal nerve, the origin of vestibulocochlear nerve can be identified and anteromedial to it, the REZ of facial nerve can be delineated (Fig. 6.83). Microvascular decompression is carried out in the operating field between the vestibulocochlear nerve superiorly and the dissected glossopharyngeal nerve inferiorly (Figs 6.84 and 6.85). It starts with gentle elevation of the compressing vascular loop from the root exit zone of the facial nerve (Figs 6.86 and 6.87). This maneuver can launch hyperexcitability in the facial monitoring that comes back to normal in a few minutes. The site of the conflict is at the REZ of facial nerve at its emergence at pontomedullary sulcus and is located at the deep inferior part of the CPA (Figs 6.84 to 6.86). Contact by the loop of the AICA at the cisternal course or at internal auditory canal is therefore only anatomical arrangement, which should not mislead the operator. The severe to profound hearing loss risk in facial nerve vascular decompression surgery is in practice reduced to zero in our last 200 cases. Vascular dissection conservatively, without pulling or deformation of the acoustic-facial pedicle is the rule. However, monitoring of the facial and cochlear nerve is used in real time to detect at the earliest any risk to their function. In typical cases, the origin of facial nerve and its subpial course is hidden by the offending artery. Using a microdissector or the bipolar forceps, the offending artery is lifted carefully away from the brainstem (Figs 6.86 and 6.87). The subpial course of facial nerve can now be seen.

Once the site for the conflict and the offending vessel/s is/are delineated, the conflict area is now insulated with pledgets of Teflon felt (Figs 6.88 to 6.90). Offending smaller vessels can be kept away by using fibrin glue apart from protecting it with Teflon pledget. Care must be taken to push the Teflon felt against the artery and not the nerve. In a compression caused by a large artery such as the vertebral artery, it is helpful to use multiple pledgets to insulate from the transmitting pulsations. There must be no compression of the nerve by the pledget. During this delicate part of the procedure, one should avoid tearing small vessels that vascularize the pons or the nerves and also avoid stretching injury to the internal auditory artery. Bipolar coagulation should not be used near the cranial

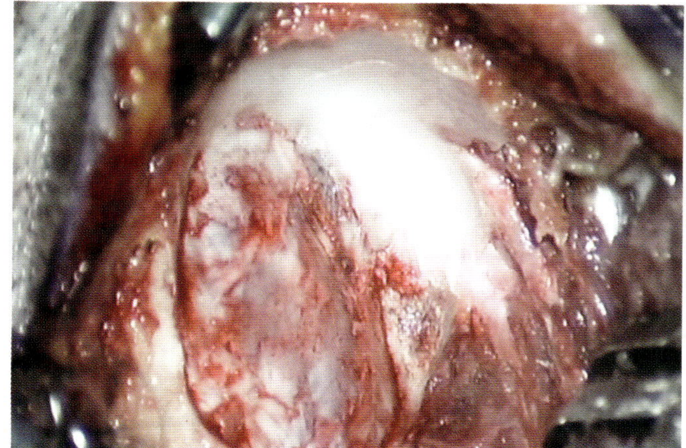

Fig. 6.76: Minimally invasive retrosigmoid approach with small craniotomy of 2 cm diameter is performed for all cases of microvascular decompression

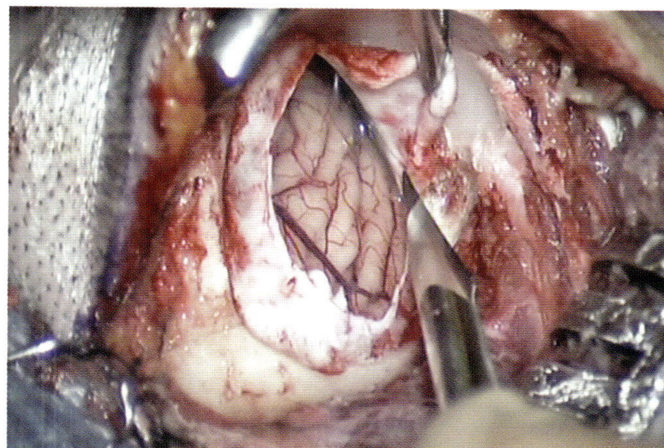

Fig. 6.77: Anteriorly based dural incision is placed to expose CPA

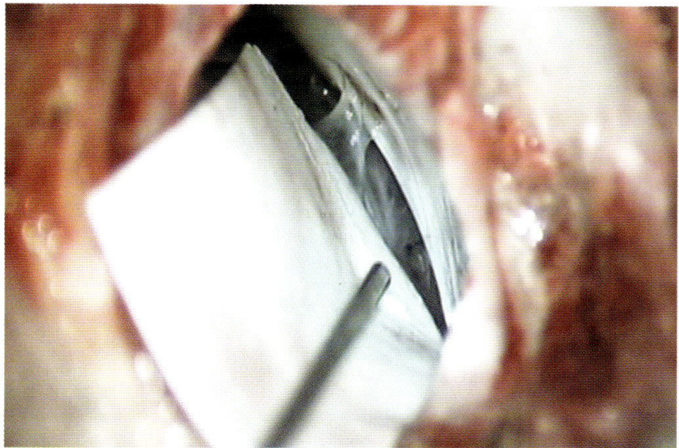

Fig. 6.78: After hyperventilation, dissection is carried out without the need for retractor

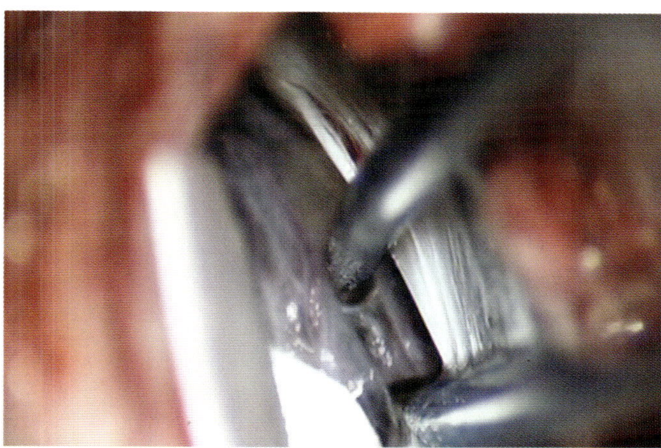

Fig. 6.79: Cisterna magna is opened to allow egress of CSF

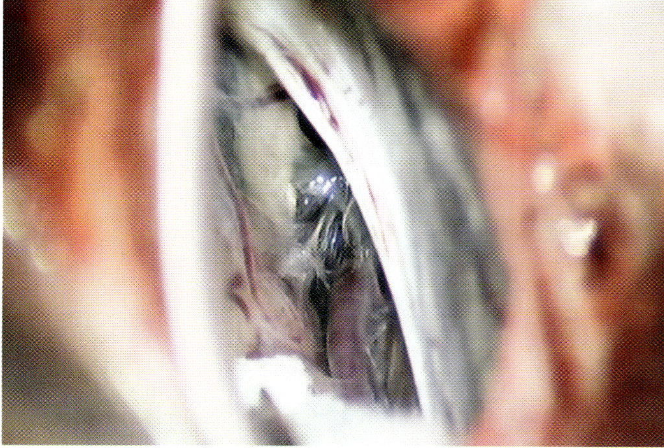

Fig. 6.80: Arachnoid draping the contents of CPA is dissected completely to provide good exposure

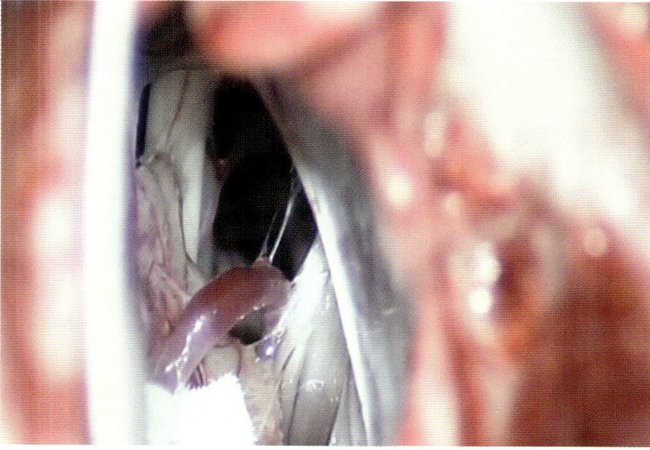

Fig. 6.81: Microscopic view of the CPA after draining of CSF and spontaneous retraction of cerebellum due to hyperventilation

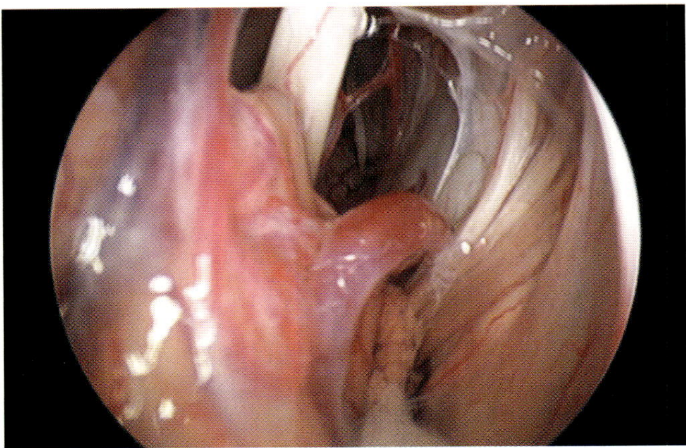

Fig. 6.82: Endoscopic view of inferior part of CPA showing acoustico-facial bundle covered medially by flocculus, lower cranial nerves closely related to PICA and choroid plexus

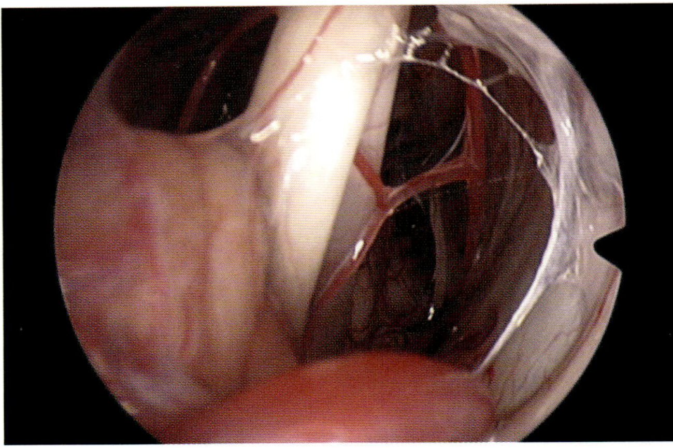

Fig. 6.83: Endoscopic view showing facial nerve in antero-inferior relation to the vestibulocochlear nerve at REZ of facial nerve

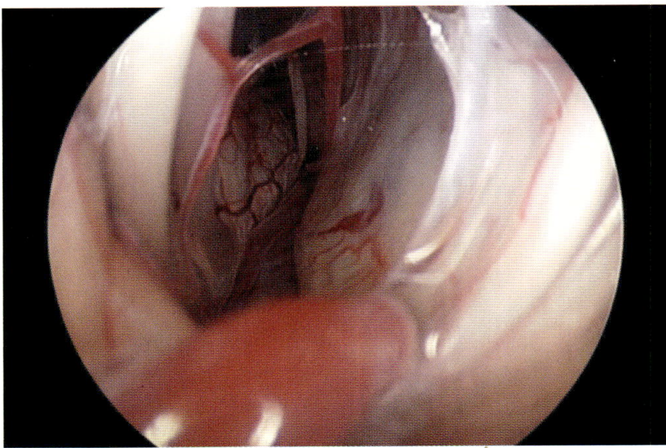

Fig. 6.84: Endoscopic view showing origin of facial nerve anteroinferior to the origin of vestibulocochlear nerve. PICA can be seen arising from vertebral artery and running perpendicular to the REZ of facial nerve

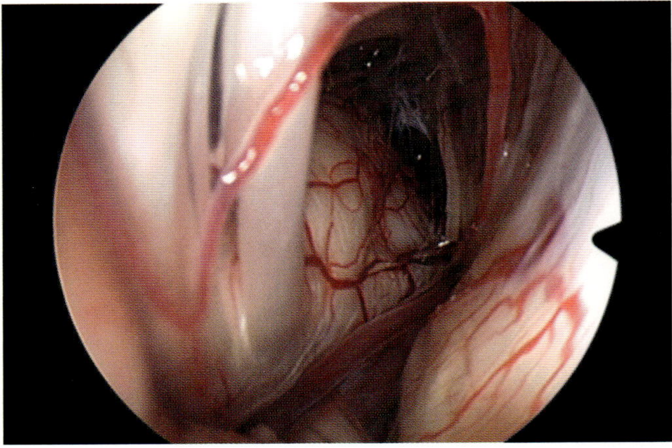

Fig. 6.85: Closer endoscopic view showing origin of facial nerve anteroinferior to the origin of vestibulocochlear nerve and PICA arising from vertebral artery and running perpendicular to the REZ of facial nerve

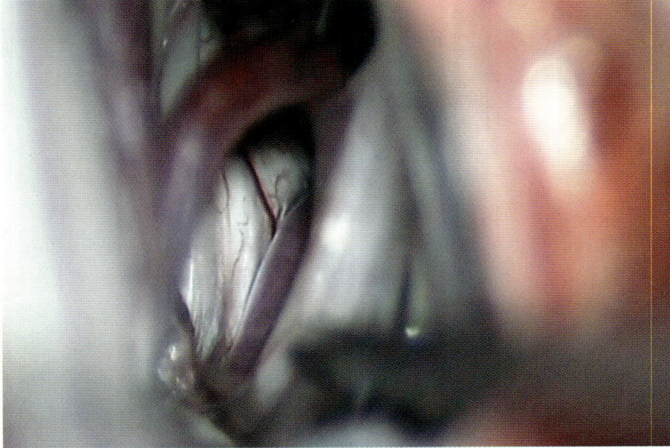

Fig. 6.86: Microscopic view showing PICA running perpendicular to the REZ of facial nerve

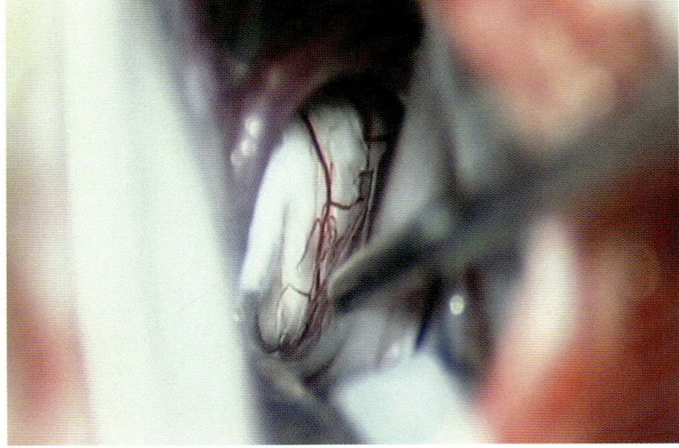

Fig. 6.87: Microscopic view showing dissection of PICA from REZ of facial nerve by bayonet shaped elevators

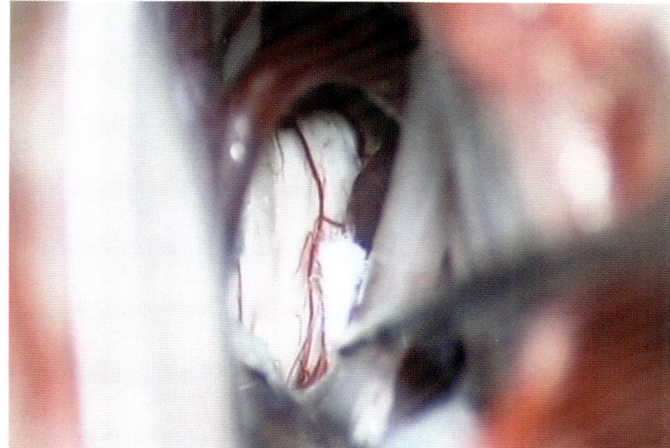

Fig. 6.88: Teflon pledget is placed separating the PICA from REZ of facial nerve

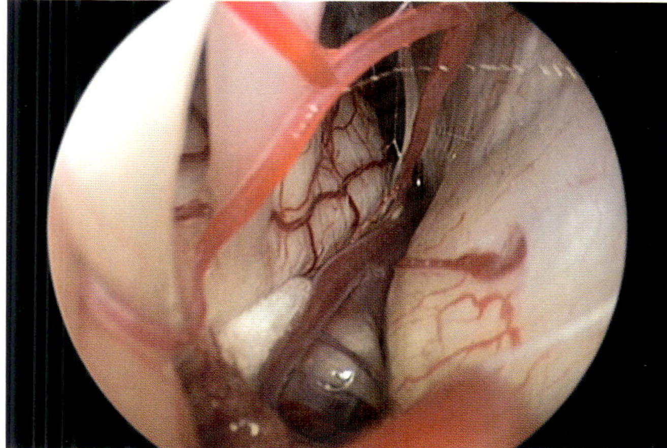

Fig. 6.89: Final endoscopic check confirming the position of Teflon insulation

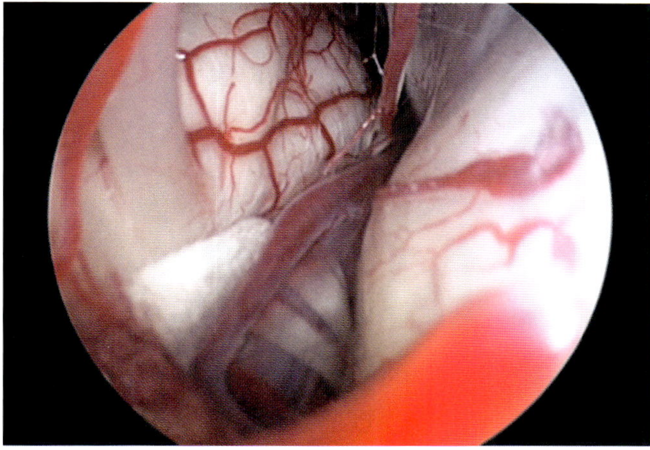

Fig. 6.90: Closure endoscopic view confirming efficacy of microvascular decompression for hemifacial spasm

nerves or over the pons and any bleeding, if it occurs has to be controlled by Surgicel and pressure over it with cottonoid. Suction cannula is the most common cause for injury to the cranial nerves and it is absolutely necessary to control the pressure in the suction with foot control and keeping the suction pressure off or at the minimum possible during the CPA procedure, especially while doing MVD. Facial nerve monitoring intraoperatively records the spontaneous ipsilateral muscle contractions. Spastic phenomena increase during handling of the facial nerve at the site of conflict and disappear gradually. Electrophysiological tests are used to ascertain the effectiveness of vascular decompression (Figs 6.1 to 6.3). The methodology is based on presence or absence of the AMR or "lateral spread" which is a hallmark of hemifacial spasm. The stimulating electrode is placed at the chin to stimulate mentalis/marginal mandibular branch of facial nerve and the recording electrodes are placed at the orbicularis oculi/oris. Before vascular decompression, a very small antidromic stimulation of the lower branch of facial nerve induces an abnormal response of the upper face and vice versa. Decompression surgery removes this AMR instantaneously in most of the cases. Finally, the endoscope is again used at the end of decompression procedure by microscope to assess and ascertain the proper positioning of the Teflon once it has been placed at the target site (Figs 6.89 and 6.90).

DIFFERENT TYPES OF CONFLICTS OBSERVED IN MVD FOR HEMIFACIAL SPASM (Fig. 6.91)

Most common site of conflict is the REZ (includes the subpial course and the initial 2 mm of its course in CPA after its origin), and most often is due to the posterior inferior cerebellar artery (PICA) alone (Figs 6.92 to 6.108) in 28% cases or along with vertebral artery (VA) (Figs 6.109 to 6.113) in 25% of patients with hemifacial spasm, because of their anatomical proximity to the REZ of facial nerve. Conflict from PICA is situated at the REZ of facial nerve at its emergence at pontomedullary sulcus and is located at the deep inferior part of the CPA (Figs 6.92 to 6.99). It can be missed by microscopic examination alone and it is advisable to always confirm with endoscope (Figs 6.100 to 6.102). Using a microdissector or the bipolar forceps, the PICA loop is dissected and lifted carefully away from the brainstem (Figs 6.103 to 6.105). The REZ of facial nerve is insulated with pledgets of Teflon (Figs 6.106 to 6.108).

If a large loop of the vertebral artery seemingly is compressing the origin of the nerve, it is important to confirm that even the PICA arising from undersurface of

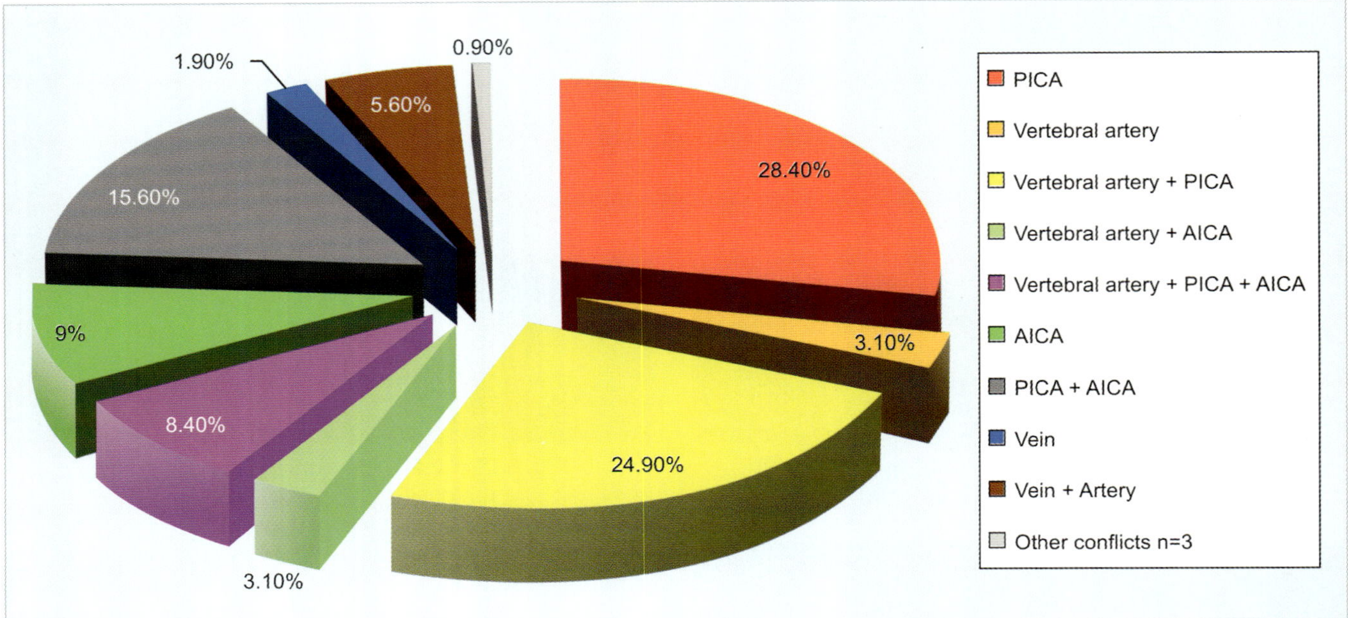

Fig. 6.91: Distribution of offending vessels in hemifacial spasm

Sources: Thesis Claire Curto.[83]

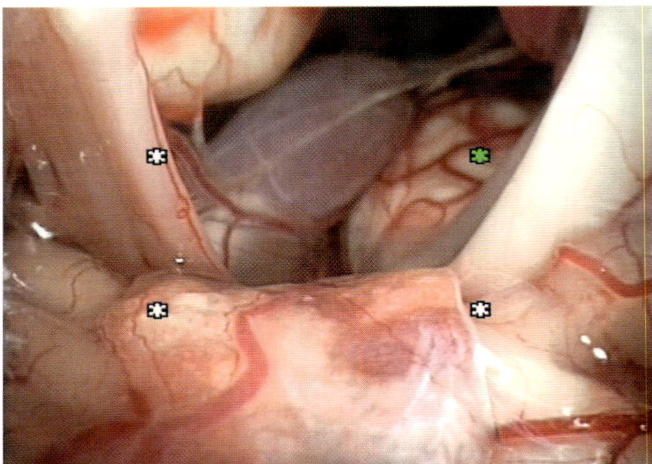

Fig. 6.92: Case 2 of left hemifacial spasm: Endoscopic view to look for the cause of vascular conflict at REZ of facial nerve

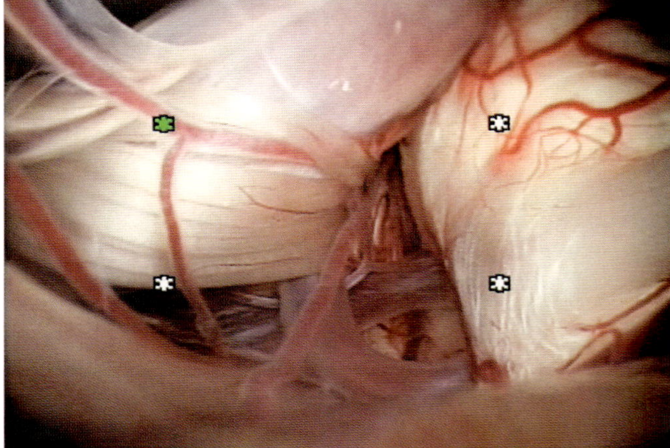

Fig. 6.93: Endoscopic view showing PICA arising from vertebral artery and forms a loop that impinges perpendicularly into the REZ of facial nerve

the vertebral artery may be causing additional compression (Figs 6.109 to 6.113).

When the two arteries, AICA and PICA, arise from a common AICA trunk (dominant AICA) from basilar artery, the division occurs at the anterior border of the facial nerve. The AICA and PICA may then form an acute angle at the anterior border of facial nerve, thereby making medial end of facial nerve highly susceptible to being entangled between the two arteries in a clamp like pressure (Figs 6.114 to 6.136 left side) or the REZ of facial nerve being compressed by acute turn of one of the arteries (Figs 6.137 to 6.141).

In case of dominant form of PICA, the AICA arises from the PICA at the root exit zone of the facial nerve and become the major offending vessel (Figs 6.142 to 6.145).

The frequency of multiple arteries causing vascular conflict is more than 50% in our series,[83] (Fig. 6.91), with following order of frequency.

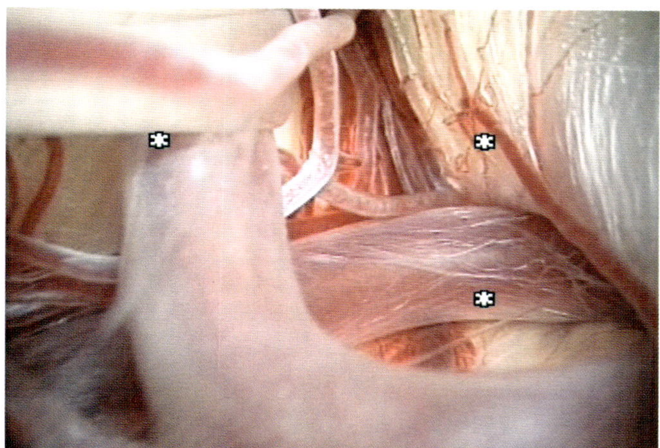

Fig. 6.94: Closer endoscopic view showing PICA loop impinging into the REZ of facial nerve causing distortion of brainstem

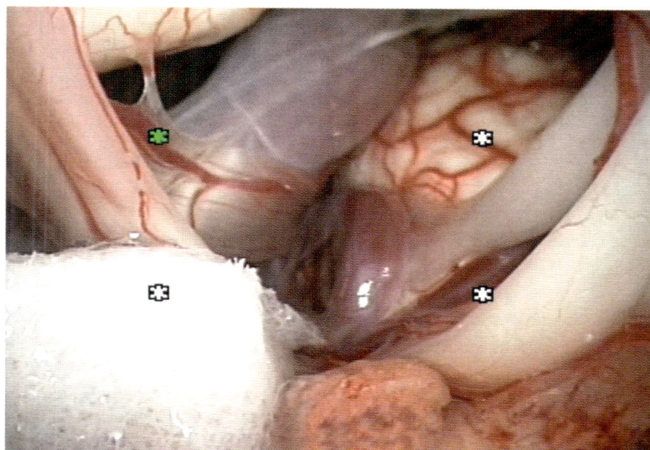

Fig. 6.95: Endoscopic view showing PICA loop dissected out of the conflicting site with REZ of facial nerve

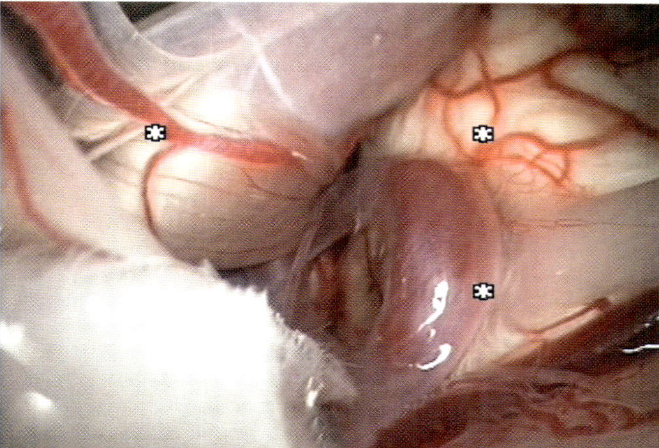

Fig. 6.96: Closer endoscopic view showing PICA loop dissected out of the conflicting site with REZ of facial nerve

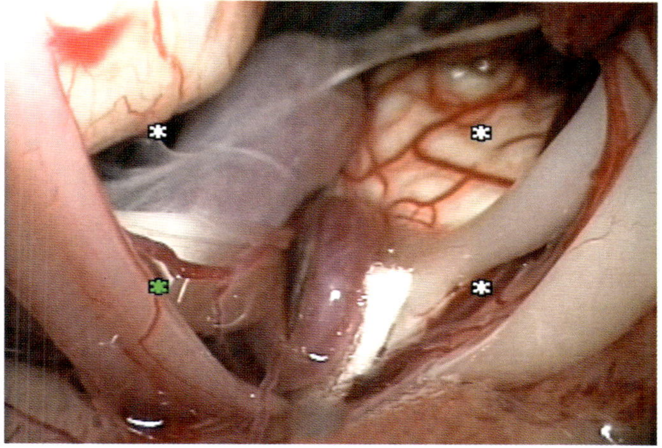

Fig. 6.97: Endoscopic view showing insulation with Teflon pledget between loop of PICA and REZ of facial nerve

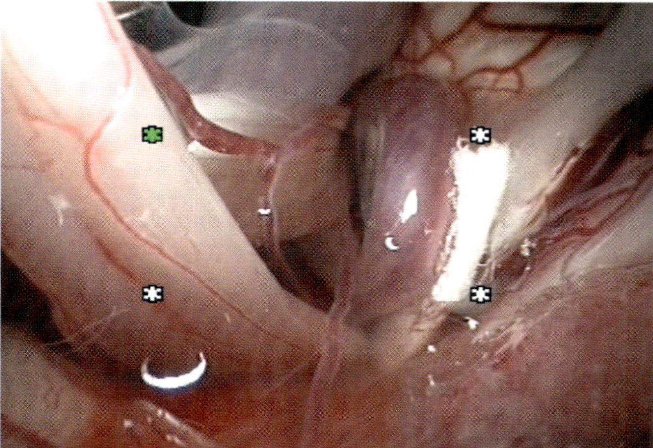

Fig. 6.98: Endoscopic view showing insulation with Teflon pledget between loop of PICA and REZ of facial nerve

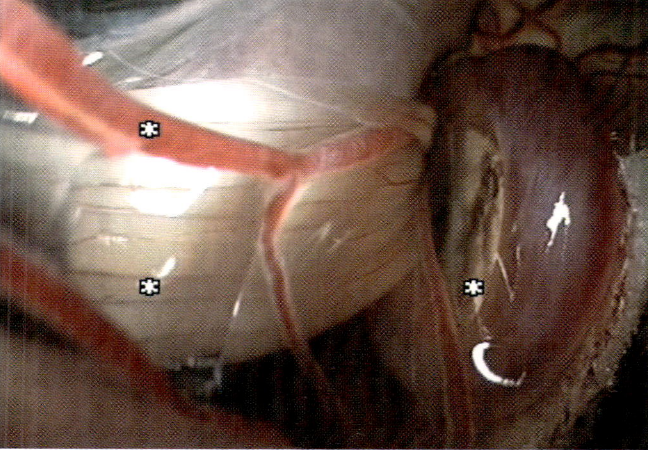

Fig. 6.99: Closer endoscopic view showing insulation with Teflon pledget between loop of PICA and REZ of facial nerve

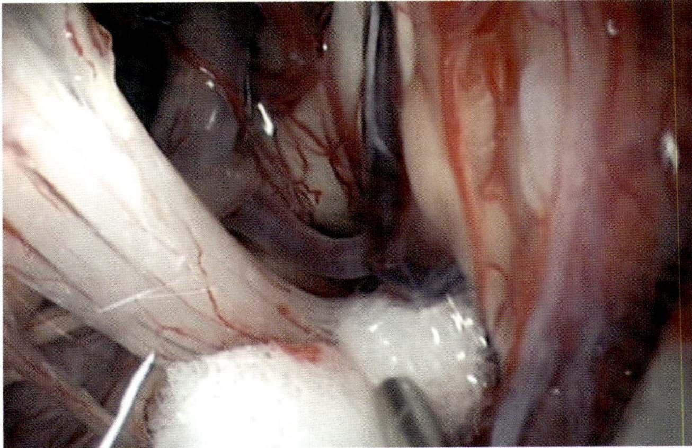

Fig. 6.100: Case 3 of left hemifacial spasm: Endoscopy to look for the cause of vascular conflict at REZ of facial nerve. Endoscopic view showing PICA arising from vertebral artery and traversing toward REZ of facial nerve. Also seen is AICA close to facial nerve but not in contact with facial nerve

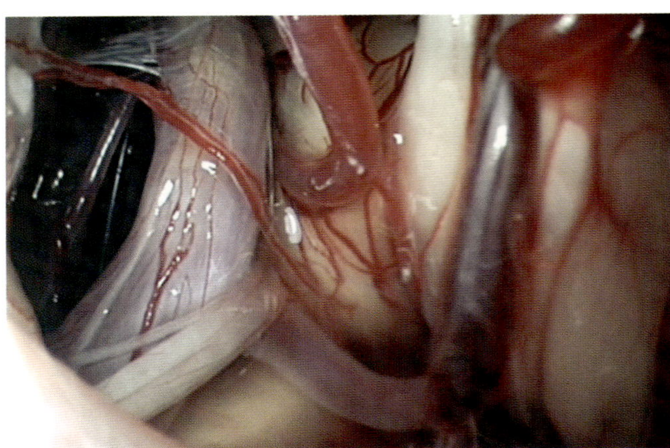

Fig. 6.101: Closer endoscopic view showing PICA arising from vertebral artery and traversing toward REZ of facial nerve which is hidden by the CSF from the foramen of Luschka. Also seen is AICA close to facial nerve but not in contact with facial nerve

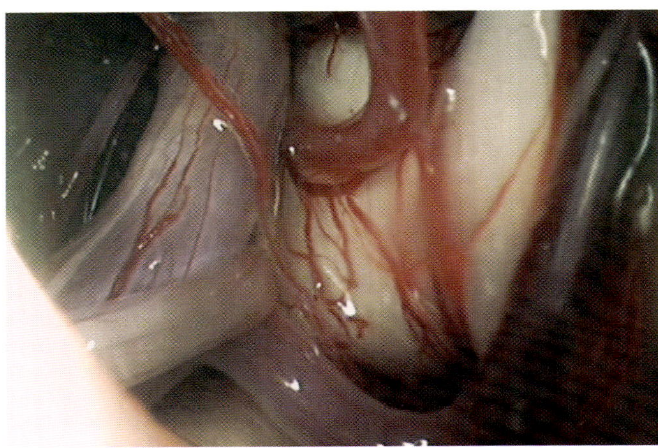

Fig. 6.102: Further closer view after suction of CSF showing PICA forming superior loop impinging into the REZ of facial nerve

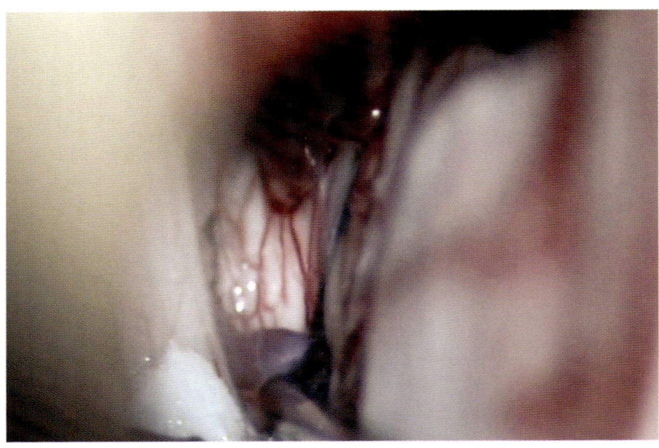

Fig. 6.103: Microscopic view showing dissection of PICA from REZ of facial nerve by bayonet shaped elevators

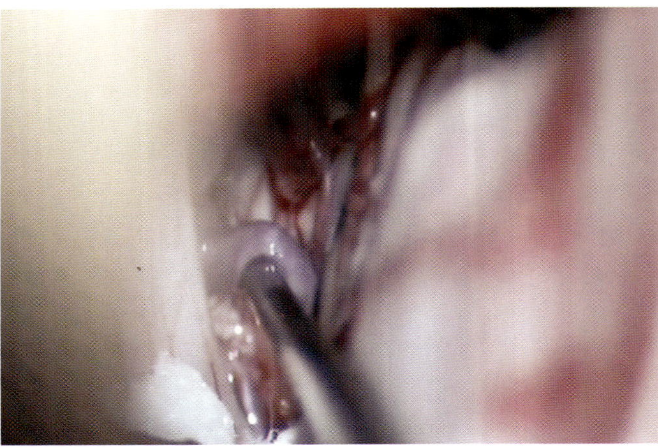

Fig. 6.104: Microscopic view showing elevation of PICA loop from REZ of facial nerve by bayonet shaped elevators

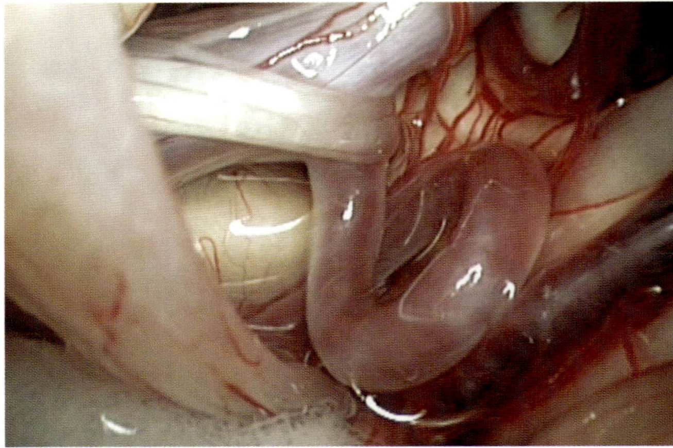

Fig. 6.105: Endoscopic view showing complete mobilization of impinging PICA loop from REZ of facial nerve

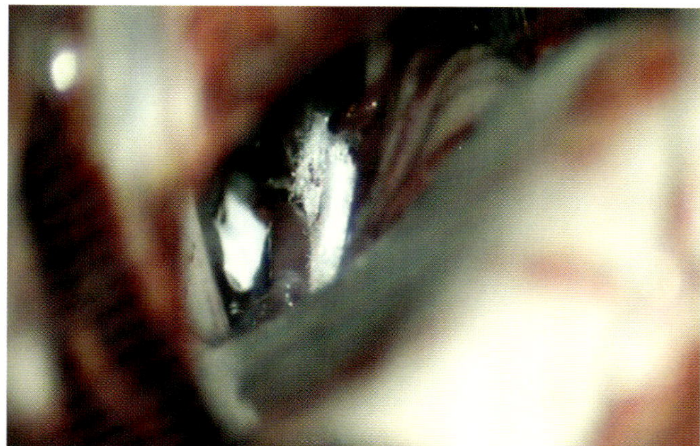

Fig. 6.106: Microscopic view showing insulation with multiple Teflon pledgets between loop of PICA, AICA and REZ of facial nerve

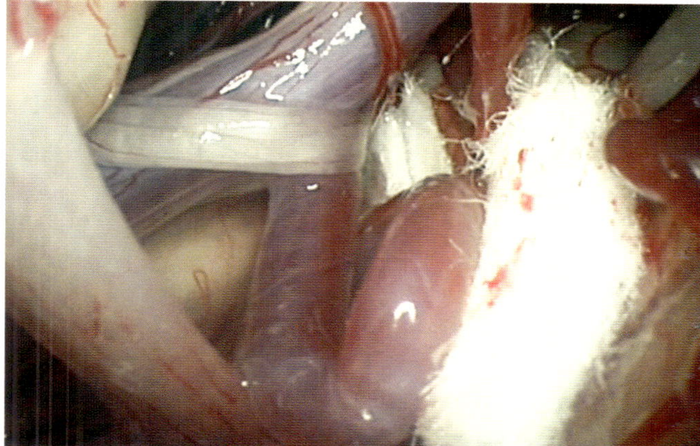

Fig. 6.107: Endoscopic view showing insulation with multiple Teflon pledgets between loop of PICA, AICA and REZ of facial nerve

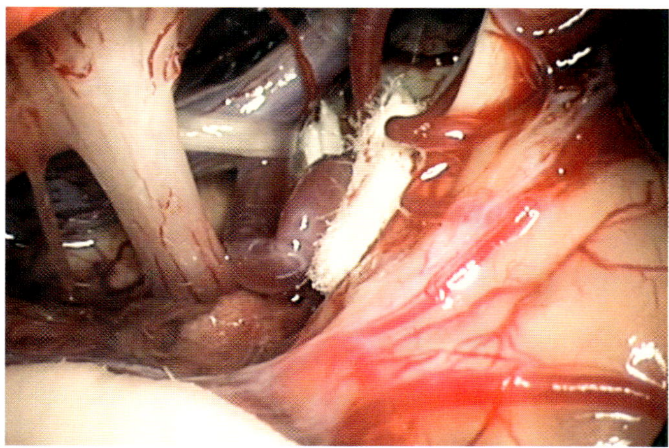

Fig. 6.108: Endoscopic view showing insulation with multiple Teflon pledgets between loop of PICA, AICA and REZ of facial nerve

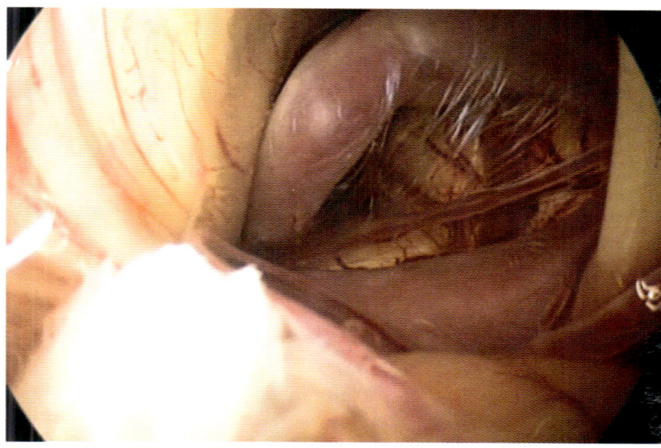

Fig. 6.109: Case 4 of left hemifacial spasm: Endoscopy to look for the cause of vascular conflict at REZ of facial nerve. Endoscopic view showing vertebral artery traversing toward and completely covering REZ of facial nerve

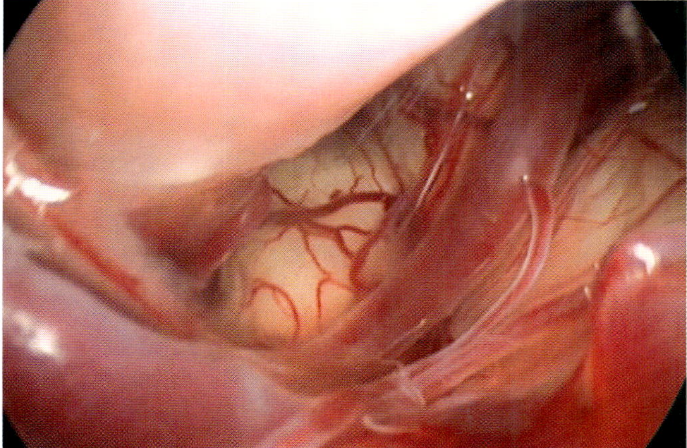

Fig. 6.110: Endoscopic view under the vertebral artery showing PICA arising from its undersurface and crossing the REZ of facial nerve. It could be easily missed, if not looked for purposefully

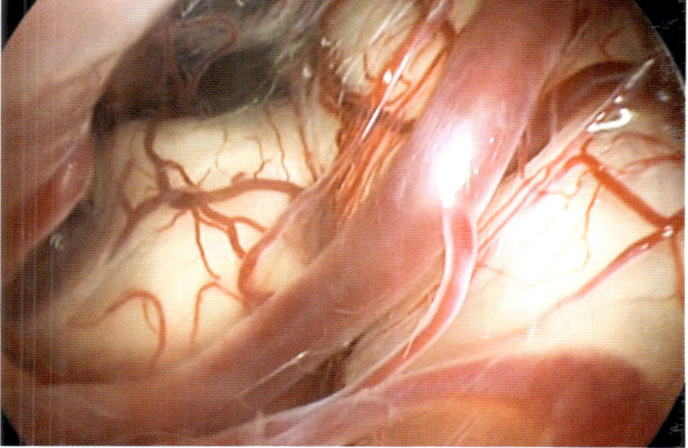

Fig. 6.111: Further closer view in REZ of facial nerve showing its relation with PICA

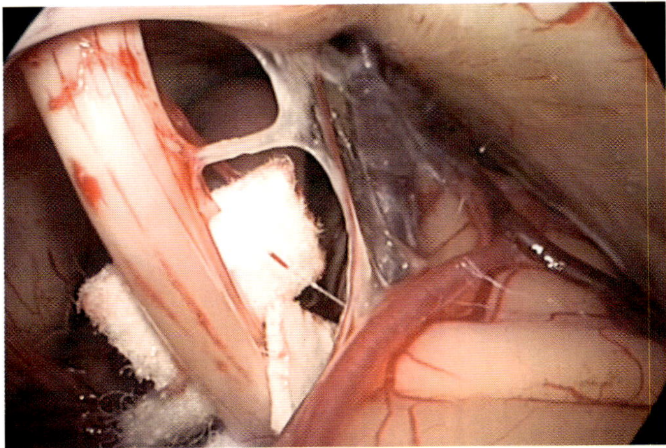

Fig. 6.112: Endoscopic view showing insulation with multiple Teflon pledgets between loop of PICA, VA and REZ of facial nerve

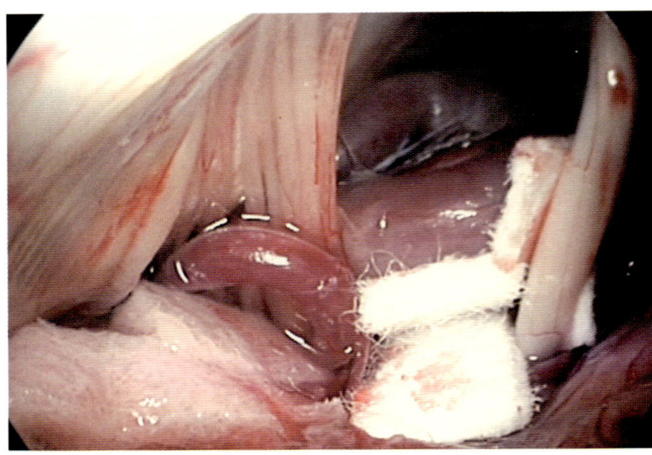

Fig. 6.113: Endoscopic view showing insulation with multiple Teflon pledgets between loop of PICA, VA and REZ of facial nerve

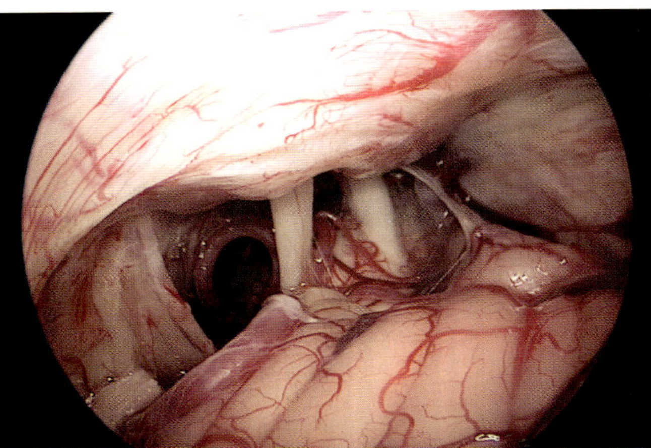

Fig. 6.114: Case 5 of left hemifacial spasm: Endoscopy to look for the cause of vascular conflict at REZ of facial nerve

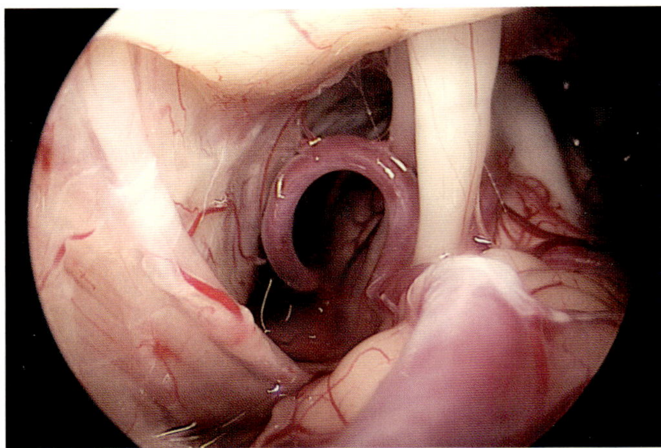

Fig. 6.115: Endoscopic view showing dominant AICA traversing toward REZ of facial nerve

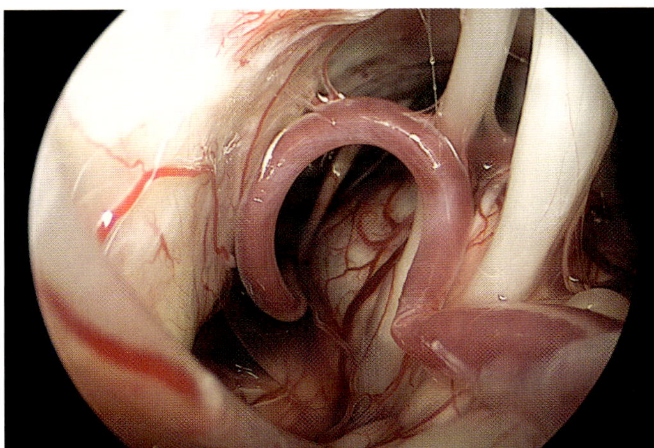

Fig. 6.116: Closer endoscopic view showing dominant AICA traversing toward facial nerve and giving rise to smaller AICA branch and continuing as PICA

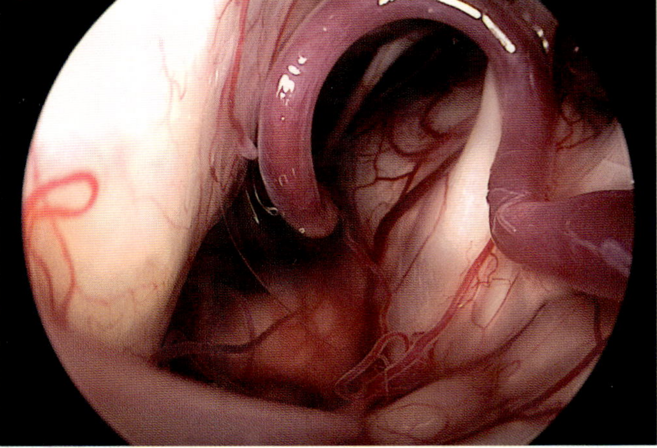

Fig. 6.117: Endoscopic view showing REZ of facial nerve free of any arterial loop around it

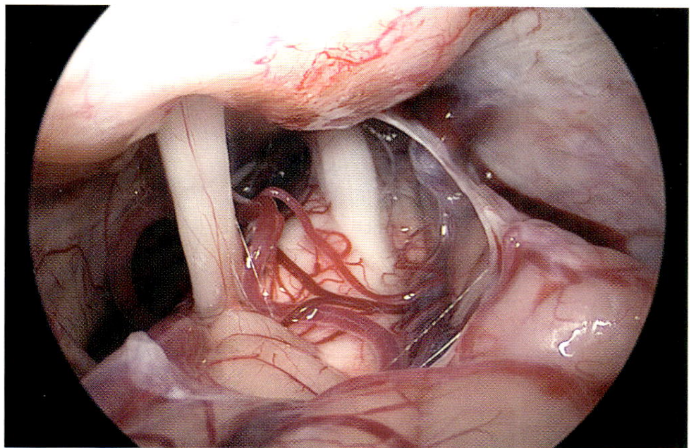

Fig. 6.118: Endoscopic view showing vestibulocochlear nerve bundle and trigeminal nerve

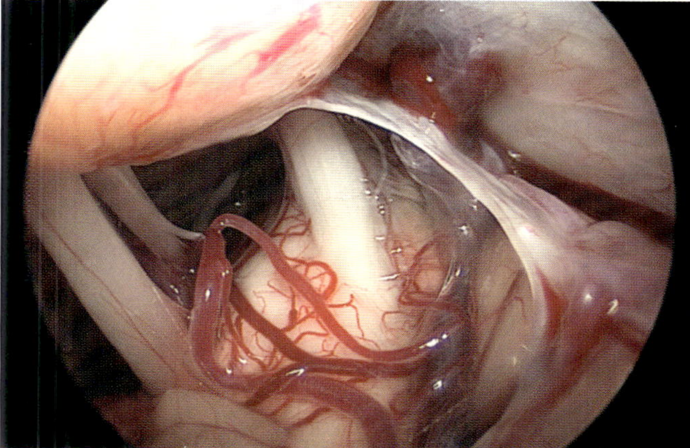

Fig. 6.119: Endoscopic view showing vestibulocochlear nerve and the facial nerve with arterial loop in between them

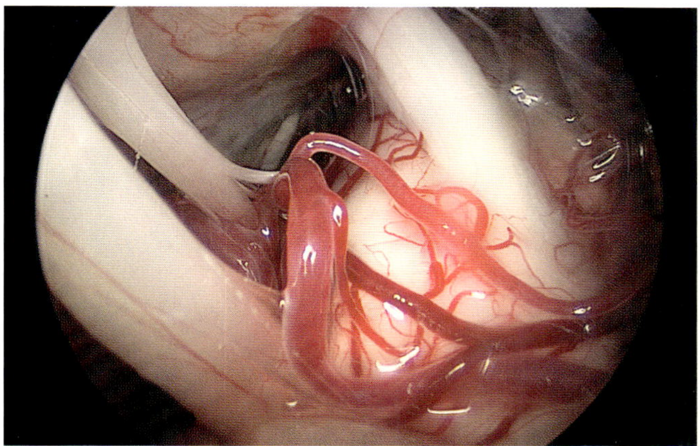

Fig. 6.120: Endoscopic view showing vestibulocochlear nerve and the facial nerve with arterial loop in between them

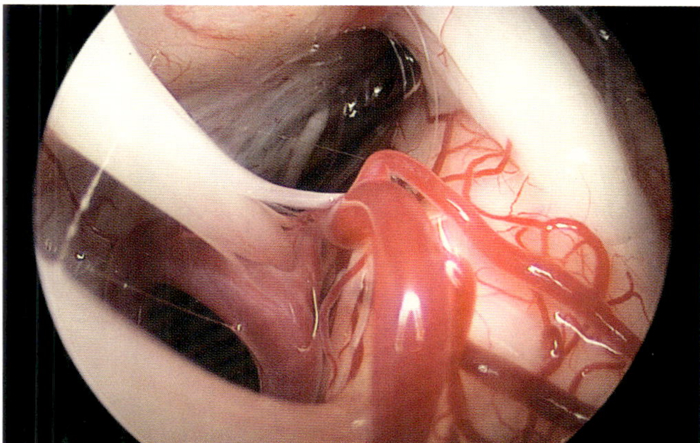

Fig. 6.121: Closer endoscopic view showing dominant AICA traversing between vestibulocochlear and facial nerve and giving rise to smaller AICA branch and continuing as PICA

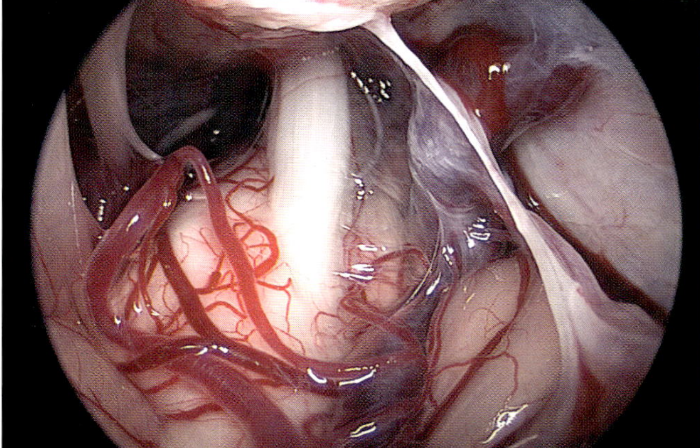

Fig. 6.122: Endoscopic view showing vestibulocochlear, facial and trigeminal nerve. We always rule out associated arterial loop compressing the trigeminal nerve in cases of hemifacial spasm and to decompress even the trigeminal nerve if vascular contact is present

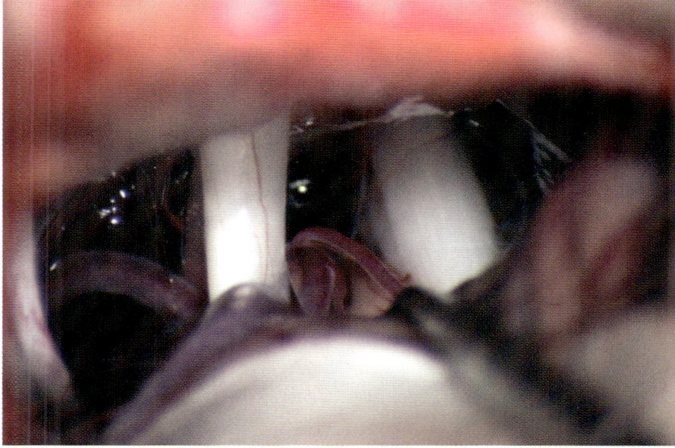

Fig. 6.123: Microscopic view showing exposure in the above mentioned case

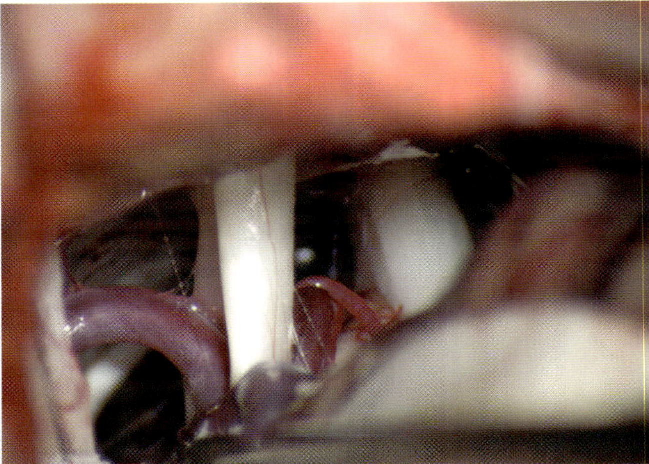

Fig. 6.124: Microscopic view showing delineation of dominant AICA near facial nerve

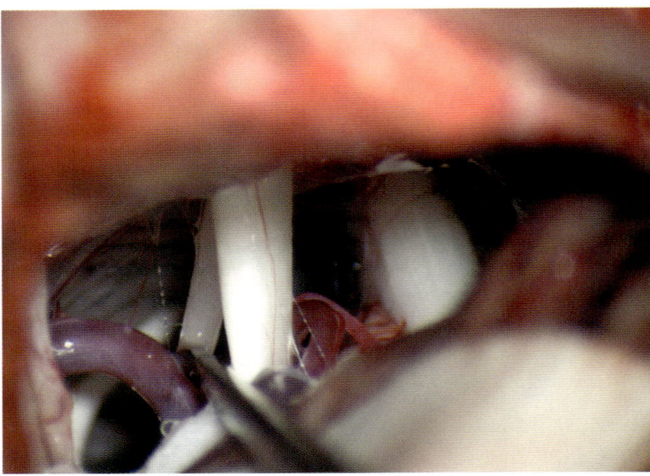

Fig. 6.125: Microscopic view showing elevation of AICA loop from facial nerve by bayonet shaped elevators

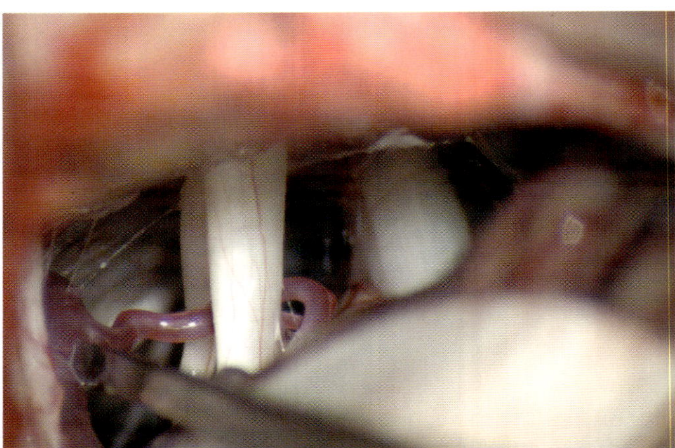

Fig. 6.126: Microscopic view showing elevation of AICA loop from facial nerve by bayonet shaped elevators

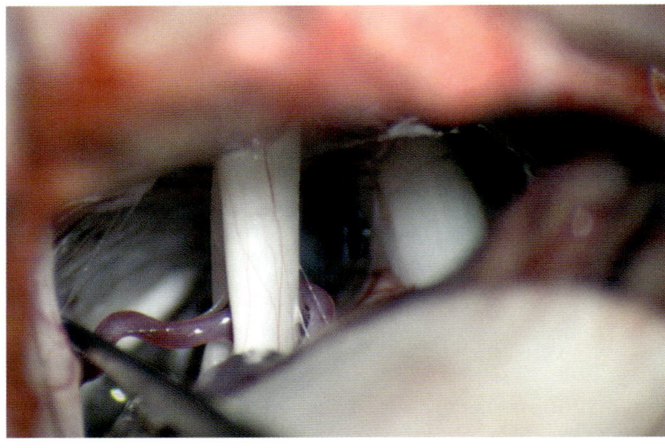

Fig. 6.127: Microscopic view showing elevation of AICA loop from facial nerve by bayonet shaped elevators

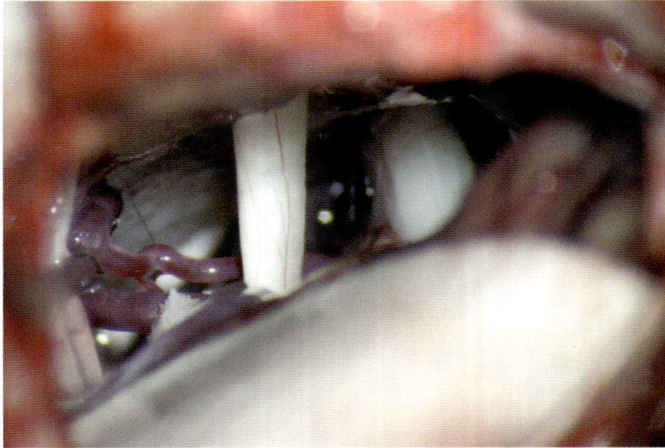

Fig. 6.128: Microscopic view showing elevated AICA loop being gently held by suction cannula while preparing to put Teflon pledget

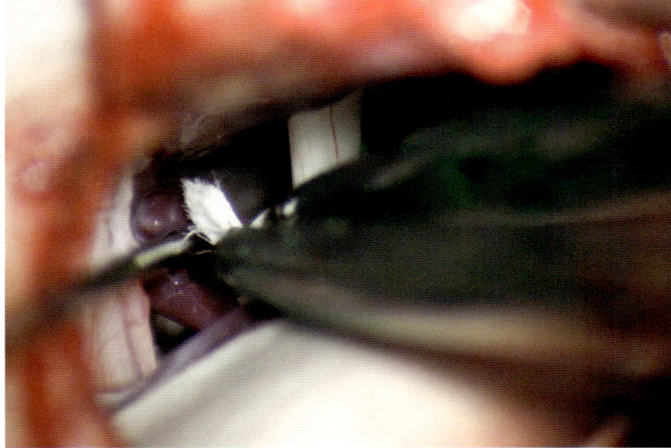

Fig. 6.129: Microscopic view showing elevated AICA loop being gently held by suction cannula while keeping Teflon pledget

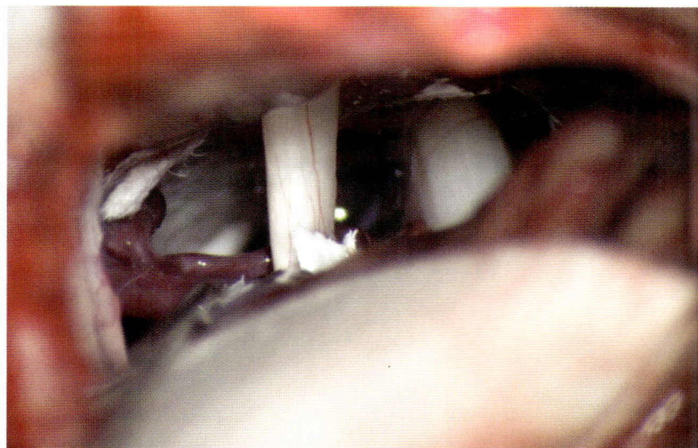

Fig. 6.130: Microscopic view showing elevated AICA loop being adhered to adjacent temporal bone with fibrin glue while reinforcing with Teflon pledget

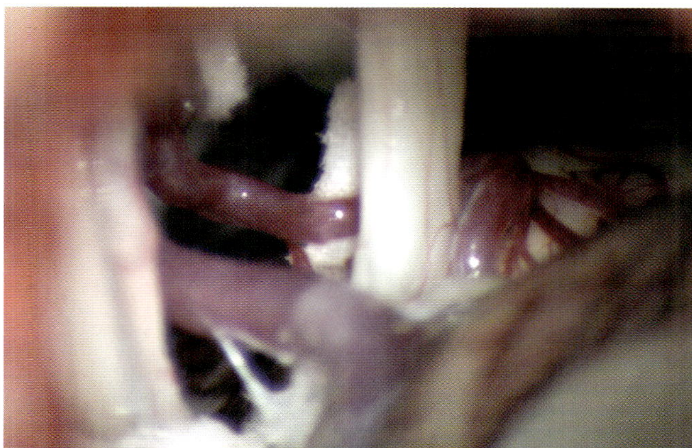

Fig. 6.131: Microscopic view showing separation of AICA loop from facial nerve by Teflon pledget

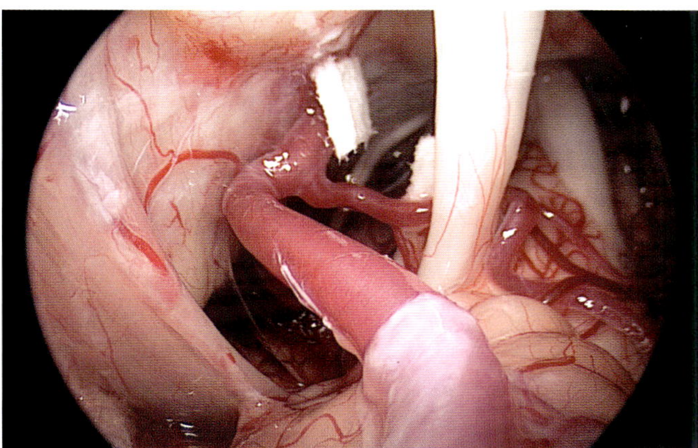

Fig. 6.132: Endoscopic view showing elevated AICA loop being adhered to adjacent temporal bone with fibrin glue while reinforcing with Teflon pledget and separation of AICA loop from facial nerve by Teflon pledget

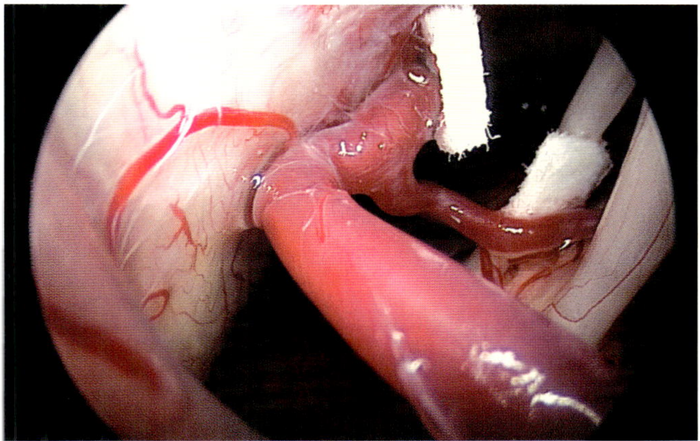

Fig. 6.133: Endoscopic view showing elevated AICA loop being adhered to adjacent temporal bone with fibrin glue while reinforcing with Teflon pledget and separation of AICA loop from facial nerve by Teflon pledget

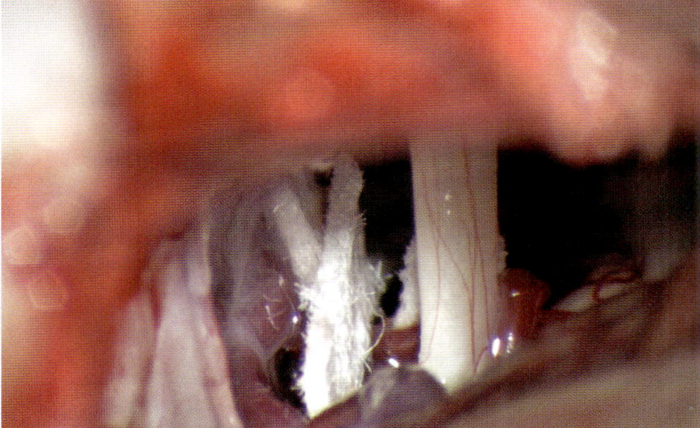

Fig. 6.134: Microscopic view showing elevated AICA loop being adhered to adjacent temporal bone with fibrin glue while reinforcing with multiple Teflon pledgets

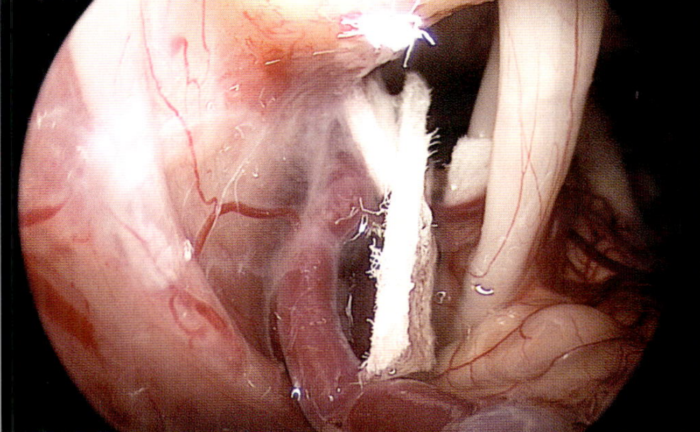

Fig. 6.135: Endoscopic view showing elevated AICA loop being adhered to adjacent temporal bone with fibrin glue while reinforcing with multiple Teflon pledgets and separation of AICA loop from facial nerve by Teflon pledget

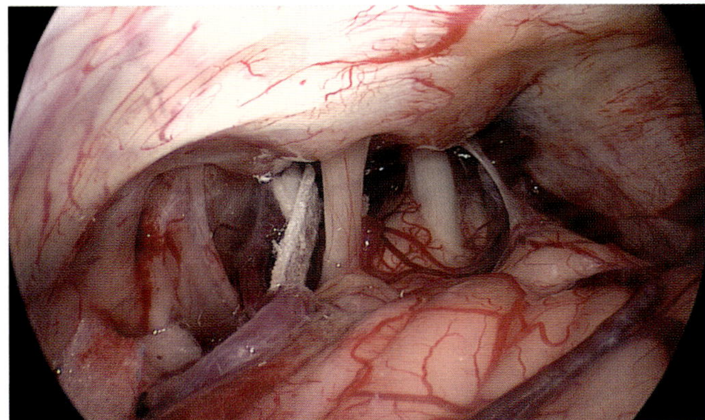

Fig. 6.136: Final endoscopic view showing microvascular decompression for left hemifacial spasm due to dominant AICA

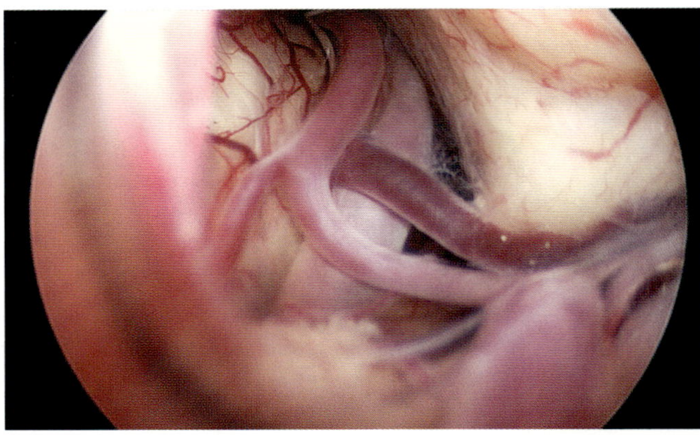

Fig. 6.137: Case 6 of right hemifacial spasm: Endoscopy to look for the cause of vascular conflict at REZ of facial nerve. Endoscopic view showing dominant AICA giving rise to AICA and PICA with former traversing toward REZ of facial nerve

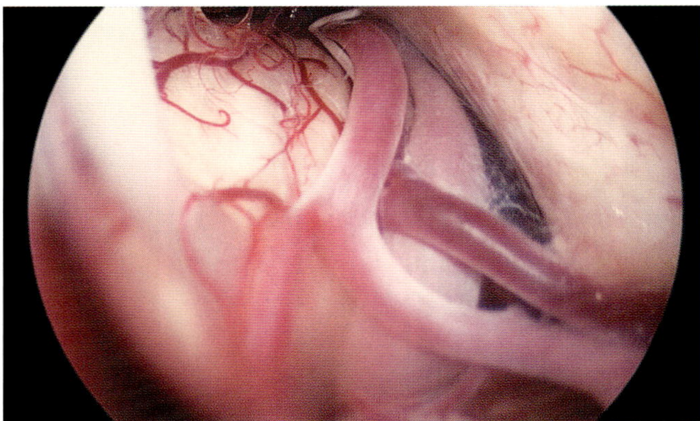

Fig. 6.138: Closer endoscopic view showing dominant AICA traversing with contact perpendicular to REZ of facial nerve

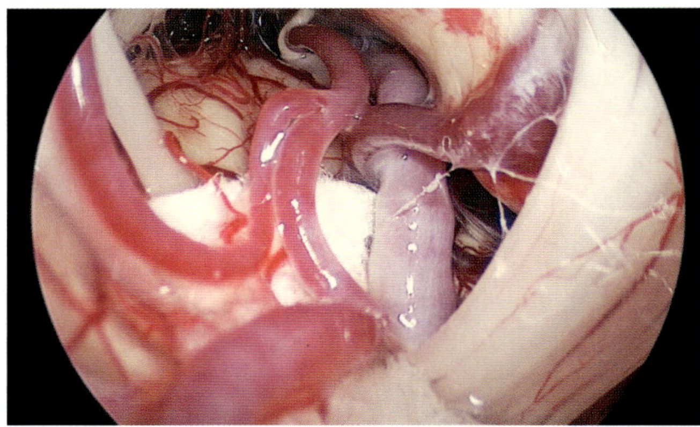

Fig. 6.139: Endoscopic view showing elevation of dominant AICA with its AICA and PICA branches and separation of AICA loop from facial nerve with multiple Teflon pledgets

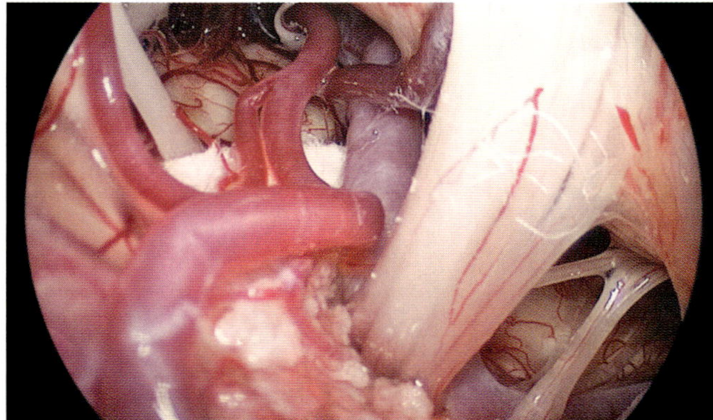

Fig. 6.140: Endoscopic view showing elevation of dominant AICA with its AICA and PICA branches and separation of AICA loop from facial nerve with multiple Teflon pledgets

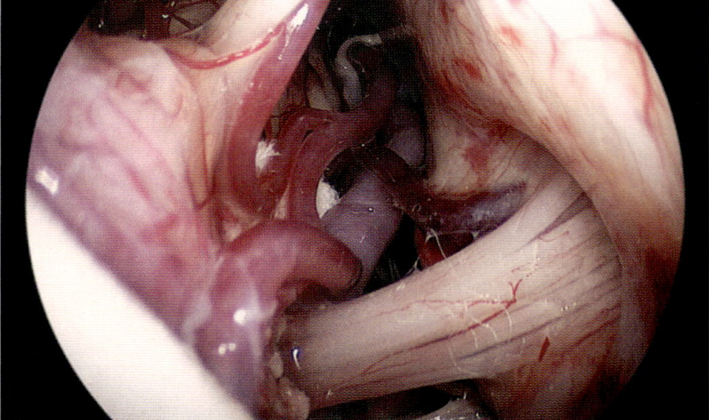

Fig. 6.141: Final endoscopic view showing elevation of dominant AICA with its AICA and PICA branches and separation of AICA loop from facial nerve with multiple Teflon pledgets

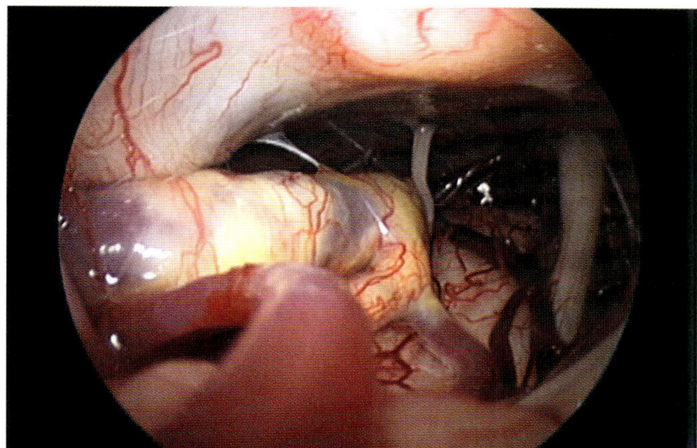

Fig. 6.142: Case 7 of left hemifacial spasm: Endoscopic view showing smaller atherosclerotic ipsilateral vertebral artery giving rise to dominant PICA

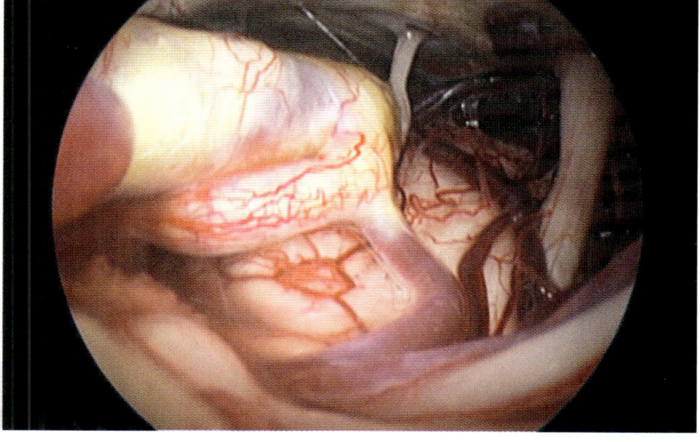

Fig. 6.143: Endoscopic view showing smaller atherosclerotic ipsilateral vertebral artery giving rise to dominant PICA which traverses toward REZ of facial nerve

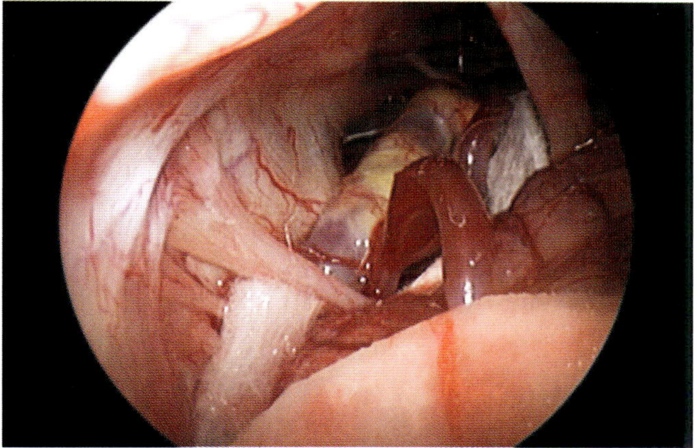

Fig. 6.144: Endoscopic view showing elevation of dominant PICA with its AICA and PICA branches and its separation from facial nerve with multiple Teflon pledgets

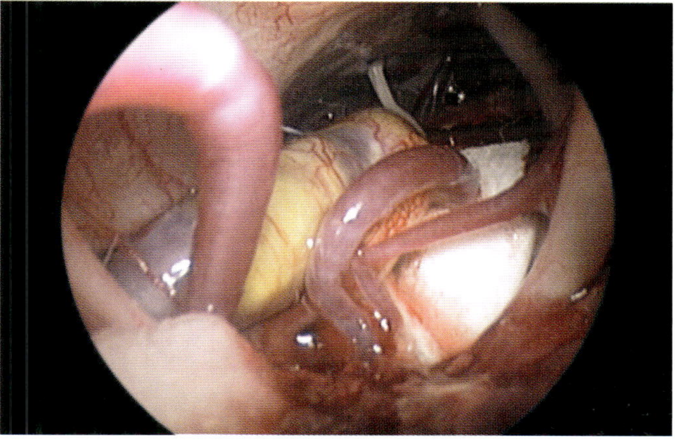

Fig. 6.145: Endoscopic view showing elevation of dominant PICA with its AICA and PICA branches and its separation from facial nerve with multiple Teflon pledgets

Vertebral artery and PICA (Figs 6.109 to 6.113): 24.9%

AICA and PICA (Figs 6.146 to 6.149): 15.6%

Vertebral artery, PICA and AICA (Figs 6.150 to 6.165): 8.4%

Anterior inferior cerebellar artery (AICA) (9%) can be responsible for conflicts on the cisternal portion of the nerve. This type of conflict is even more difficult to operate when the AICA goes in between the facial and vestibulocochlear nerves (Figs 6.166 to 6.170), because of the difficulty to mobilize the artery without risking any hearing impairment.

Some conflicts with AICA are located within the internal auditory canal (IAC), and it is then necessary to drill the IAC to have a good view of the facial nerve. Pieces of Teflon are most of the time too large to be interposed in such cases and Neuropatch (Braun®) can be used instead (Figs 6.171 to 6.177).

Rarely, the cause for hemifacial spasm is underlying space occupying lesion of CPA, which may secondarily cause pressure over the REZ of facial nerve directly or by displacement of the neighboring artery (Figs 6.178 to 6.182).

Conflicts of the Youth

Hemifacial spasm occurs more in middle aged and elderly people, in whom atherosclerosis and hypertension modify vascular walls and alter intravascular blood flow, thus contributing to abnormal nervous stimulation. Nevertheless hemifacial spasm can affect young people, before the age of 30. Several causes can be suggested: thick arachnoid membrane, narrower posterior fossa or anomaly of the facial nerve (plexiform rootlets).

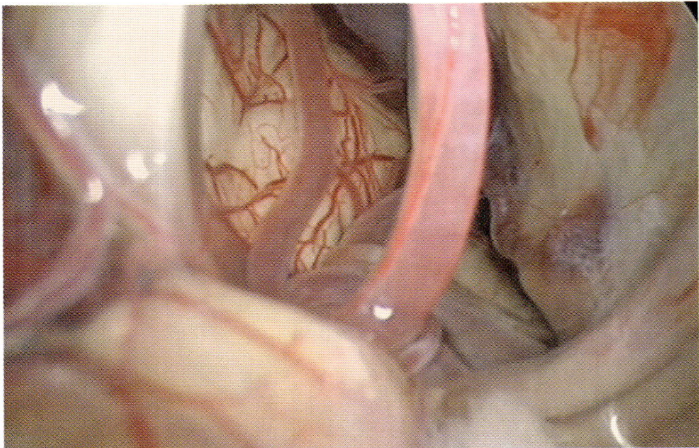

Fig. 6.146: Case 8 of right hemifacial spasm: Endoscopic view showing AICA causing compression at the REZ of facial nerve

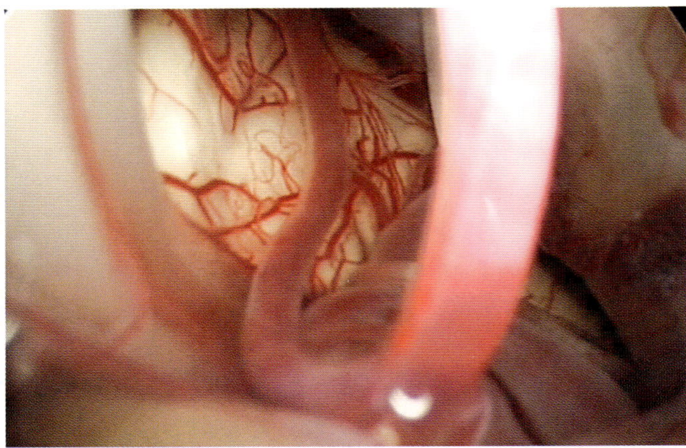

Fig. 6.147: Closer endoscopic view showing AICA causing compression at the REZ of facial nerve

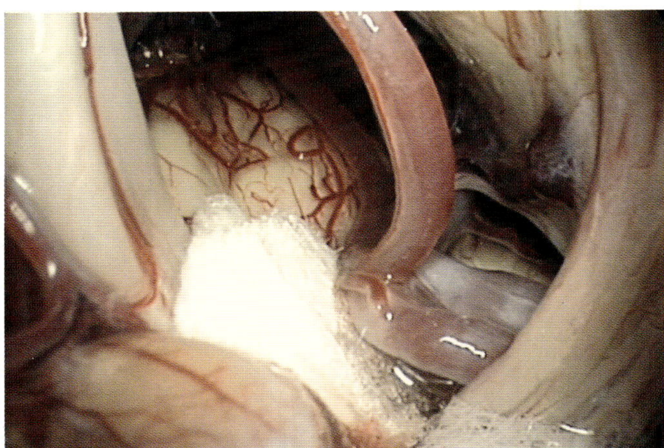

Fig. 6.148: Endoscopic view showing elevation of AICA and PICA (which was an additional source of compression at REZ of facial nerve: from facial nerve and their separation with multiple Teflon pledgets

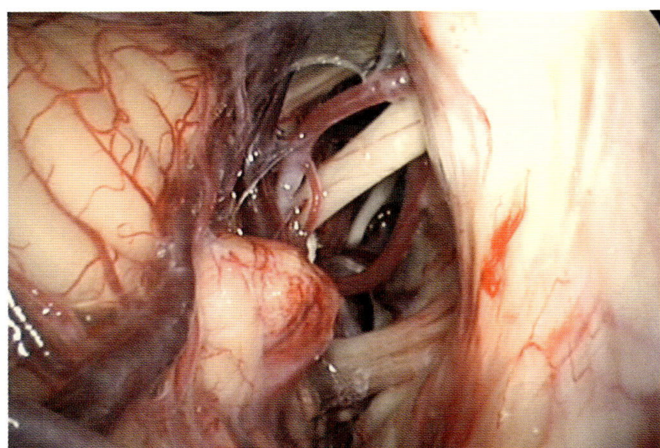

Fig. 6.149: Final endoscopic view showing microvascular decompression for left hemifacial spasm due to combination of AICA and PICA

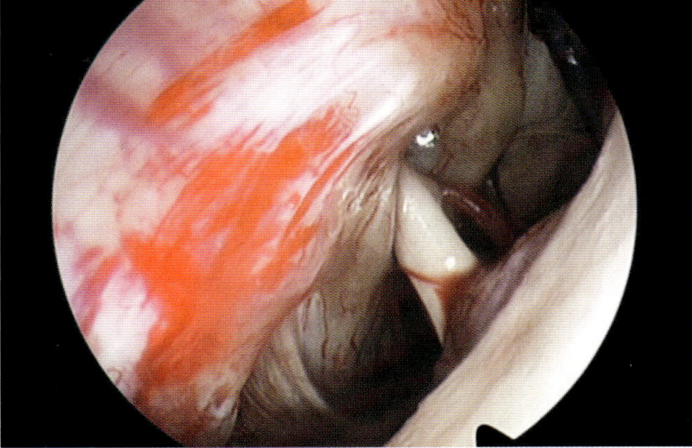

Fig. 6.150: Case 9 of left hemifacial spasm: Endoscopic view showing AICA loop extending into the porus of IAC

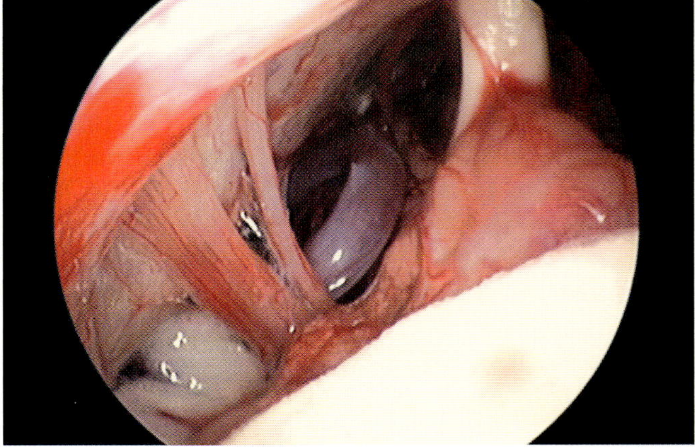

Fig. 6.151: Inferior endoscopic view between vestibulocochlear and lower cranial nerves to find the cause for hemifacial spasm. Ipsilateral vertebral artery is seen

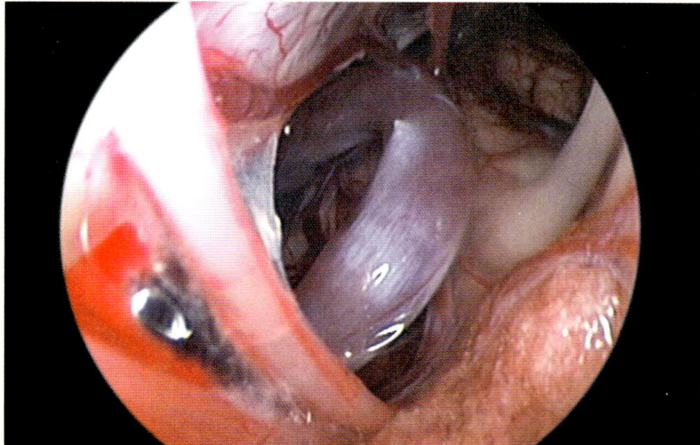

Fig. 6.152: Endoscopic view showing ipsilateral vertebral artery giving rise to PICA and both of them in contact with REZ of facial nerve

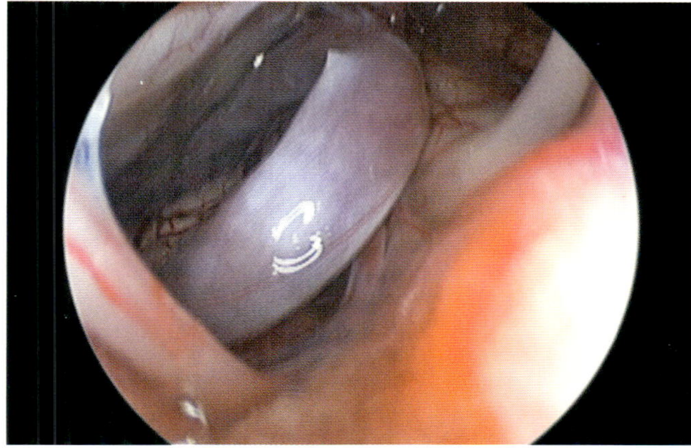

Fig. 6.153: Closer endoscopic view showing ipsilateral vertebral artery giving rise to PICA and both of them in contact with REZ of facial nerve

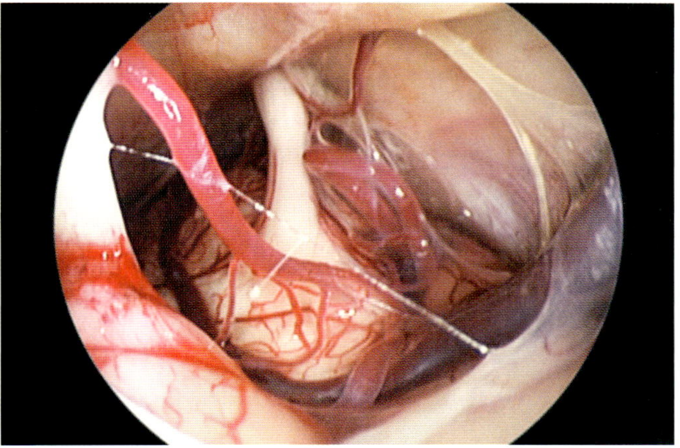

Fig. 6.154: Endoscopic view showing SCA in contact with trigeminal nerve in the same case of hemifacial spasm

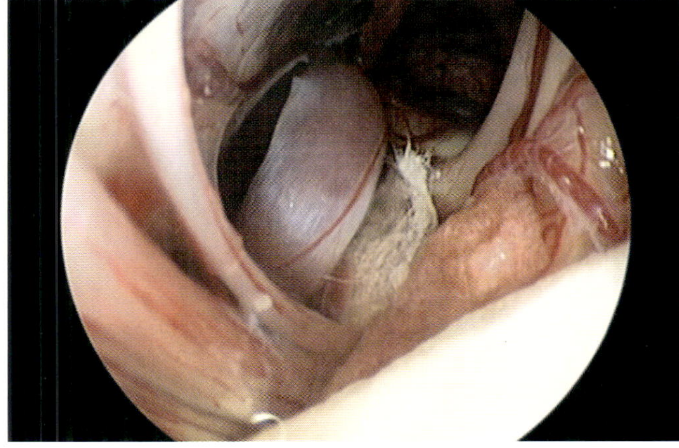

Fig. 6.155: Endoscopic view showing separation of vertebral artery along with PICA arising from its undersurface form their contact with REZ of facial nerve by Teflon pledget

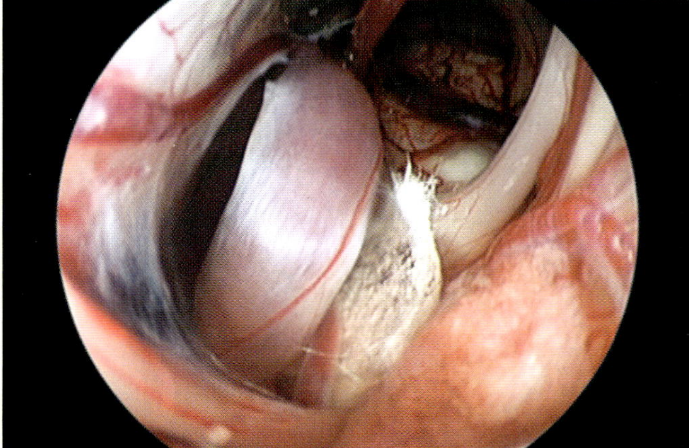

Fig. 6.156: Closer endoscopic view showing separation of vertebral artery along with PICA arising from its undersurface form their contact with REZ of facial nerve by Teflon pledget

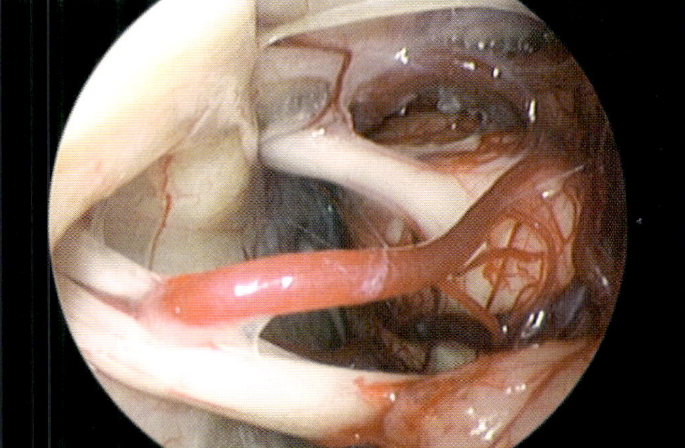

Fig. 6.157: Endoscopic view showing separation of SCA in contact with trigeminal nerve. Also seen is the loop of AICA passing between vestibulocochlear and facial nerves and causing their distortion

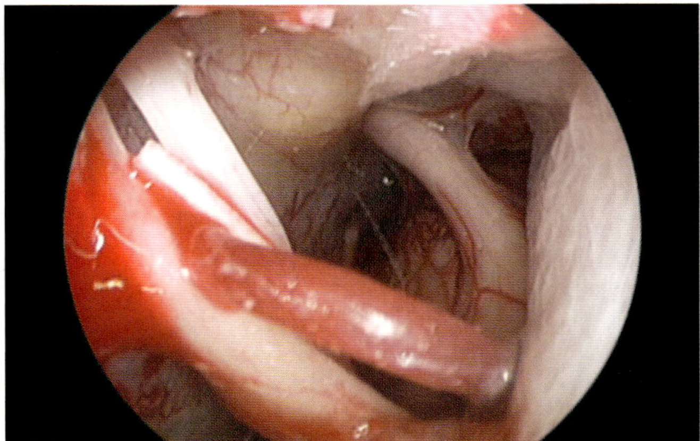

Fig. 6.158: Endoscopic view showing separation of loop of AICA from the facial nerve by Neuropatch placed between AICA loop and facial nerve

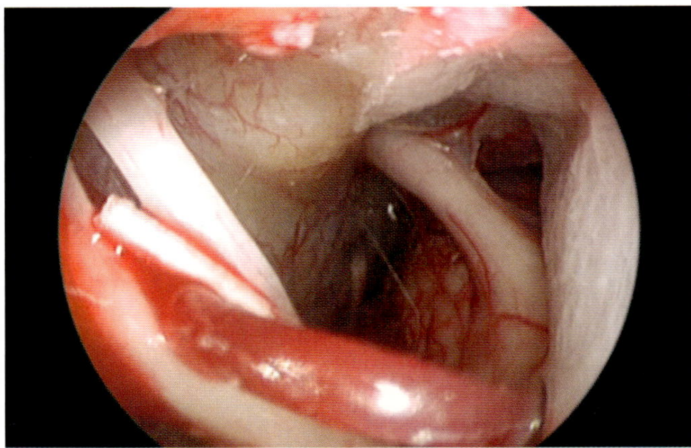

Fig. 6.159: Closer endoscopic view showing separation of loop of AICA from the facial nerve by Neuropatch placed between AICA loop and facial nerve

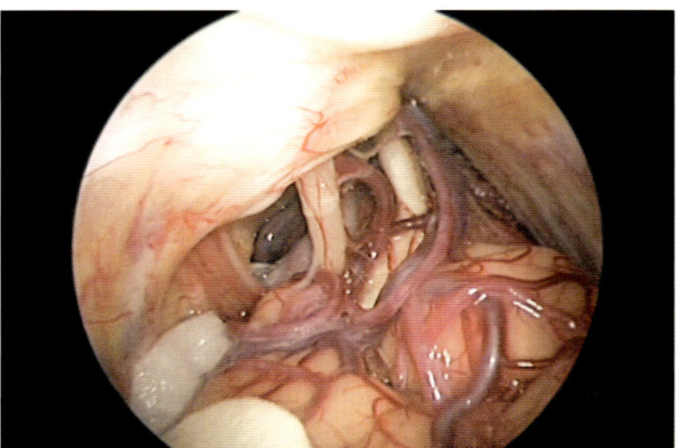

Fig. 6.160: Case 10 of left hemifacial spasm: Endoscopic view showing general view of left CPA with all its contents

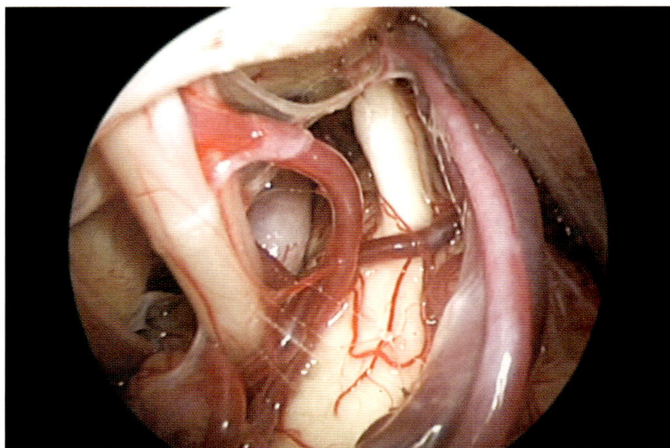

Fig. 6.161: Endoscopic view showing AICA loop extending between vestibulocochlear and facial nerves into the porus of IAC

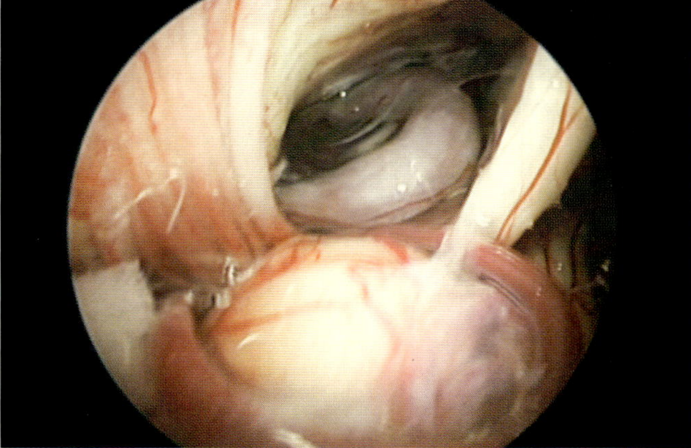

Fig. 6.162: Inferior endoscopic view between vestibulocochlear and lower cranial nerves showing vertebral artery with PICA near REZ of facial nerve

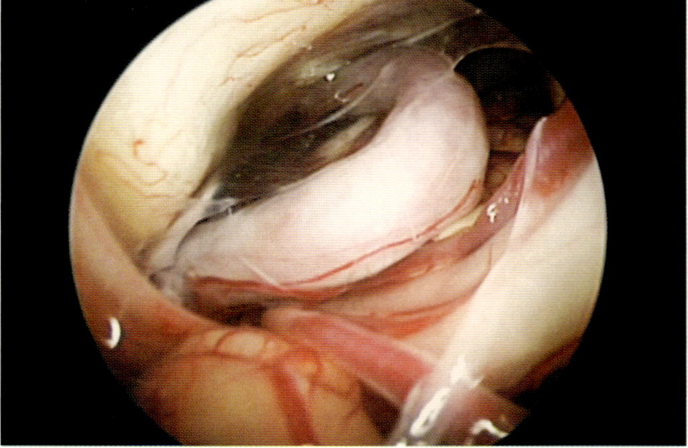

Fig. 6.163: Endoscopic view showing vertebral artery with PICA near REZ of facial nerve

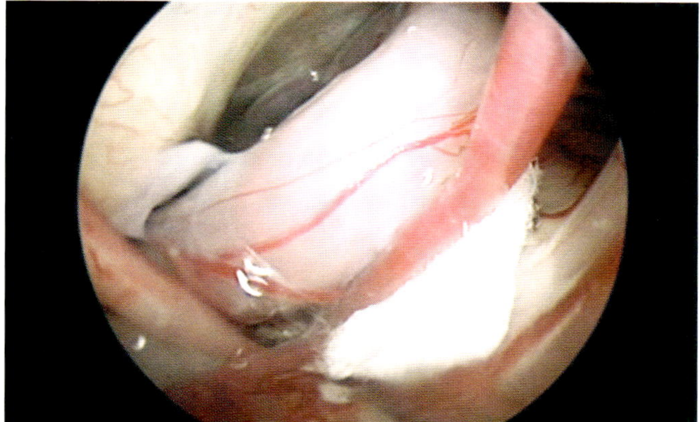

Fig. 6.164: Endoscopic view showing separation of vertebral artery along with PICA arising from its undersurface form their contact with REZ of facial nerve by Teflon pledget

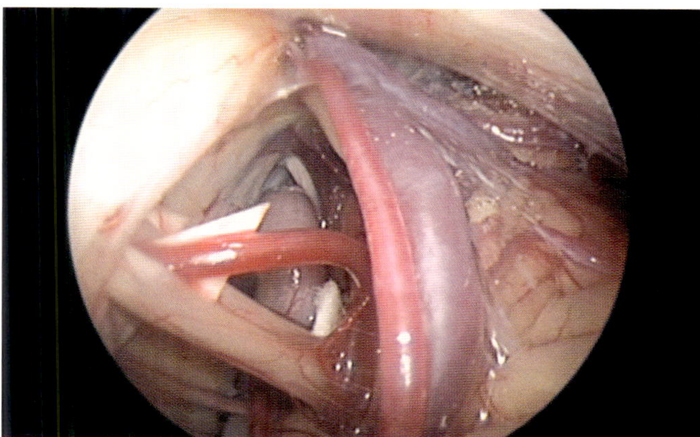

Fig. 6.165: Endoscopic view showing separation of loop of AICA from the facial nerve in its cisternal course by Neuropatch placed between AICA loop and facial nerve

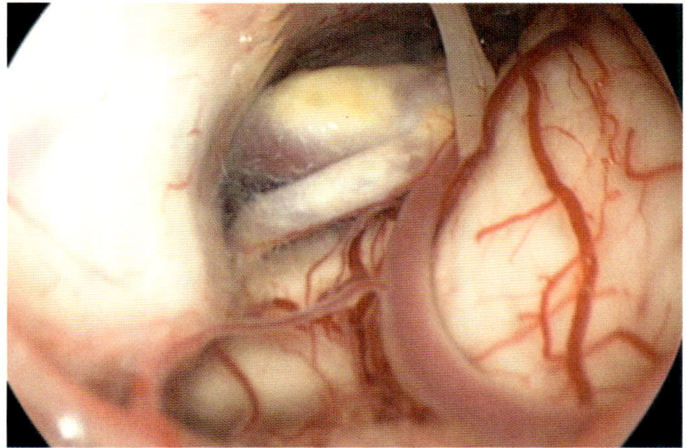

Fig. 6.166: Case 11 of left hemifacial spasm: Endoscopic view showing smaller atherosclerotic ipsilateral vertebral artery not giving rise to PICA and dominant AICA arising from basilar artery causing compression of trigeminal nerve at its REZ

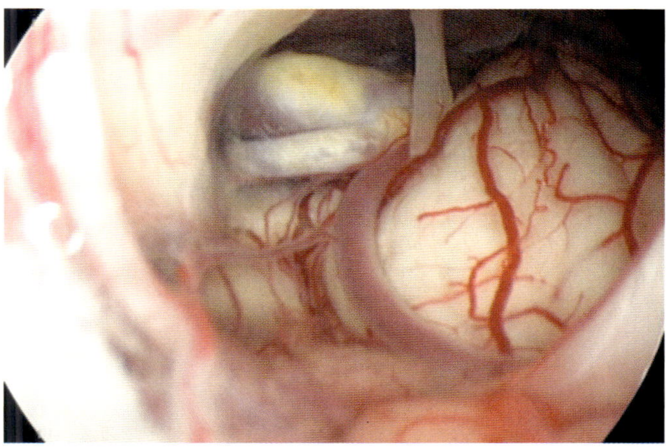

Fig. 6.167: Endoscopic view showing AICA arising from basilar artery causing compression of facial nerve at its REZ

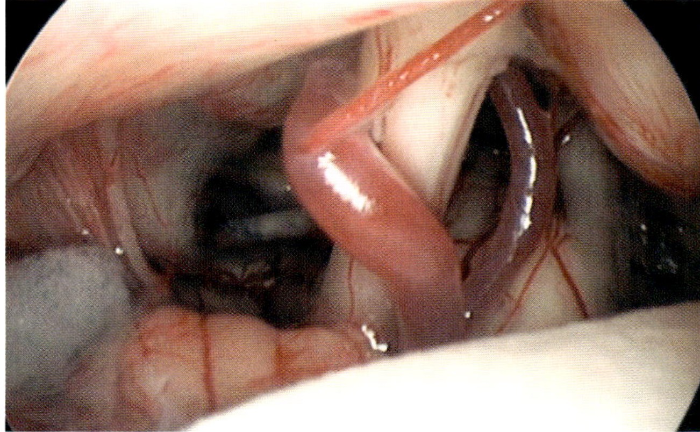

Fig. 6.168: Endoscopic view showing meatal segment of AICA loop along with labyrinthine artery causing additional compression of facial nerve in its cisternal segment

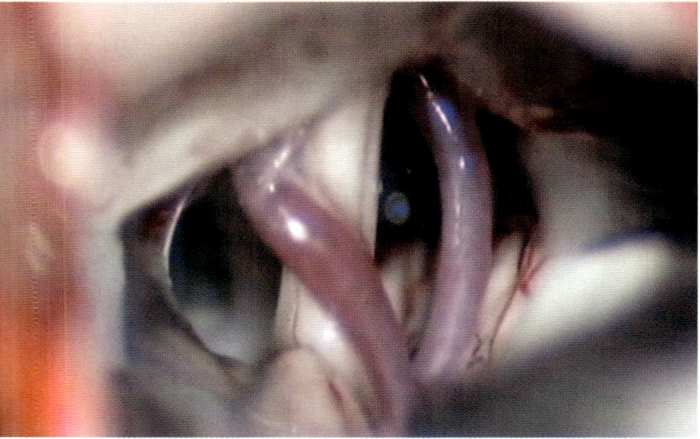

Fig. 6.169: Microscopic view showing meatal segment of AICA loop along with labyrinthine artery causing additional compression of facial nerve in its cisternal segment

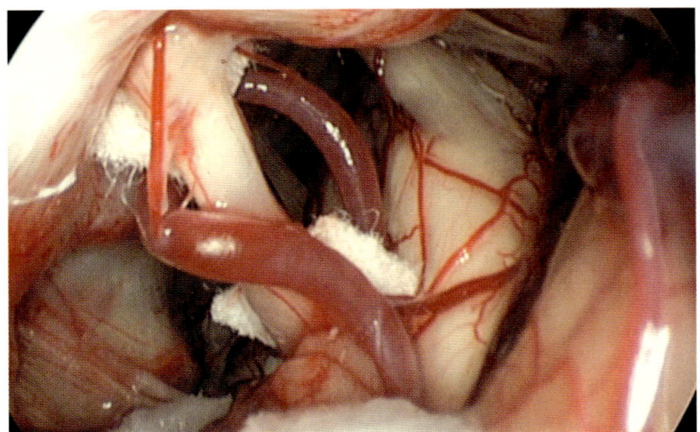

Fig. 6.170: Endoscopic view showing separation of AICA loop from facial nerve by Neuropatch pledgets

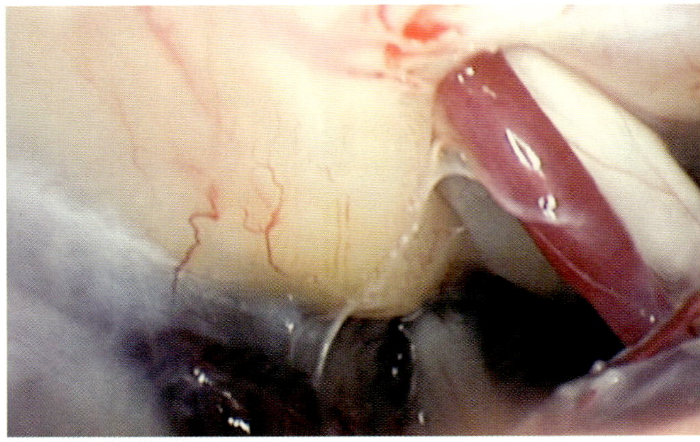

Fig. 6.171: Case 12 of right hemifacial spasm: Endoscopic view showing meatal segment of AICA loop entering within the porus and causing compression of contents of IAM. There was no obvious cause of compression at REZ of facial nerve

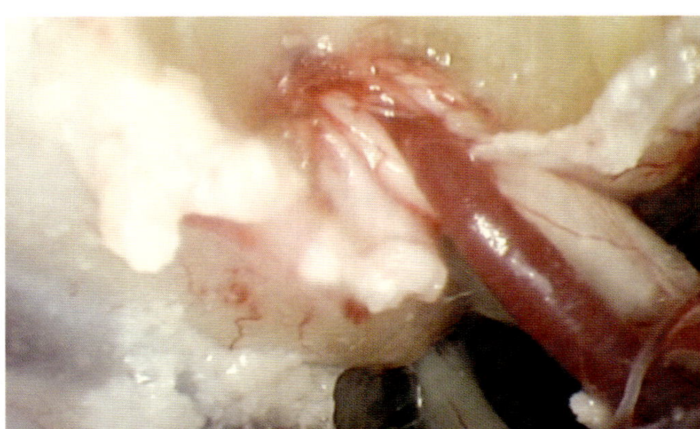

Fig. 6.172: Endoscopic view showing meatal segment of AICA loop entering within the porus and causing compression of facial nerve. The IAM has been drilled open to attempt decompression of facial nerve

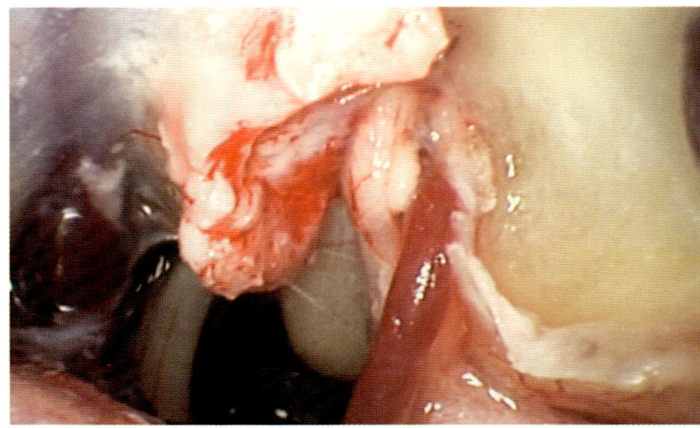

Fig. 6.173: Decompression of facial nerve in IAM segment by AICA loop entering in IAM by drilling open the IAM and placing Teflon pledget between facial nerve and AICA

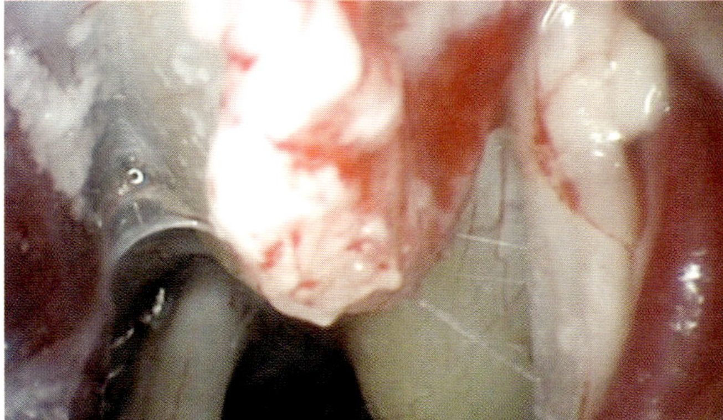

Fig. 6.174: Closer endoscopic view showing decompression of facial nerve in IAM segment by AICA loop by placing Teflon pledget between them

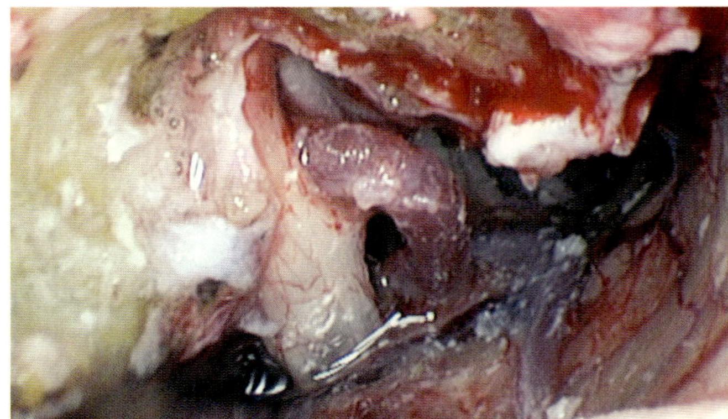

Fig. 6.175: Case 13 of left hemifacial spasm: Endoscopic view showing meatal segment of AICA loop entering within the porus and causing compression of facial nerve. The IAM has been drilled open to attempt decompression of facial nerve. There was no other obvious cause of compression at REZ of facial nerve

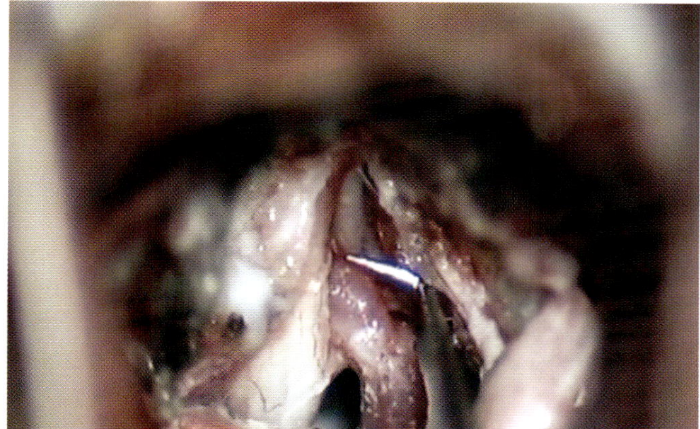

Fig. 6.176: Microscopic view showing decompression of facial nerve in IAM segment by AICA loop by placing Neuropatch pledget between them.

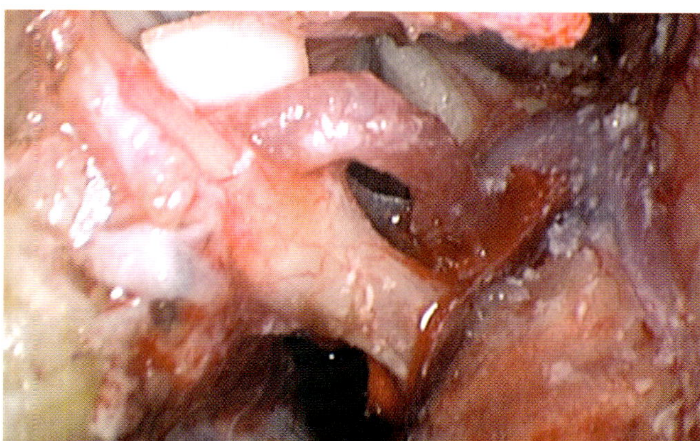

Fig. 6.177: Endoscopic view showing decompression of facial nerve in IAM segment by AICA loop by placing Neuropatch pledget between them.

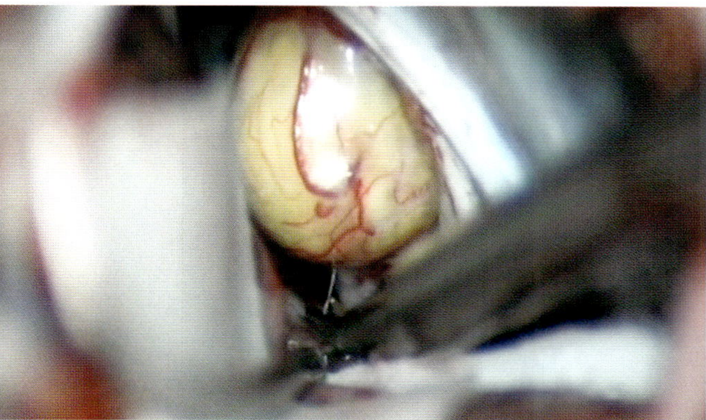

Fig. 6.178: Case 13 of right hemifacial spasm: Microscopic view showing compression of facial nerve at REZ due to displacement of PICA loop toward REZ by glossopharyngeal schwannoma

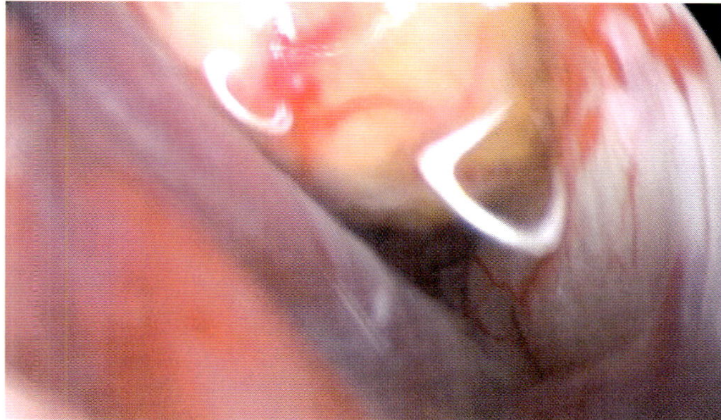

Fig. 6.179: Endoscopic view showing displacement of PICA loop toward facial nerve REZ by glossopharyngeal schwannoma

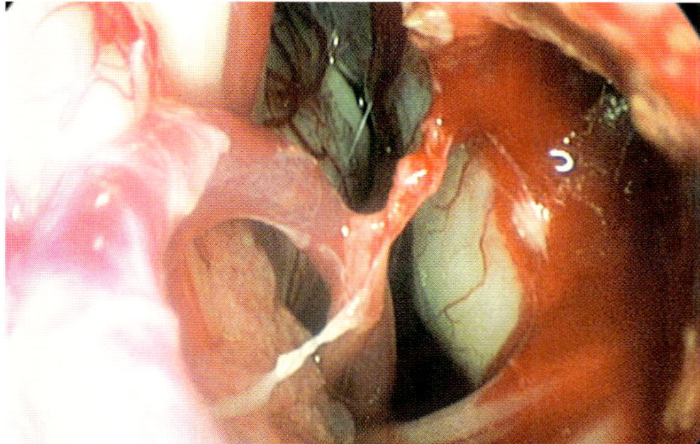

Fig. 6.180: Endoscopic view after removal of glossopharyngeal schwannoma showing compression of facial nerve at REZ due to displacement of PICA loop toward REZ. Also seen is jugular foramen after removal of glossopharyngeal nerve along with its tumor.

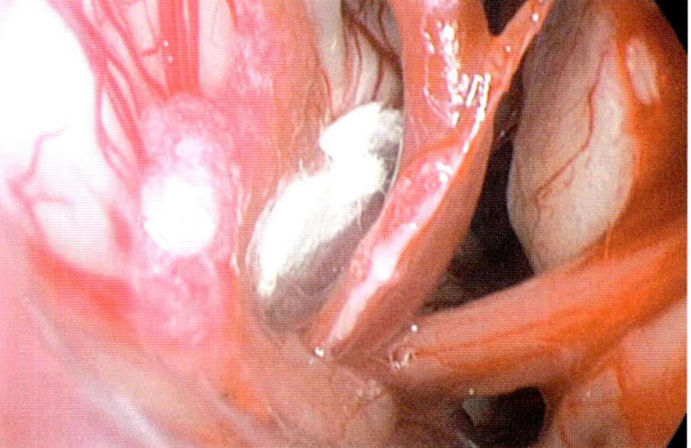

Fig. 6.181: Endoscopic view showing decompression of facial nerve at REZ from PICA by Teflon pledget.

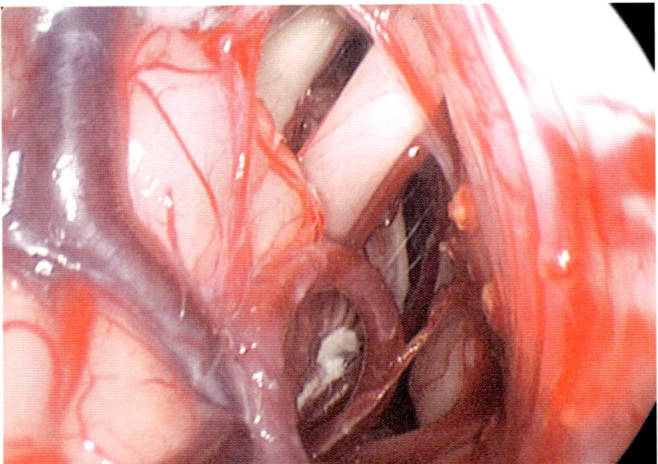

Fig. 6.182: Final endoscopic view showing decompression of facial nerve at REZ from PICA by Teflon pledget

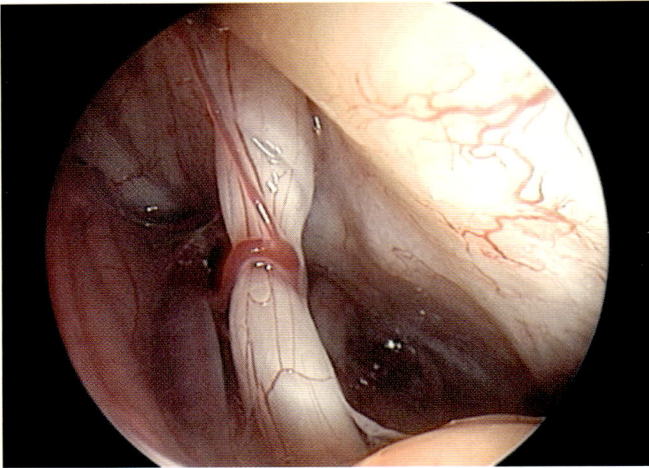

Fig. 6.183: Endoscopic view showing meatal loop of AICA along with its subarcuate branch causing nutcracker type of compression over the vestibulocochlear nerve

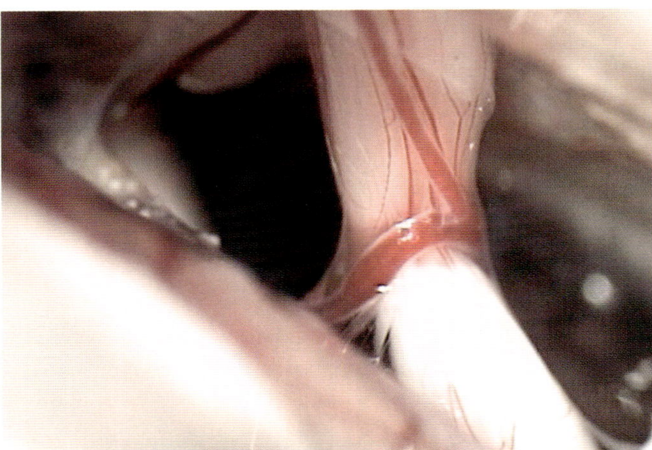

Fig. 6.184: Microscopic view showing meatal loop of AICA along with its subarcuate branch causing nutcracker type of compression over the vestibulocochlear nerve

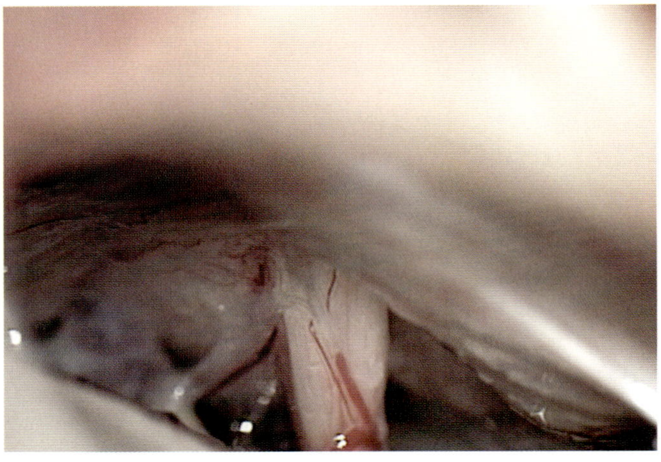

Fig. 6.185: Microscopic view showing coagulation of subarcuate branch with bipolar cautery

Venous conflicts: An isolated venous conflict is rare and is reported between 0.4 and 4.1% in literature and 1.9% in our study.[83] The difficulty is in identifying the vein that is pathological and in deciding how to deal with it (whether to interpose Teflon, coagulate it or preserving it).

In conclusion, in our cases or MVD for HFS,[83] a vascular decompression procedure was performed on PICA in 77%, on vertebral artery in 40% and on AICA in 36%.

MICROVASCULAR DECOMPRESSION OF THE VESTIBULOCOCHLEAR NERVE

The transitional zone or REZ of the eighth nerve varies in its location along the course of nerve in its cisternal course. Consequently, the sites of the vascular conflicts can occur anywhere along the nerve from the brainstem to the internal auditory canal. There are different types of contact between the vessel and the vestibulocochlear nerve:

1. *Nutcracker type of contact*: The conflict includes one or more offending vessels (AICA and subarcuate artery or AICA and PICA) above and below the nerve which is entangled between them (Figs 6.183 to 6.188).
2. *Simple contact*: The conflict is by a loop of the AICA (Fig. 6.189) and a single point of contact over the nerve. A special finding is a long subarcuate artery stretching posteriorly the nerve at its entrance into the internal auditory canal (Figs 6.190 to 6.191).

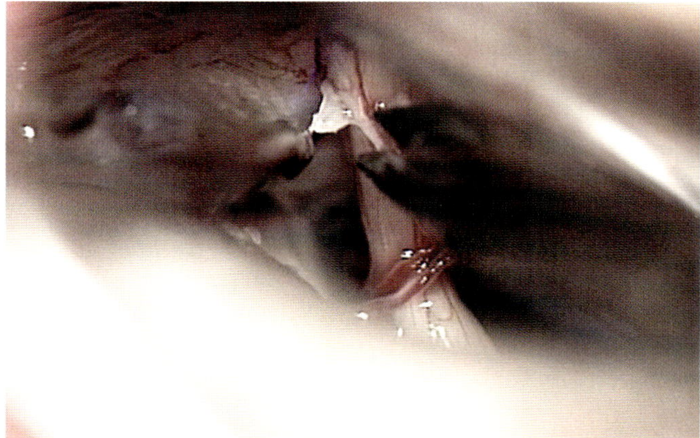

Fig. 6.186: Microscopic view showing division of subarcuate branch with bayonet scissors

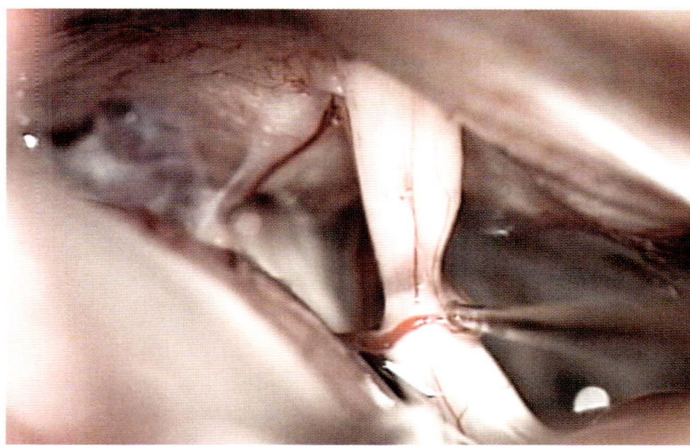

Fig. 6.187: Microscopic view showing mobilization of AICA loop after dividing the subarcuate branch. Distinct segment of demyelination is seen in the part of vestibulocochlear nerve compressed by AICA loop

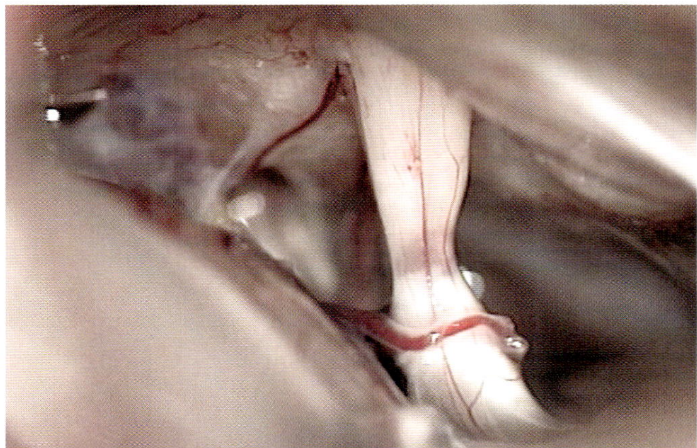

Fig. 6.188: Final picture showing segment of demyelination seen in the part of vestibulocochlear nerve compressed by AICA loop after its mobilization

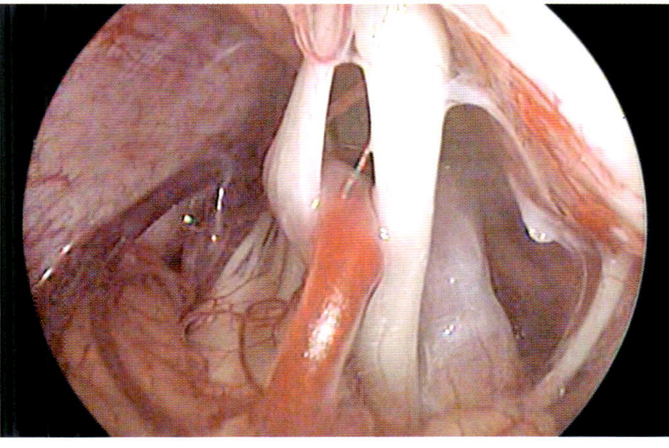

Fig. 6.189: Endoscopic view showing meatal loop of AICA causing single contact compression over the vestibulocochlear nerve

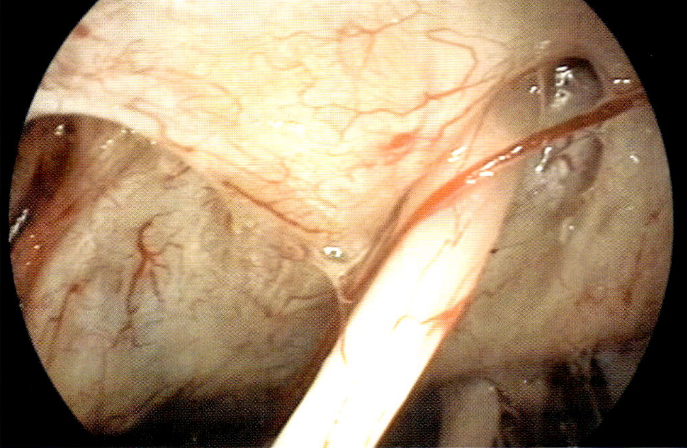

Fig. 6.190: Endoscopic view showing subarcuate artery causing single contact compression over the vestibulocochlear nerve

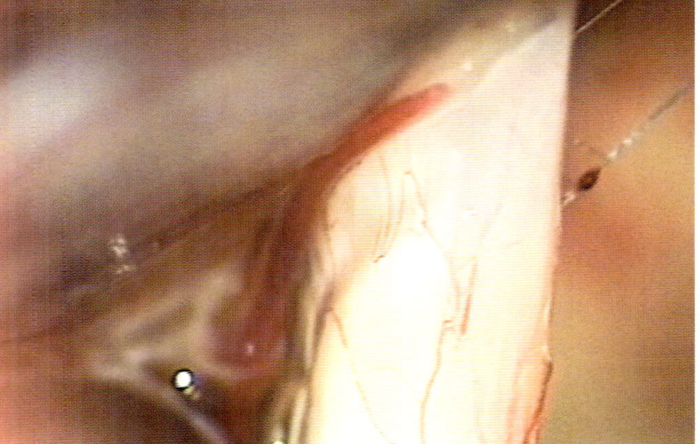

Fig. 6.191: Endoscopic view showing subarcuate artery causing single contact compression over the vestibulocochlear nerve eading to its distortion and focal demyelination

3. *Multiple contacts*: The conflict includes different points of contact by several loops of the AICA around the REZ of the nerve, in its cisternal and/or intracanalicular course.
4. *Vein contact*: The venous structure is an inconstant and aberrant inferior cerebellar vein, part of a developmental venous anomaly, and the contact is along the REZ of the nerve and at the Luschka foramen.

Vascular decompression for disabling tinnitus is particularly delicate because of the risk of hearing loss and the course of the anterior inferior cerebellar artery responsible for the conflict. Indeed, this artery is involved in 60% of cases, and in half of these cases, it has a route between the VII and VIII making illusory any possibility of decompression. In addition, the vascular loop within the internal auditory canal requires its opening by drilling, which increases the risk of hearing without leading to mobilization of the artery that can be fixed by a labyrinthine artery. Monitoring of the cochlear nerve is a means of early warning from direct trauma by the decrease in amplitude and longer waves. The offending vessels characteristically induce pressure and distort the cochlear nerve at any place along its course. REZ of cochlear nerve is variable with mean of 8.3 mm away from its exit from pontomedullary junction and often up to porus and within IAC. The compressive effect is most commonly due to sharp angled loops at areas of vessel bifurcations. Two other typical aspects are when the loop pinches the nerve, or when the subarcuate artery constricts the nerve. Using the 4 mm 30° endoscope, a panoramic view of all the CPA structures is obtained. The tip of the endoscope is passed above and below the acoustico-facial bundle to identify the precise location and course of the offending vessels.

Vascular decompression for disabling positional vertigo is still controversial. The vascular compressive neuropathy should induce vestibular nerve irritation that results to hyperactivity and hyperexcitability of the nuclei and central nuclear dysfunction. We are convinced of the reality of the conflict and neurovascular surgical decompression is the logical solution, but has an uncertain outcome. The vestibular neurotomy seems more reasonable for its high percentage of good results. But the section of the vestibular nerve, in the case of a hyperexcitable nerve could represent the equivalent of a sensory deafferentation with neurosensory sequelae as persistent balance problems.

MICROVASCULAR DECOMPRESSION FOR GLOSSOPHARYNGEAL NEURALGIA

The posterior inferior cerebellar artery often distorts the lower cranial nerves asymptomatically. The intervention is thus determined by the presence of an ectatic vertebral artery, as part of glossopharyngeal neuralgia. In our five cases out of six that we operated for glossopharyngeal neuralgia, the PICA was in close contact and distorting the glossopharyngeal nerve (Figs 6.192 to 6.198) and was often fixed to the nerve by fibrous tissue. These fibrous adhesions had to be carefully sectioned to separate both neurovascular components giving normal straight course to the nerve and mobilizing the artery (Figs 6.199 to 6.202).

The position that vertebral artery tends to take after mobilization and interposition of Teflon felt occasionally does not eliminate the distortion of cranial nerves. Section of the glossopharyngeal nerve can then be performed, resulting in only minimal neuromuscular sequelae. This was done in our one case out of total of six.

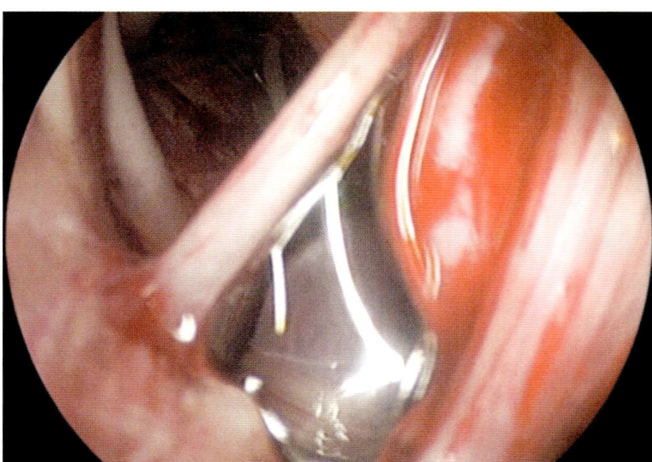

Fig. 6.192: Case 1 of glossopharyngeal neuralgia: Endoscopic view showing view of distorted glossopharyngeal nerve

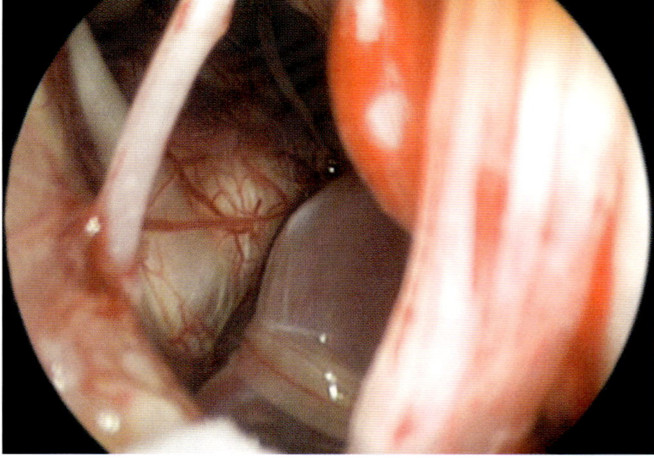

Fig. 6.193: Endoscopic view showing distorted glossopharyngeal nerve with compression of its REZ by PICA arising out of VA

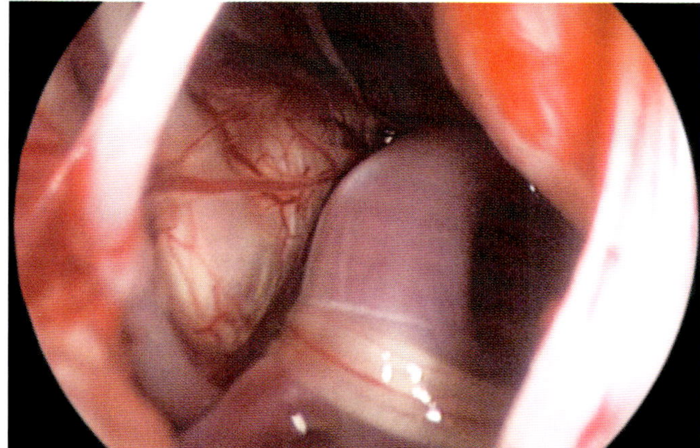

Fig. 6.194: Closer endoscopic view showing compression of REZ of glossopharyngeal nerve by PICA arising out of VA.

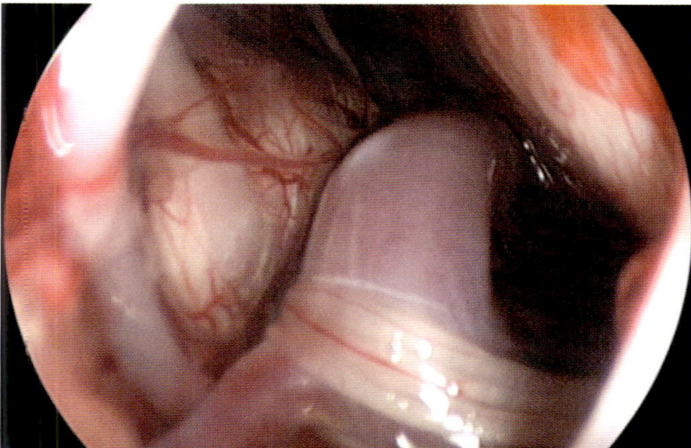

Fig. 6.195: Closer endoscopic view showing compression of REZ of glossopharyngeal nerve by PICA arising out of VA

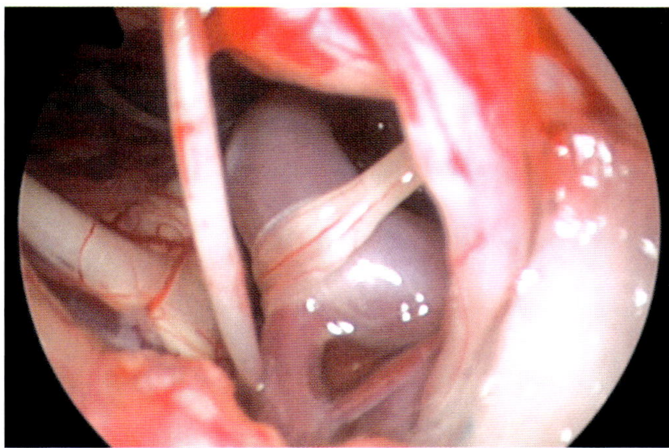

Fig. 6.196: Endoscopic view showing mobilization of PICA loop from its contact with glossopharyngeal nerve

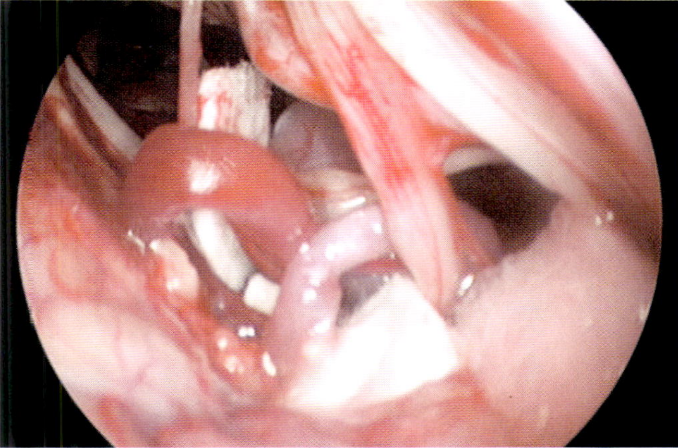

Fig. 6.197: Endoscopic view showing mobilization of PICA loop from its contact with glossopharyngeal nerve and insulation of later by Teflon pledgets

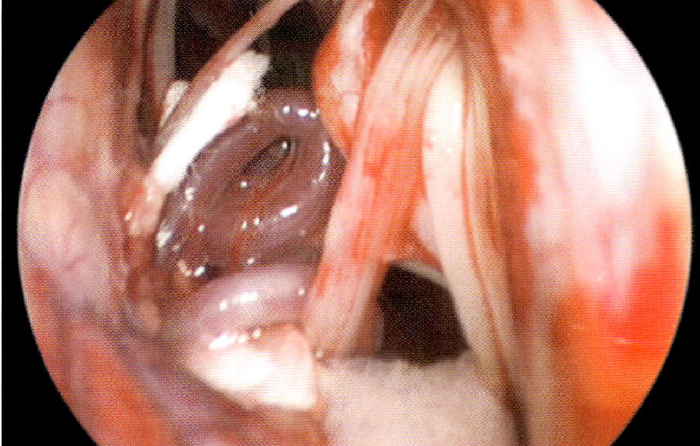

Fig. 6.198: Final endoscopic view showing mobilization of PICA loop from its contact with glossopharyngeal nerve and insulation of later by Teflon pledgets

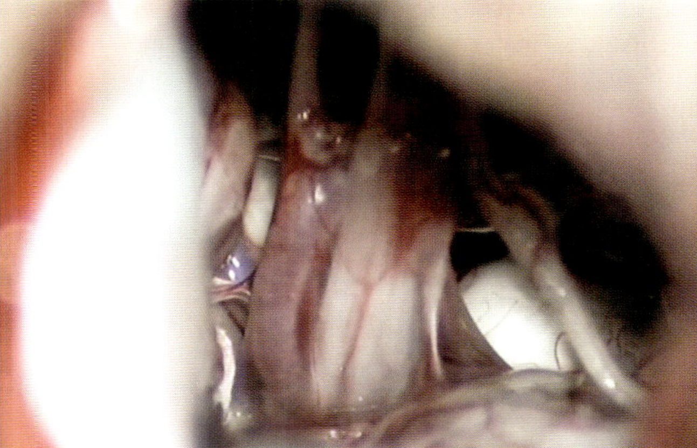

Fig. 6.199: Case 2 of glossopharyngeal neuralgia: Microscopic view showing compression of glossopharyngeal nerve by PICA with fibrous adhesions between them

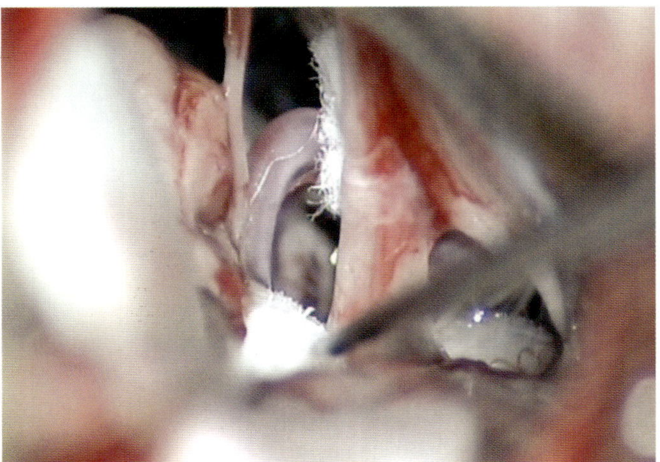

Fig. 6.200: Microscopic view showing division of fibrous adhesions between glossopharyngeal nerve and PICA and insertion of Teflon pledgets to decompress the glossopharyngeal nerve from PICA

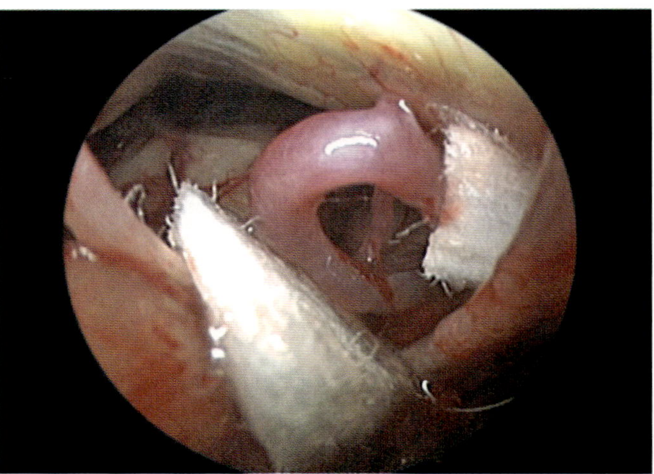

Fig. 6.201: Endoscopic view showing mobilization of PICA loop from its contact with glossopharyngeal nerve and insulation of later by Teflon pledgets. Note the contact of PICA with vagal nerve rootlets are also insulated with Teflon

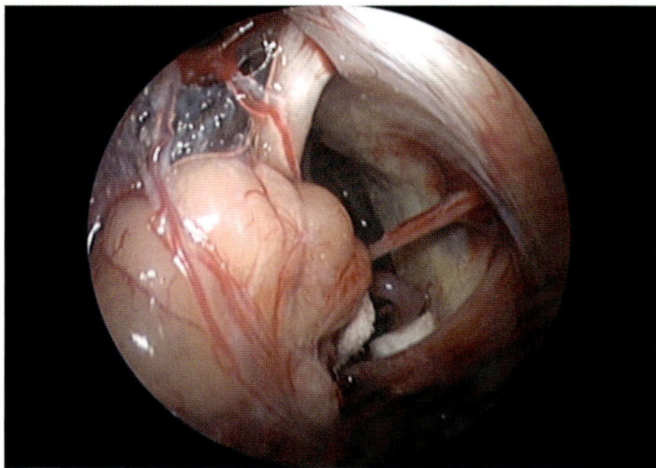

Fig. 6.202: Final endoscopic view showing mobilization of PICA loop from its contact with glossopharyngeal nerve and insulation of later by Teflon pledgets. Note the contact of PICA with vagal nerve rootlets are also insulated with Teflon

RESULTS AFTER MICROVASCULAR DECOMPRESSION SURGERY

Microvascular decompression has become an accepted surgical technique for the treatment of trigeminal neuralgia, hemifacial spasm and glossopharyngeal neuralgia because of their good surgical outcomes. Disabling tinnitus and vertigo has not been able to match the similar successful results consistently probably due to multiple etiologies for same and inability to effectively screen out the ones exactly caused by vascular compression. The results as regards to mortality have been consistently good with less 0.4% in most of the recent studies, and none in our experience of over 30 years. The morbidity in terms of CSF leak and hearing loss have been going down over the years of experience and with intraoperative monitoring in most of the centers. Senior author (JM) has been performing MVD for the various vascular syndromes by endoscope-assisted MIRA since 1993 and has records for 919 patients till June 2011. It includes 565 MVD for hemifacial spasm, 284 for trigeminal neuralgia, 63 for tinnitus/vertigo and 7 for glossopharyngeal neuralgia.

The results will be presented individually for each vascular syndrome and the data presented are analyzed at that respective time in different studies including our own series.

SURGICAL RESULTS OF MVD FOR TRIGEMINAL NEURALGIA

Surgical approaches to pain management are performed when medication cannot control pain or patients cannot tolerate the adverse effects of the medication. Microvascular decompression (MVD) was generally performed in the past when the patient is healthy and relatively young. Nowadays there is no age limit thanks to minimally invasive surgery with low morbidity. The oldest patient in our series was 87 years old. Tables 6.1 to 6.3 demonstrate the cure rate of MVD for trigeminal neuralgia, cause for neurovascular compression and complications of MVD for trigeminal neuralgia respectively in different studies.

Factors Affecting Recurrence

Barker and Janetta[31] found four factors predicting long-term relief from trigeminal neuralgia after MVD was identified: immediate postoperative relief; male sex; absence of venous compression of the trigeminal-root entry zone and duration of preoperative symptoms of less than 8 years. Sindou et al.[34] found severe focal arachnoiditis and low degree of compression of nerve during the surgery as the only negative predictive factor and older patients and severe distortion of the nerve root as the only positive predictive factor with statistical significance and found no association with sex, venous etiology and preoperative duration of symptoms. Sindou found delayed improvement in pain relief in 13% patients after more than 3 months of surgery. Concerning the surgical technique, Sindou et al. had better outcome when the prosthesis used to maintain the offending vessel apart was not touching the trigeminal root, i.e., when MVD achieved a real decompression (rather than a neocompression). Broggi et al.[84] found the preoperative period of symptoms more than 7 years as the only factor significantly influencing the recurrence of pain. Kassam et al.[35] and Mooij et al.[86] both compared the results of MVD in typical and atypical TN and concluded that the results are significantly better with typical TN.

In our experience, the association of trigeminal neuralgia and temporomandibular algo-dystrophia represents the

Table 6.1: Cure rates of MVD for trigeminal neuralgia

Author	*No. of Patients with Long-term f/u*	*Mean Years of Follow-up*	*% Cured at 1 Year after First Operation**	*Recurrence at 1 Year*	*% Cured after Revision Operation*	*Cure Rate over Long-term*
Barker et al.[31]	1155	6.2	84	24	88	70% at 10 years
Sindou et al.[34]	362	7.2	84.8	NA	NA	73.2% at 15 years (Prediction)
Kondo et al.[32]	281	> 7 years	92.9–96.7	6.5–10.1	NA	80.3–82.5
Kassam et al.[35]#	969	5	84.1 (14.1 with occasional medicines)	13.7	NA	73.7% at 5 years (extra 6.8% with occasional medicines)
Broggi et al.[84]	148	3.2	75.7	15.6	78	78% at 3.2 years
Sun et al.[85]	61	6.7	–	16	NA	75
Mooij et al.[86]	156	9.7	73	19	NA	73
Our results (unpublihsed data till 2007)	205	> 5 yrs	86	15	91	88

*Complete relief or more than 75% reduction in pain at 1 year, not recuiring medicines. If the data include patients with intermittent pain and occasional use of medicines, the success rate improves much more.
#Only typical trigeminal neuralgia cases with long-term follow-up were included.

Table 6.2: Causes for neurovascular compression in trigeminal neuralgia

Author	*SCA Alone (%)*	*AICA Alone (%)*	*Vertebral/ Basilar A. (%)*	*Vein Alone (%)*	*Multiple combination (%)*	*Remarks*	*No Vascular Contacts*
Barker et al.[31]	75	10	3	13	56	Nonspecific small artery (15%)	0
Sindou et al.[34]	74.3	6.1	5.1	3.3	42.8	–	4.7
Mooij et al.[86]	66	NA	NA	9	14.1	Tumor in 1.9%	6
Our results[82]	46	2.5	2	11	34	–	–

Table 6.3: Complications of MVD for trigeminal neuralgia

Author	Mortality (%)	CSF Leak Rate (%)	Severe Sensory Hearing Loss (%)	Facial Paresis Transient (T)/ Permanent (P) (%)	Neurological Complications (%)	Remarks
Barker et al.[31]	0.15	1.5	1.1	0.7 (T) 0.08 (P)	1	–
Sindou et al.[34]	0.44	–	1.9	0.83	0.27	Trochlear nerve palsy 0.83%
Broggi et al.[84]	0	4.8	3.2	1.2 (T), 1.2 (P)	1.2	Transient diplopia 2.4%, trigeminal hypoesthesia 3.5%
Sun et al.[85]	0	NA	1.5	0	0	3% trigeminal anesthesia & dysasthesia
Mooij et al.[86]	0	NA	2.6 (partial), 0.6 severe	0.6 (P)	0.6	Lower cranial nerves palsy 0.6%

major negative factor. Other negative criteria for recurrence are male sex, previous percutaneous treatment, location of the conflict at the Meckel's cave entrance and represents accessory pejorative factors. The causes for neurovascular compression are shown in Table 6.2.

Complications (Table 6.3)

Mortality reported in most of the large series is 0.3% or less. Nowadays it is practically reduced to zero. The operative risk is inherent in any surgery. Morbidity is very limited and is reduced further with minimally invasive techniques. In the past, Janetta reported hearing impairment in 2% of cases, delayed facial paralysis in 0.1% of cases. In our recent case series, hearing and facial function were preserved in all patients. Sindou reported occipital nerve neuralgia in 0.6%. It should be noted that the headache after decompression surgery for trigeminal neuralgia is rarely reported. CSF leak and aseptic meningitis are still present as transient complication in 3–8% of cases.

Remarks on Our Results

We performed surgery for trigeminal vascular decompression from 1994. Before that period, TN resistant to medical treatment was treated by trigeminal ganglion rhizotomy with good results, hence our reluctance to change technique. In a series of 206 cases till 2007 (unpublished data), 121 women (59%), 85 men (41%), surgery was performed at a mean age of 57 years ranging from 32 to 83 years. We had 29 patients requiring revision surgery due to failure in reduction of pain or recurrent pain in a period of 12 years (in 14%). The recurrence occurred either immediately after surgery, between the third and sixth months (23 patients). All patients with recurrence underwent revision surgery with the following results. About 14 of them had recurrence due to fibrous tissue inducing new neurovascular conflict. Seven of these patients had success after revision surgery and 7 had failures even after surgery and were advised percutaneous ablative procedures. Six patients had Teflon displacement and all were successfully treated by revision surgery. Three patients had Teflon granulomas that were treated successfully after revision surgery. Six patients had initial failure to improve after surgery in the immediate postoperative period and on revision surgery 2 of these 6 cases had aberrant vein that was ablated with 1 success and 1 failure. Four patients with no improvement after initial surgery had no explanation even after revision surgery and we performed partial rhizotomy (2 successes, 2 failures).

SURGICAL RESULTS OF MVD FOR HEMIFACIAL SPASM

Surgical care for patients suffering from hemifacial spasm has to be efficient, with a low morbidity, as always in treatment for a functional disease. Tables 6.4 to 6.6 demonstrate the cure rate of MVD, cause for neurovascular compression and complications of MVD in hemifacial spasm respectively in different studies.

Our Results

In our series of 553 cases (unpublished data), 95% of the patient had complete relief of their hemifacial spasm, including the improvement in 11% cases after revision surgery. In literature, the success of the procedure varies from 83 to 97%.[47,53–56,83,86–92]

The results at the primary surgery was 83% of success rate and 17% had unsatisfactory results.[83] Out of 326 patients analyzed with a minimum follow-up of 6 months,[83] 83% had success (271 cases), 2% had improvement and 15% had failure after the primary surgery.

For the vast majority of patients, the successful result is immediate and occurs within the first week, while in 25% of cases it is delayed with a progressive decrease in spasms in 2–6 months. In successful results, the hemifacial spasm disappears immediately within 1 week of surgery in 75%

Table 6.4: Cure rate of MVD for hemifacial spasm

Author	*No. of Patients with Long f/u*	*Mean Years of Follow-up*	*% Cured after First Operation**	*Delayed Recurrence*	*% Cured after Revision Operation*	*Cure Rate over Long-term*
Barker et al.[47]	612	10	NA	NA	NA	86
Sindou et al.[55]	147	7	NA	NA	NA	87
Kondo et al.[32]	461	12	97.4	6.9–8.9	NA	84.2–89
Huh et al.[87]	1582	2.6	94.6	0.4	95.4	90.3
Park et al.[88]	236	1.5	NA	NA	NA	93.6
Our results[83]	326	Range 6 months –8 years	83.2	0.35	93.6	93.25

*Complete relief or more than 90% reduction at 1 year.

Table 6.5: Cause for neurovascular compression in hemifacial spasm

Author	*PICA Alone*	*VA Alone*	*PICA + VA*	*AICA Alone*	*Other Multiple Combinations*	*Vein Alone*
Barker et al.[47]	68.2	24.2	NA	35.3	20.4	2.9
Sindou et al.[55]	60.8	21.4	NA	54.3	13	4.1
Samii et al.[54]	72.5	27	NA	26.2	1.4	0.7
Park et al.[88]	35.6	15.7	NA	74.2	NA	0.4
Our study[83]	37.2	11.6	32.4	8.1	8.8	1.3

Table 6.6: Complications of MVD for hemifacial spasm

Author	*Mortality*	*CSF Leak Rate (%)*	*Sensory Hearing Loss Transient (T)/ Permanent (P) (%)*	*Facial Paresis Transient (T)/ Permanent (P) (%)*	*Neurological Complications Including Meningitis, CPA Hematoma (%)*	*Lower Cranial N Palsy Transient (T)/Permanent (P) (%)*
Barker et al.[47]	0.1	2.9	3.2	4.2	0.1	NA
Sindou et al.[55]	0	7	1.6 (P), 14 (T)	1.3	0	0.7 (P)
Samii et al.[54]	0.7	4.8	15.9	2.7	2.7	NA
Huh et al.[87]	0	1.1	5.1(T), 2.1(P)	17.4(T), 1.2(P)	2.3	Lower cranial N palsy 2.7(T), 0.1(P)
Park et al.[88]	NA	NA	0.8	9.3	NA	NA
Our results[83]	0	4.9	3.2(T), 0.6(P)	0.3	2.7%	NA

and the successful result is delayed in 25% of patients, up to average of 6 months after first surgery, with 2 cases improving after a longer period of 12 and 18 months. The explanation for this delay is not clear. The hypothesis is that it corresponds to the time needed for hyperactivity of the nucleus to decrease.[55,89] The distortion of the brainstem by the offending vessels is a predictive factor of such delayed recovery.

About 51 patients underwent reoperation which increased the overall successful results at 94%. The percentage of success rate at the revision surgery is the same as the primary surgery without additional side effects. The reoperations were highly instructive. The main cause, in spite of an accurate endoscopic assessment of the CPA, was a "missed" arterial conflict.

- A posterior inferior cerebellar artery, which was a circular loop and thus offered a double fulcrum on the root of the facial nerve.
- An anterior inferior cerebellar artery in contact with the facial nerve in a normal anatomic position.
- An asymptomatic associated vascular compression of the trigeminal nerve.
- A vein in intimate contact with the root of the facial nerve that had not been coagulated in primary surgery.
- No known causes and the Teflon position were changed.

The results of MVD for hemifacial spasm are stable over time. This represents a very significant difference compared with the long-term follow up of patients with trigeminal neuralgia. Out of 565 patients with hemifacial spasm, only two patients developed a distant recurrence, 5 and 11 years later. On another hand, two patients presented few transitory recurrences during crisis of rheumatoid inflammatory disorder.

One point must be emphasized regarding the intraoperative monitoring of the facial nerve. Immediate intraoperative disappearance of AMR allows to increase the success rate of the surgery as all the cases operated that had the AMRs disappear during the surgical procedure of decompression had successful results, confirming its efficiency. When the AMR persist, the surgeon must check the effectiveness of the decompression and must look for simultaneous multiple conflicts. This data confirm the criteria defined by Moller and lead us to recommend intraoperative electrophysiological tests on facial nerve as an indispensable complementary tool in the MVD of patients suffering of hemifacial spasm.

Thus, to increase the success rate during the surgical vascular decompression of the facial nerve, the surgeon must ensure to recognize multiple arterial conflicts using endoscopic procedure, to control the adhering vein at the facial nerve root, to isolate the facial nerve from any vascular contact and to check the efficiency of vascular decompression with facial nerve monitoring.

Surgical efficiency can be highlighted in Figures 6.203 and 6.204 which show preoperative and postoperative quality of life evaluation on 326 patients operated and with at least 2 years follow up using HFS questionnaire developed by Tan et al.[91] This validated score evaluates from 0 to 4 (not affected to very affected) eight criteria of quality of life: driving, reading, TV watching, depressive mood, shunning of visual contacts, embarrassment caused by the condition, worry about others' reaction, sleeping impairment.

Figure 6.203 shows preoperative quality of life (includes telephonic/questionnaire survey of 326 patients)[83]

Figure 6.204 shows postoperative quality of life (includes telephonic/questionnaire survey of 326 patients)[83]

Complications

Morbidity was low in our study (around 4%), essentially due to CSF leak (3%, 11 patients out of 326 analyzed), hearing impairment to deafness in 0.6%, secondary transient facial weakness can occur by dormant viral resurgence after 10–14 days, and postoperative headache or Arnold neuralgia are uncommon. No mortality has been deplored in our experience.

The facial nerve through the posterior approach is not exposed and we have not observed immediate postoperative facial paralysis as it is reported to be transient or permanent in 3–20% in published series.[47,54–56,87,88] The only case of postoperative facial paralysis was in a particular case of revision surgery performed previously at another center with unsuccessful result and auditory nerve trauma; where the Dacron used for insulation was embedded in the root exit zone. The dilemma was to let the Dacron undisturbed and subsequently have persistent hemifacial spasm or to remove it with some injury to the facial nerve. The hemifacial spasm was cured with a facial weakness of the inferior branches. Delayed facial weakness after MVD of facial nerve can occur in up to 3% of cases. We observed delayed facial palsy at the 2nd or 3rd week, all being transient in nature without any long-term sequelae. The onset of weakness after operation is consistent in its timing, occurring on average 12 days after the procedure. The etiology of this complication is viral resurgence, and the palsy completely resolves within a month with a medical treatment with oral steroids and antiviral agents

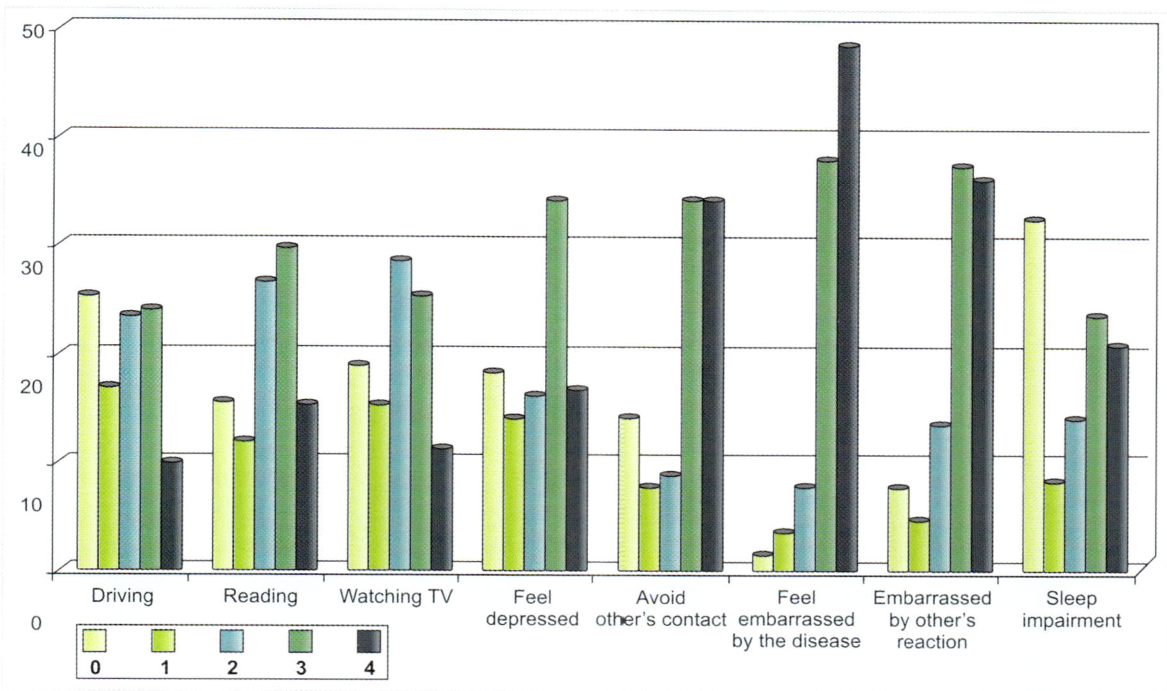

Fig. 6.203: Preoperative quality of life (includes telephonic/questionnaire survey of 326 patients)[83] in patients with hemifacial spasm

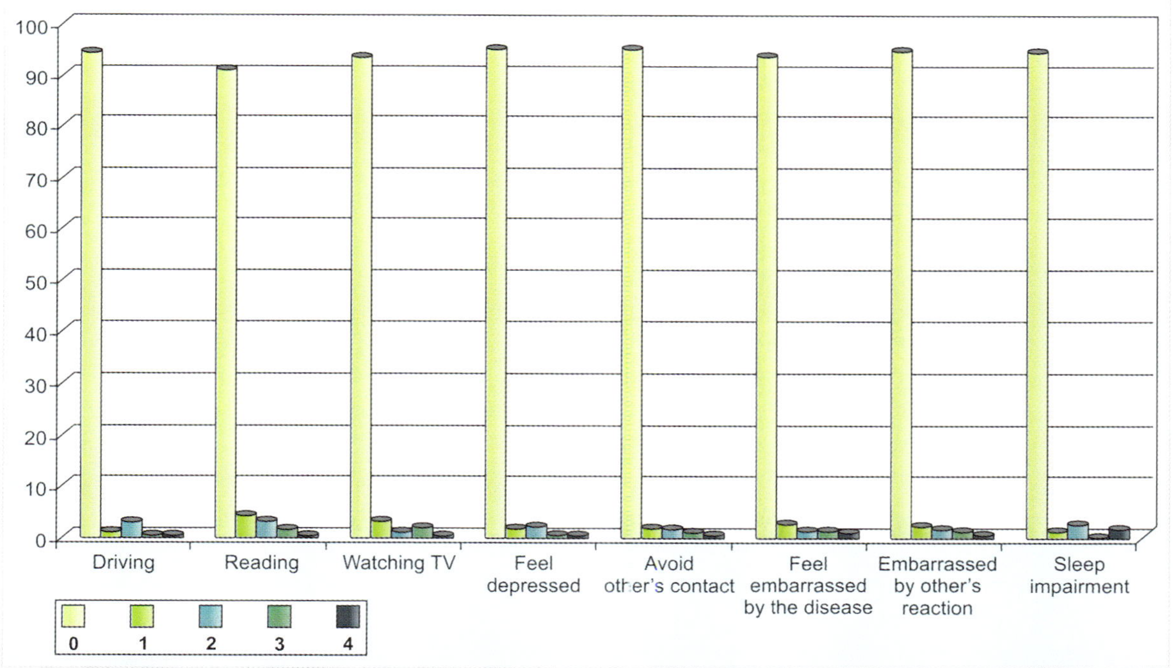

Fig. 6.204: Postoperative quality of life (includes telephonic/questionnaire survey of 326 patients)[83] in patients with hemifacial spasm

for 10 days.[93] The hearing impairment is the operative risk reported in all series. For us, this incident occurred in 5% of our first 116 cases (3 severe to profound permanent, 2 moderate transient hearing losses). There was no hearing impairment over the last 5 years. The use of intraoperative cochlear monitoring is an additional procedure to control the auditory pathway.

Safe handling of arterial loops is essential, so as not to cause spasm of them, particularly with regard to the anterior inferior cerebellar artery. Irrigation of the arteries with a solution of papaverine prevents ischemia related to spasm (Sindou et al.[90]). Obviously any direct trauma, traction or suction of the cochlear nerve should be prevented. The endoscopic maneuvers must be done carefully keeping in mind the potential risk of heating effect of the tip of the endoscope on the neural structures and especially the more fragile auditory nerve.

Conclusion

Hemifacial spasm is a very disabling disease with an impact on patients' self-image and the quality of life. Its pathophysiology remains unclear, probably involving vascular compression responsible for nervous deformity in the CNS segment of facial nerve, leading to intrinsic modifications of vascular walls contributing to focal demyelination and ectopic stimulation of facial nerve and a nuclear hyperactivity. The diagnosis is clinical, radiological examination by MRI allows eliminating differential diagnosis and gives surgeons a precise vascular mapping of the CPA, thanks to the use of high-resolution sequences T2 CISS sequences. The most common neurovascular conflicts occur between facial nerve at its root entry zone and the vertebral artery and/or the posterior inferior cerebellar artery. Surgical treatment based on neurovascular decompression combining the use of operating microscope, perioperative endoscope and facial nerve monitoring is the only curative treatment. It is efficient and has a very low morbidity rate. The good results obtained are long lasting and patients rapidly go back to the socio-professional lives they expected.

RESULTS AFTER MVD FOR UNILATERAL INCAPACITATING TINNITUS

The literature has sufficient data to prove that MVD can cure severe incapacitating tinnitus in carefully selected patients.[59,61,94–97] However, the success rate of this procedure is inferior to that of MVD for hemifacial spasm or trigeminal neuralgia, mainly because of the anatomic difficulty in isolating the offending vessels sometimes, in addition to the multitude of other confounding etiologies for tinnitus. Following MVD for tinnitus, a "good" result is considered as a patient who had a total resolution or a significant decrease in tinnitus.[59,61,94] The frequency of "good" results in the literature has ranged from 33 to 77% with more success in women than in men.[61] Some authors have performed revision surgeries before obtaining these final results of 77%.[94] The only report that exceeded this range was by Okamura et al.[95] who had 94% good results following the surgery. However, their selection criteria were much more flexible than the ones that we used for our patients, and they included cases of low-frequency fluctuating hearing loss and intermittent tinnitus.

As for the offending vessels and their relation to the results of MVD, it seems that when the vertebral artery was the offender, decompression gave the best results, compared to AICA or PICA decompression.[59]

Some authors have found a relation between the duration and character of the tinnitus and the postoperative results,[61] while we found no such relation.[59] We believe that ABR returns to normal in some patients who had good results for the tinnitus[59] and that hearing loss may also improve partially.[95]

Our Results[59]

Between 1994 and 2008, 60 patients with tinnitus underwent endoscope-assisted MVD. Among them 43 patients had a long-term follow up, 22 women and 21 men. The average age was 57 years old, ranging from 37 to 71 years old. The mean duration of tinnitus before surgery was 3.2 years (1–8 years).

Tinnitus

In the immediate postoperative period (7 days following surgery), we have found the following results:

- Total relief in 16/43 patients (37%)
- Marked improvement in 11/43 patients (26%)
- No improvement in tinnitus in 16/43 patients (37%).

At 2 months postoperatively, the results are the following:

- Total relief in 9 patients (21%)
- Marked improvement in 14 patients (33%)
- No improvement in 19 patients (44%)
- Worsening in 1 patient (2%).

At 2 years postoperatively, the results are the following:

- Total relief in 9 patients (21%)
- Marked improvement in 13 patients (31%)
- No improvement in 19 patients (44%)
- Worsening in 2 patients (4%).

The characteristics of the tinnitus (pulsatile nature, pitch, persistence or intermittency) are very labile parameters that were not quantified. In our series, the results did not change significantly with time after 2 months postoperatively. This is not consistent with the data of other authors who mention some improvement up to 1 year.

POSTOPERATIVE HEARING

It is reasonable to believe that when pulsatile compression on the cochlear nerve is released; hearing loss due to such compression might be improved. We considered that there is an improvement in hearing if there is a gain superior or equal to 5 dB over a minimum of 3 standard frequencies of the audiogram. As such, we found that 12 patients had an improvement of hearing over 3 or more frequencies. On the preoperative audiograms, we notice that the high frequencies were mostly altered (4000 and 8000 Hz). We found that the improvement by more than 5 dB over these 2 frequencies is present in 17 patients, but this improvement did not reach statistical significance ($p > 0.05$). Hearing remained unchanged in 20 subjects. On the other hand, eight patients presented a 5–10 dB worsening of their hearing, and one patient a more significant loss of more than 30 dB. Two causes might explain this complication: the manipulation of the arteries, or the thermal effect from the light of the tip of the endoscope. Two other patients had in the year following the surgery a loss of hearing: one patient had a sudden hearing loss 11 weeks after the surgery, which never recovered, and another patient had a fluctuating hearing loss.

Correlation Between Tinnitus and Hearing

There exists a significant statistical correlation between the resolution of the tinnitus and the improvement in hearing. In fact, a 5 dB improvement over at least three frequencies of the audiogram is statistically associated with a resolution of the tinnitus (Fisher exact test) ($p = 0.034$ for an improvement over three frequencies, $p = 0.009$ over four frequencies, and $p = 0.050$ over five frequencies). In addition, the sum of the auditory gains over the seven tested frequencies (250, 500, 1000, 2000, 4000, 6000 and 8000 Hz) is statistically different in the patients without any postoperative tinnitus compared to those who still have tinnitus. These former patients present an average sum of auditory gain of 20 dB ($p = 0.039$).

Correlation Between Tinnitus and ABR

The ABR returned to normal (I–III < 0.2 ms relative to the nonoperated side) in all patients who had successful results (total relief and marked improvement patients).

Correlation Between Tinnitus and VNG

Out of our 43 patients, only one had vestibular test normalization with relief of tinnitus.

Vascular Structures Responsible for the Conflict

We have grouped the causes of cochlear nerve compression into the following groups:

- AICA only: 18/43 (39%) (Fig. 6.9)
- AICA and PICA (pinching the nerve): 4/43 (9%)
- PICA with or without Vertebral artery: 12/43 (28%)
- Subarcuate artery ("hugging" the cochlear nerve): 7/43 (19%)
- Vein: 2/43 (5%) (when present, the cause-effect is questionable).

Though it might be difficult to predict the clinical results in relation to the incriminated vessel, it seems that the seven patients whose conflicts were related to the subarcuate artery had the best results. Among the seven operated cases, four had a total resolution of tinnitus, two had a decrease in tinnitus and one had no change. On the other hand, in cases of an aberrant vein or a vascular loop inside the internal auditory canal, there was no improvement at all. For the other cases, no statistical correlation was found between the incriminated vessel and the postoperative result.

Complications

In the surgeries of cochlear nerve decompression, no neurological sequelae were present postoperatively. There was no facial paralysis. There was one case of a profound hearing loss in the immediate postoperative period, probably related to a thermal heating effect from the tip of the endoscope. This happened in the earlier stages of our development of this technique. Two other hearing loss cases occurred in the first year after surgery. In one case, a sudden hearing loss appeared and did not recover despite an adequate medical treatment. In the other case, a fluctuating hearing loss occurred, with vertigo, establishing the diagnosis of Ménière's disease that manifested itself 6 months postoperatively.

Conclusion

When the neurovascular conflict is proven, decompression represents the only real treatment for these cases of tinnitus. This hypothesis is supported by the comparable management of hemifacial spasm and trigeminal neuralgia. Our patient selection criteria are unilateral tinnitus, positive offending vascular loop on MRI and retrocochlear ABR abnormalities. Out of 43 patients operated on by MVD of the cochlear nerve, the result was relief of tinnitus in 21% and decrease in its intensity in 31% of patients. There a significant statistical correlation between the resolution of tinnitus and the postoperative audiological evaluation confirming the concept of compression of the cochlear nerve. The failures of the VIIIth cranial nerve MVD must be analyzed with respect to the complex process of patient selection not yet definitively defined; the surgical findings which can limit the efficacy of the surgical procedure and the duration of the tinnitus with a central component.

In total, based on our experience with the MVD surgery using the minimally invasive endoscope-assisted retrosigmoid approach, we can reduce the patient morbidity whatever the patient age is, but we did not succeed in increasing the rate of successful results above 50%. MVD of the auditory cranial nerve is less rewarding when compared to MVD of the trigeminal or the facial cranial nerves. This can be explained first by the difficulty in making a certain diagnosis, and second, by the complexity of the offending vascular loop anatomy which could limit the surgical maneuver.

CONCLUSION

In our neuro-otological experience (1117 retrosigmoid approach surgeries for indications like vascular compression syndromes and vestibular neurotomy), we have very little morbidity. This should be the rule in the functional surgical indications. The most common surgical causes of incomplete cure are misjudgment of the real offending vessel and incomplete or improper replacement of the conflict vessel. The use of endoscope intraoperatively enhances the chances of visualization of offending vessels without increasing the amount of retraction of cerebellum and thus reducing the chances of complications like hearing loss and facial weakness. When there are multiple vessels running closely to the nerve, a real offending vessel that compressed REZ should be accurately diagnosed. If that is not possible, as usually is the case, all the conflicting vessels (even vein) should be decompressed. If prosthesis was inappropriately inserted, decompression of REZ may not be satisfactory or it may cause recompression. One of the most common causes of recurrence is adhesions between the nerve at REZ and Teflon pledget leading to recompression. To avoid such incomplete cure or recurrences, Teflon should not be inserted between REZ and offending vessel as much as possible, but away from REZ, preferably between offending vessel and the brainstem. Furthermore, we have lately used fibrofatty subcutaneous tissue, especially in trigeminal neuralgia, to prevent recompression with Teflon pledgets in certain difficult situations. The loop of the offending vessel can be fixed to nearby dura with the use of fibrin glue. Intraoperative monitoring of the facial and cochlear nerve function by antidromic stimulation improves the value of monitoring as it gives real time information and thus helps in better prevention of these complications. The absence of AMR or lateral spread intraoperatively should be pursued in all cases of hemifacial spasm for increasing the success of MVD.

REFERENCES

1. De Ridder D, Møller A, Verlooy J, Cornelissen M, De Ridder L. Is the root entry/exit zone important in microvascular compression syndromes? Neurosurgery. 2002;51:427–34.
2. Katusic S, Beard CM, Bergstralh E, Kurland LT. Incidence and clinical features of trigeminal neuralgia: Rochester, Minnesota, 1945–1984. Ann Neurol. 1990;27:89–95.
3. Auger RG, Whisnant JP. Hemifacial spasm in Rochester and Olmsted County, Minnesota, 1960 to 1984. Arch Neurol. 1990;47:1233–4.
4. Fraioli B, Esposito V, Ferrante L, Trubiani L, Lunardi P. Microsurgical treatment of glossopharyngeal neuralgia: case reports. Neurosurgery. 1989;25:630–2.
5. Jannetta PJ. Microsurgery of cranial cross-compression. Clin Neurosurg. 1979;26:607–15.
6. Leclercq TA, Hill CL, Grisoli F. Retromastoid microsurgical approach to vascular compression of the eighth cranial nerve. Laryngoscope. 1980;90:1011–7.
7. Ryu H, Yamamoto S, Sugiyama K, Nishizawa S, Nozue M. Neurovascular compression syndrome of the eighth cranial nerve: can the site of compression explain the symptoms? Acta Neurochir (Wien). 1999;141:495–501.
8. Møller AR. Vascular compression of cranial nerves: Part II—Pathophysiology. Neurol Res. 1999;21:439–43.
9. Nielsen VK. Pathophysiology of hemifacial spasm, I: ephaptic transmission and ectopic excitation. Neurology. 1984;34:418–26.
10. Love S, Coakham H. Trigeminal neuralgia: pathology and pathogenesis. Brain. 2001;124:2347–60.
11. Møller AR. Cranial nerve dysfunction syndromes: pathophysiology of microvascular compression. In: Barrow DL (Ed.). Neurosurgical topics book 13: surgery of cranial nerves of the posterior fossa. Park Ridge: AANS; 1993, pp 105–29.
12. Ferguson JH. Hemifacial spasm and the facial nucleus. Ann Neurol. 1978;4:97–103.
13. Fromm GH. Pathophysiology of trigeminal neuralgia. In: Fromm GH, Sessle BJ (Eds.). Trigeminal neuralgia. Boston: Butterworth Heinemann; 1991, pp 105–30.
14. Møller AR, Janetta PJ. Microvascular decompression of hemifacial spasm; intraoperative electrophysiological observations. Neurosurgery. 1985;16:612–8.

15. Adams CBT. Microvascular compression. An alternative view and hypothesis. J Neurosurg. 1989;57:1-12.
16. Girard N, Poncet M, Caces F, Tallon Y, Chays A, Martin-Bouyer P, Magnan J, Raybaud C. Three dimensional MRI of hemifacial spasm with surgical correlation. Neuroradiology. 1997;39(1):46-51.
17. Elaini S, Miyazaki H, Rameh C, Deveze A, Magnan J. Correlation between magnetic resonance imaging and surgical findings in vasculo-neural compression syndrome. Int Adv Otol. 2009;5(Suppl):1-23.
18. Tash R, DeMerrit J, Sze G, et al. Hemifacial spasm: MR imaging features. AJNR Am J Neuroradiol. 1991;12:839-42.
19. Tien RD, Wilkins RH. MRA delineation of the vertebro-basilar system in patients with hemifacial spasm and trigeminal neuralgia. AJNR Am J Neuroradiol. 1993;14: 34-6.
20. Adler CH, Zimmerman RA, Savino PJ, et al. Hemifacial spasm: evaluation by magnetic resonance imaging and magnetic resonance tomographic angiography. Ann Neurol. 1992;32:502-6.
21. Hosoya T, Watanabe N, Yamaguchi K, et al. Three-dimensional MRI of neurovascular compression in patients with hemifacial spasm. Neuroradiology. 1995;37:350-2.
22. Du C, Korogi Y, Nagahiro S, et al. Hemifacial spasm: three dimensional MR images in the evaluation of neurovascular compression. Radiology. 1995;197:227-31.
23. Dandy WE. Concerning the cause of trigeminal neuralgia. Am J Surg. 1934;24:447-55.
24. Gardner WJ, Milkos MV. Response of trigeminal neuralgia to decompression of sensory root: discussion of cause of trigeminal neuralgia. JAMA. 1959;170:1773-6.
25. Gardner WJ. Concerning the mechanism of trigeminal neuralgia and hemifacial spasm. J Neurosurg. 1962;19: 947-58.
26. Jannetta PJ, Rand RW. Transtentorial gasserian rhizotomy in trigeminal neuralgia by microsurgical technique. Bull Neurol Soc (Los Angeles). 1966;31:93-9.
27. Jannetta PJ. Arterial compression of the trigeminal nerve at the pons in patients with trigeminal neuralgia. J Neurosurg. 1967;26:159-62.
28. Jannetta PJ. Microsurgical approach to the trigeminal nerve for tic douloureux. Prog Neurol Surg. 1976;7:180-200.
29. Andre NA. Observations. College et de l'Academie Royale de Chirargie. Paris: Delaguette; 1756. Cited by: Rose FC in Trigeminal neuralgia. Arch Neurol. 1999;56:1163-4.
30. Katusic S, Beard CM, Bergstralh E, Kurland LT. Incidence and clinical features of trigeminal neuralgia, Rochester, Minnesota, 1945-1984. Ann Neurol. 1990;27:89-95.
31. Barker FG 2nd, Jannetta PJ, Bissonette DJ, Larkins MV, Jho HD. The long-term outcome of microvascular decompression for trigeminal neuralgia. N Engl J Med. 1996;334:1077-83.
32. Kondo, Akinori. Follow-up results of microvascular decompression in trigeminal neuralgia and hemifacial spasm. Neurosurgery. 1997;40(1):46-52.
33. Miyazaki H, Deveze A, Magnan J. Neuro-otologic surgery through minimally invasive retrosigmoid approach; endoscope-assisted microvascular decompression, vestibular neurotomy, and tumor removal. Laryngoscope. 2005;115(9);1612-7.
34. Sindou M, Leston J, Decullier E, Chapuis F. Microvascular decompression for primary trigeminal neuralgia: long-term effectiveness and prognostic factors in a series of 362 consecutive patients with clear-cut neurovascular conflicts who underwent pure decompression. J Neurosurg. 2007;107:1144-53.
35. Tyler-Kabara E, Kassam A, Horowitz M, Urgo L, Hadjipanayis C, Levy E, Chang Y. Predictors of outcome in surgically managed patients with typical and atypical trigeminal neuralgia: comparison of results following microvascular decompression. J Neurosurg. 2002;96: 527-31.
36. Gowers R (Ed.). Manual of diseases of the nervous system. London: J & A Churchill; 1888.
37. Hunt J. The sensory system of the facial nerve and its symptomatology. J Nerv Ment Dis. 1909;36:321-50.
38. Sicard J, Bollack M. L'hémispasme facial d'origine corticale cérébrale. Rev Neurol. 1912;24:742-3.
39. Wartenberg R. Hemifacial spasm, a clinical and pathophysiological study. New York: Oxford University Press; 1952.
40. Alajouanine T, Thurel R. Les spasmes de la face et leurs traitements. Paris: Masson; 1936.
41. Gardner WJ, Sava GA. Hemifacial spasm: a reversible pathophysiologic state. J Neurosurg. 1962;19:240-7.
42. Jannetta PJ, Hackett E, Ruby JR. Electromyographic and electron microscopic correlates in hemifacial spasm treated by microsurgical relief of neurovascular compression. Surg Forum. 1970;21:449-51.
43. Jannetta PJ. Microsurgical exploration and decompression of the facial nerve in hemifacial spasm. Curr Top Surg Res. 1970;2:217-20.
44. Auger RG, Whisnant JP. Hemifacial spasm in Rochester and Olmstead County, Minnesota, 1960 to 1984. Arch Neurol. 1990;47:1233-4.
45. Badr-el-Dine M, El-Garem H, Talaat A, Magnan J. Endoscopically assisted minimally invasive microvascular decompression of hemifacial spasm. Otol Neurotol. 2002;23:122-8.
46. Magnan J, Chays A, Caces F, et al. Place de l'endoscopie et de la decompression vasculaire dans le traitement du spasme de l'hemiface. Ann Oto-laryngol. 1994;111:153-60.
47. Barker II FG, Jannetta PJ, Bissonette DJ, et al. Microvascular decompression for hemifacial spasm. J Neurosurg. 1995;82:201-10.
48. Mauriello J, Aljian J. Natural history of treatment of facial dyskinesias with botulinum toxin: a study of 50 consecutive patients over seven years. Br Ophthalmol. 1991;75:737-9.
49. Yoshimura DM, Aminoff M, Tami TA, Scott AB. Treatment of hemifacial spasm with botulinum toxin. Muscle Nerve 1992;15:1045-9.

50. Kalra HK, Magoon EH. Side effects of the use of botulinum toxin for treatment of benign essential blepharospasm and hemifacial spasm. Opthalmic Surg. 1990;21:335–8.
51. Taylor JDN, Kraft SP, Kazdan MS, et al. Treatment of blepharospasm and hemifacial spasm with botulinum A toxin: a Canadian multicentre study. Can J Ophthalmol. 1991;26:133–8.
52. Magnan J, Caces F, Locatelli P, Chays A. Hemifacial spasm: endoscopic vascular decompression. Otolaryngol Head Neck Surg. 1997;117:308–14.
53. Kim P, Fukushima T. Observations on synkinesis in patients with hemifacial spasm. Effects of microvascular decompression and aetiological considerations. Neurosurgery 1984;60:821–7.
54. Samii M, Gunther T, et al. Microvascular decompression to treat hemifacial spasm: long-term results for a consecutive series of 143 patients. Neurosurgery. 2002;50:712–9.
55. Sindou, MP. Microvascular decompression for primary hemifacial spasm. Importance of intraoperative neurophysiological monitoring. Acta Neurochir (Wien). 2005;147:1019–26.
56. Moffat D, Durvasula V, et al. Outcome following retrosigmoid microvascular decompression of the facial nerve for hemifacial spasm. J Laryngol Otol. 2005;119: 779–83.
57. Magnan J, Chays A, Lepetre C, et al. Surgical perspectives on endoscopy of the cerebellopontine angle. Am J Otol. 1994;15:366–70.
58. Magnan J, Chays A, Cohen OM, et al. Endoscopy of the cerebellopontine angle. Am J Otol. 1995;16:115–8.
59. Guevara N, Deveze A, Buza V, Laffont B, Magnan J. Microvascular decompression of cochlear nerve for incapacitating tinnitus: pre-surgical data, surgical analyses and long-term follow-up of 15 patients. Eur Arch Otorhinolaryngol. 2008;265:397–401.
60. Reed GF. An audiometric study of two hundred cases of subjective tinnitus, Arch Otolaryngol. 1960;71:94–104.
61. Moller MB, Moller AR, Jannetta PJ, Jho HD. Vascular decompression surgery for severe tinnitus: selection criteria and results. Laryngoscope. 1993;103:421–7.
62. Jannetta P. Neurovascular cross compression in patients with hyperactive dysfunction of the eighth cranial nerve. Surg Forum. 1975;26:467–9.
63. Jannetta P, Moller M, Moller A. Disabling positional vertigo (DPV). New Engl J Med. 1984;310:1700–5.
64. Moller M. Results of microvascular decompression (MVD) of the eighth nerve as treatment of disabling positional vertigo (DPV). Ann Otol Rhinol Laryngol. 1990;99:724–9.
65. McCabe B, Gantz B. Vascular loop as a cause of incapacitating dizziness. Am J Otol. 1989;10(2):117–20.
66. Schwaber M, Hall J. Cochleovestibular compression syndrome: clinical features and audiovestibular findings. Laryngoscope. 1992;102:1021–9.
67. Brackmann D, Kesser A, Day JD. Microvascular decompression of the vestibulocochlear nerve for disabling positional vertigo. The House ear clinic experience. Otol Neurotol. 2001;22:882–7.
68. Bergsneider M, Becker D. Vascular compression syndrome of the vestibular nerve. A critical analysis. Otolaryngol Head neck Surg. 1995;112:118–23.
69. Schwaber M. Vascular compression syndromes. In: Jackler R, Brackmann D (Eds.). Neurotology. Mosby. 1993; 881–903.
70. Herzog J, Bealey S, Meyer J. Vascular loop of the internal auditory canal: a diagnostic dilemma. Am J Otol. 1997;18:26–31.
71. Makins A, Nikolopoulos T, Ludman C, O'Donoghue G. Is there a correlation between vascular loops an unilateral auditory symptoms. Laryngoscope. 1998;108:1739–42.
72. Sakaki T, Morimoto T, Miyamoto S, et al. Microsurgical treatment of patients with vestibular and cochlear symptoms. Surg Neurol. 1987;27:141–6.
73. Magnan J, El Garem H, Deveze A, Lavieille J. The value of endoscopy in the surgical management of vertigo. Mediterr J Otol. 2006;2:1–8.
74. Harris W. Persistent pain in lesions of the peripheral and central nervous system. Brain. 1921;44:557–71.
75. White J, Sweet WH. A forty year experience: pain and the neurosurgeon. Springfield, IL: Charles C Thomas; 1969, pp 265–302.
76. Fraioli B, Esposito V, Ferrante L, et al. Microsurgical treatment of glossopharyngeal neuralgia: case reports. Neurosurgery. 1989;25:630–2.
77. Kandan SR, Khan S, Jeyaretna DS, Lhatoo S, Patel NK, Coakham HB. Neuralgia of the glossopharyngeal and vagal nerves: long-term outcome following surgical treatment and literature review. Br J Neurosurg. 2010;24:441–6.
78. Sindou M, Keravel Y. Neurosurgical treatment of vago-glossopharyngeal neuralgia. Neurochirurgie. 2009;55:231–5.
79. Rushton JG, Stevens JC, Miller RH. Glossopharyngeal (vagoglossopharyngeal) neuralgia: a study of 217 cases. Arch Neurol. 1981;38:201–5.
80. McLaughlin MR, Jannetta PJ, Clyde BL, et al. Microvascular decompression of cranial nerves: lessons learned after 4400 operations. J Neurosurg. 1999;90:1–8.
81. El-Garem H, Badr-El-Dine M, Talaat AM, Magnan J, Endoscopy as a tool in minimally invasive trigeminal neuralgia surgery, Otol Neurotol 2002:23(2):132-5.
82. Balansard C, Meller R, Bruzzo M, Chays A, Girard N, Magnan J. Trigeminal neuralgia: results of microsurgical and endoscopic-assisted vascular decompression. Annales d'oto-laryngologie et de chirurgie cervico faciale. 2003;120(6):330–7.
83. Curto CL, Magnan J. Hemifacial spasm. Thesis. Aix Marseille University, Marseille, France.
84. Broggi G, Ferroli P, Franzini A, Servello D, Dones I. Microvascular decompression for trigeminal neuralgia: comments on a series of 250 cases, including 10 patients with multiple sclerosis. J Neurol Neurosurg Psychiatr. 2000;68:59–64.
85. Sun T, Saito SH, Nakai O, Ando T: Long-term results of microvascular decompression for trigeminal neuralgia with reference to probability of recurrence. Acta Neurochir 1994; 126:144–148.

86. Oesman C, Mooij J. Long-term follow-up of microvascular decompression for trigeminal neuralgia. Skull Base 2011; 21: 313–322.
87. Huh R, Han I, Moon J, Chang J, Chung S. Microvascular decompression for hemifacial spasm: analyses of operative complications in 1582 consecutive patients. Surgical Neurology 2008; 69: 153–157.
88. Park J, Kong D, Lee J. Hemifacial spasm: neurovascular compressive patterns and surgical significance. Acta Neurochirur 2008; 150: 235–241.
89. Goto Y, Matsushima T, et al. Delayed effects of the microvascular decompression on hemifacial spasm: a retrospective study of 131 consecutive operated cases. Neurol Res. 2002;24:296–300.
90. Sindou M, Keravel Y. Neurosurgical treatment of primary hemifacial spasm with microvascular decompression. (In French) Neurochirurgie. 2009;55:236–247.
91. Tan E, Fook-Chong S, et al. Validation of a short disease specific quality of life scale for hemifacial spasm: correlation with SF-36. J Neurol Neurosurg Psychiatr. 2005;76:1707–10.
92. Badr-El-Dine M, El-Garem H, Talaat A, Magnan J. Endoscopically assisted minimally invasive microvascular decompression of hemifacial spasm. Otol Neurotol. 2002;23(2):122–8.
93. Lovely T, Getch C, Jannetta P. Delayed facial weakness after microvascular decompression of cranial nerve VII. Surg Neurol. 1998;50:449–52.
94. Brookes GB. Vascular decompression surgery for severe tinnitus. Am J Otol. 1996;17:569–76.
95. Okamura T, Kurokawa Y, Ikeda N, Abiko S, Ideguchi M, Watanabe K, Kido T. Microvascular decompression for cochlear symptoms. J Neurosurg. 2000;93:421–6.
96. Ryu H, Yamamoto S, Sugiyama K. Neurovascular compression syndrome of the eight cranial nerve. What are the most reliable diagnostic signs? Acta Neurochir (Wien). 1998;140:1279–86.
97. Vasama JP, Moller MB, Moller AR. Microvascular decompression of the cochlear nerve in patients with severe tinnitus. preoperative findings and operative outcome in 22 patients. Neurol Res. 1998;20:242–8.

7 Hearing Preservation Surgery for Acoustic Neuroma

INTRODUCTION

The ultimate principle of acoustic neuroma surgery is complete removal of tumor without producing additional neurological damage. This principle and the fact that acoustic neuroma (AN) is a vestibular schwannoma provide the basis for the preservation of residual hearing and facial nerve function. Thanks to the continuous advances in imaging assessment, acoustic neuroma is detected at its earlier so-called otologic stage. More and more often it appears as a tumor of the vestibulocochlear nerve bundle without the signs of brainstem compression. Nowadays more emphasis is on the refinement of steps for optimization of preserving the preoperative hearing level.

The various options for treatment of AN include surgical excision, stereotactic radiation therapy and observation with serial magnetic resonance imaging (MRI). Currently, no randomized, prospective clinical trial has compared the three treatment options and there are no clearly accepted, evidence-based, best practices for managing AN.[1] While surgery is the uncontroversial option for large tumors with brainstem compression and hydrocephalus, the decision making is still controversial in patients with smaller acoustic tumors, especially less than 2 cm. All three options are potentially useful, and unbiased provision of information to help them decide on a path of treatment is mandatory for proper informed consent. Fortunately, stereotactic radiotherapy protocols[2–5] and surgical techniques[6–10] have evolved in the past 30 years resulting in more safety for patients. Most of the studies in literature are retrospective and did not adhere to consistent and validated standards for hearing preservation, facial nerve function, or balance disturbance, especially for the literature involving radiotherapy. Most surgical complications occur within the first week of resection, whereas some radiotherapy complications may occur many years after treatment is complete. The patients are informed about the risks and benefits of all the three options.

The advantages of radiotherapy are avoidance of surgery and its related morbidity, and theoretical chance of mortality (though it is rare nowadays). Also with modern radiotherapy options, the chances for hearing preservation and facial neuropathy are same as good centers for surgery. Following radiotherapy, there are occasional cases, fortunately extremely rare, of immediate intracranial hypertension, accelerated hydrocephalus or explosive evolution in the long term,[11–13] suggesting great caution in both young and elderly patients. There may be viable tumor cells following radiation therapy and may show growth after a dormant period. There are rare but real chances of getting the tumor malignant over the years.[14,15] The reported incidence of malignant conversion is growing (0.3%)[4] with increasing literature on radiotherapy. Therefore, undergoing radiotherapy means living with the tumor, though in dormant form and permission to undergo regular imaging for the life time.

Observation followed by serial follow-up MRI[16,17] is a choice that we leave to the patient. We suggest this approach to medically unfit or elderly (more than 70 years) patients or in case of a small tumor that is a few mm in size. Till date, we do not have a way to predict which patients have growing tumor. So this choice means a delay of the problem in considerable number of patients for the moment when surgical conditions can be less favorable and hearing preservation results, worse. The monitoring is done by MRI after 1 year (6 months is too short a period to see obvious growth of the tumor size), and then repeated every year. Any significant increase in size will then be in favor of a surgical excision.

As surgeons, we are of course biased toward surgical options. Our first reported hearing preservation surgery by retrosigmoid approach for AN was in 1980[18] and we have been striving to improve the results over time with significant success.[6] With surgery, there are risks for associated complications most common among them being the cerebrospinal fluid (CSF) leak (less than 3% in our cases). The incidence for permanent facial palsy after surgery in reputed centers (including ours) and after radiotherapy is not much different (around 3% for small to medium tumors less than 2.5 cm). Whatever the therapy adopted, monitoring, surgery or radiotherapy, the preservation of useful hearing should never prevail over facial function.

OUR TREATMENT PHILOSOPHY IN ACOUSTIC NEUROMA SURGERY

Our personal preference is for translabyrinthine approach for larger tumors with poor hearing (speech discrimination score of less than 50% irrespective of pure tone averages) where hearing preservation is not of much clinical use for the patient. In all the patients of AN eligible for hearing preservation (speech discrimination score better than 70% and pure tone averages better than 50 dB), we prefer the retrosigmoid approach, irrespective of its proximity to the fundus or vestibule. Hearing preservation surgery for AN has been attempted since 1968[19,20] with successful hearing preservation in a small percentage (around 20–30%) using either middle fossa or retrosigmoid approach.[18-22] The hearing preservation rates have significantly improved in the past decade[8-10] and this is increasing with the help of intraoperative direct cochlear nucleus monitoring.

Retrosigmoid approach allows a minimally invasive access that means minimal morbidity, even in elderly patients.[23] This "keyhole" approach compared to the traditional suboccipital approach, offers a control of all neurovascular structures crossing the cerebellopontine angle (CPA). The retrosigmoid approach presents remarkable advantages: immediate and accurate identification of tumor, internal auditory canal (IAC) and adjacent neurovascular structures. Moreover, it allows excellent preservation of facial nerve function as the facial nerve is deeper than the tumor plane. Lastly, it offers hearing preservation from 18% to 75%.[24-37] The disadvantage is the legendary gravity of the posterior suboccipital approach, which suggests retrosigmoid approach as not allowing direct control of the lateral fundus part of the internal auditory meatus (IAM) without opening the labyrinth and has been reported as a technique of higher risk for residual tumor.[38,39] Actually, it was demonstrated that risk depends more on the operator than on the approach. Endoscopy-assisted surgery for removal of tumor from the lateral end of fundus of IAM has drastically improved the complete tumor removal with preservation of hearing.[40,41] In our study of 106 patients, out of 3 patients suspected of having residual tumor, after MRI monitoring after a median duration of four years, only one presented a tumor fragment necessarily requiring revision surgery. The surgical revision was performed by retrosigmoid approach with no alteration of hearing and facial function for the patient. The disadvantages of classical retrosigmoid approach are greater incidence of headache or CSF leak, which has not been the case with minimally invasive retrosigmoid approach (MIRA) (CSF leak rate of 3% and virtually no headache). Most of our cases did not require intensive care therapy, which means excellent cost–benefit ratio.

Middle fossa approach in selected intracanalicular tumors has remarkable percentage of hearing preservation reported by some authors.[8-10] The disadvantage of middle fossa approach is comparably lower preservation of facial nerve function and relative difficulty in removing tumors with substantial extension into the cerebellopontine angle (CPA) (though it can be overcome with extended approach after dividing superior petrosal sinus).

Indication

Our indications were related to tumor size and the preoperative hearing threshold. In intracanalicular neuromas and ANs less than 2 cm in CPA with preservable hearing, we prefer the retrosigmoid approach. In neuromas greater than 2 cm in CPA, we prefer the translabyrinthine approach. But there may be unusual cases where hearing preservation is most important for patients such as unilateral hearing or bilateral neuromas where we may prefer combined retrosigmoid with presigmoid retrolabyrinthine approach in larger tumors.

To grade the tumor stages and to compare results we use Zini Magnan's classification,[42] which is a modification of Tos's classification.[43] This grading is based on MRI studies and intraoperative data.

- Stage 1: Intracanalicular tumor (Figs 7.1 to 7.4).
- Stage 2: Small tumor, up to 10 mm, in CPA, no contact with the brainstem (Figs 7.5 to 7.9).

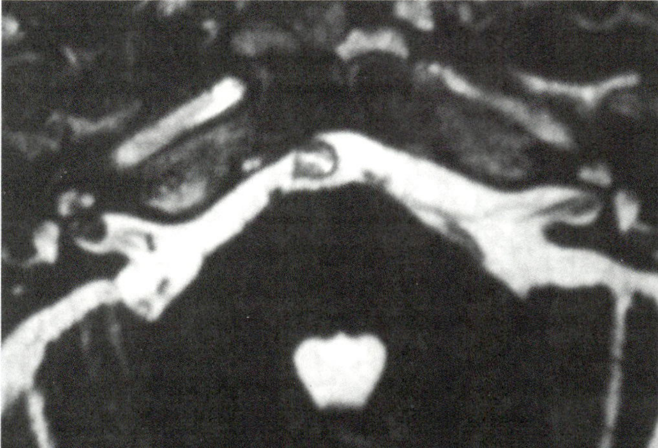

Fig. 7.1: MRI T2 sequence picture showing Stage 1 intracanalicular AN tumor occupying the fundus of right internal auditory meatus

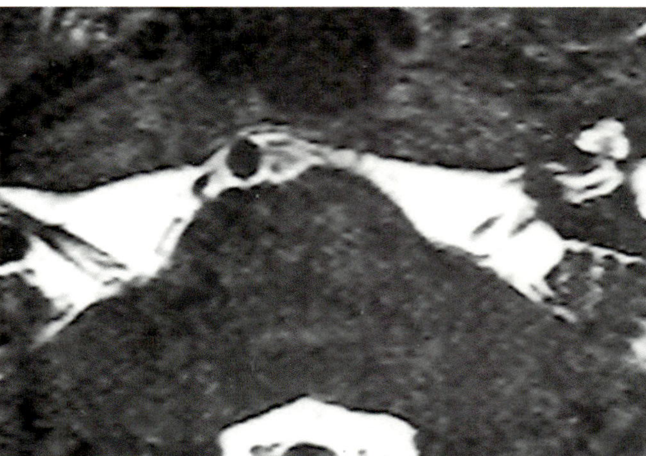

Fig. 7.2: MRI T2 sequence picture showing Stage 1 intracanalicular AN tumor with the fundus of left internal auditory meatus free of tumor

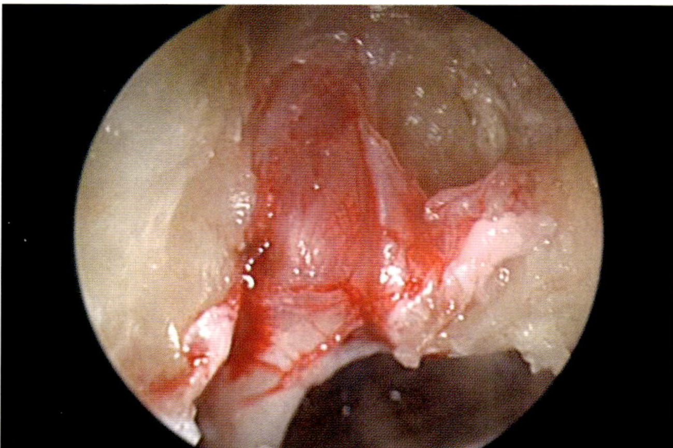

Fig. 7.3: Endoscopic view of Stage 1 intracanalicular AN tumor after drilling of internal auditory meatus

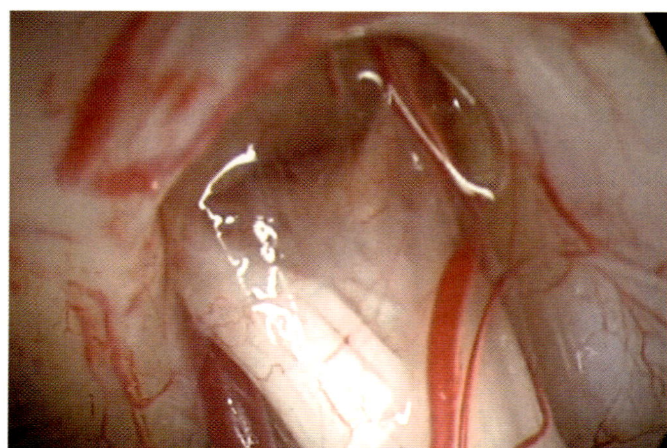

Fig. 7.4: Endoscopic view of Stage 1 intracanalicular AN tumor

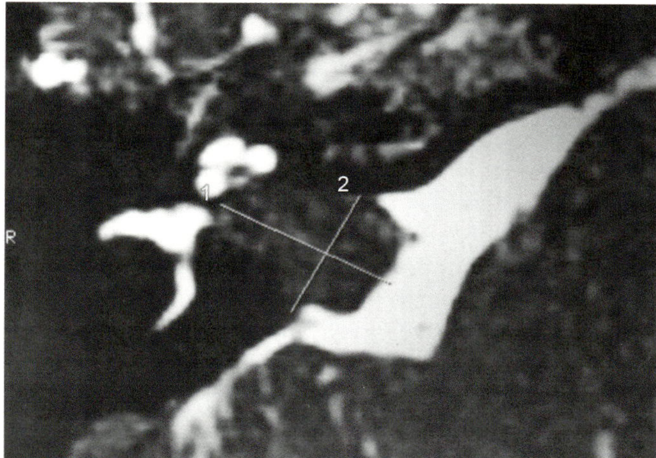

Fig. 7.5: MRI T2 sequence picture showing Stage 2 AN tumor occupying the fundus of internal auditory meatus

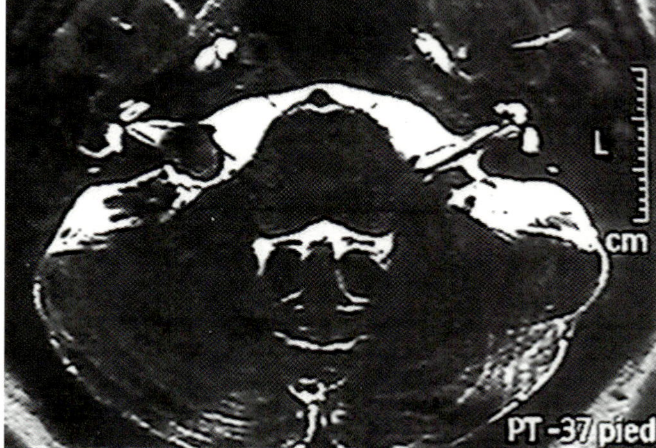

Fig. 7.6: MRI T2 sequence picture showing Stage 2 AN tumor with the fundus of internal auditory meatus free of tumor

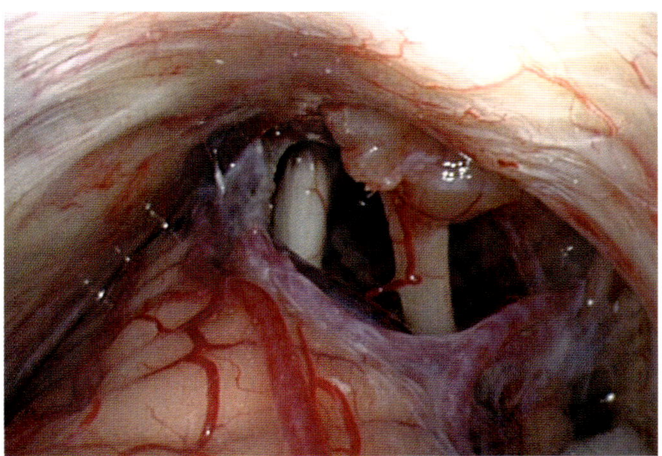
Fig. 7.7: Endoscopic view of Stage 2 AN tumor in CPA, with no contact with the brainstem

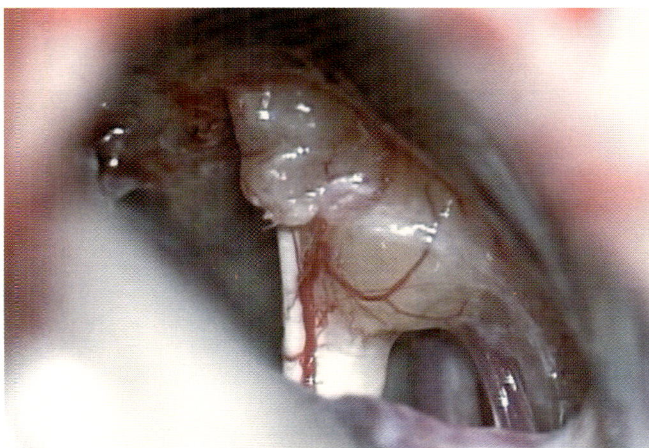
Fig. 7.8: Microscopic view of Stage 2 AN tumor in CPA, with no contact with the brainstem

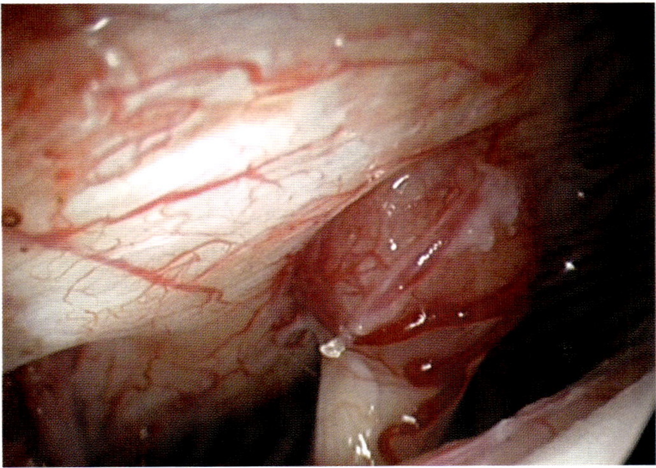
Fig. 7.9: Endoscopic view of Stage 2 AN tumor in CPA, with no contact with the brainstem

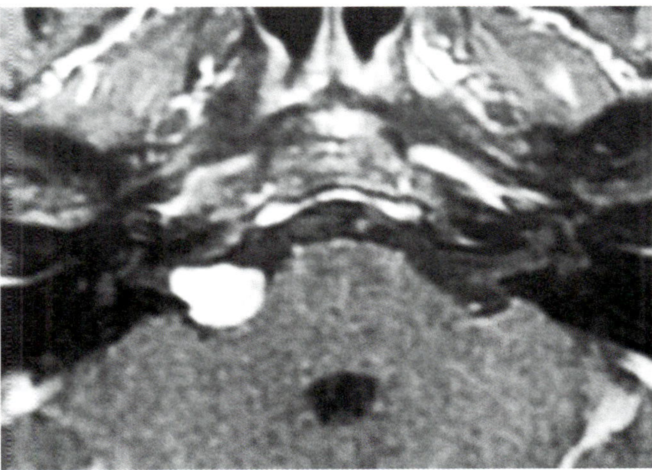
Fig. 7.10: Magnetic resonance imaging T1 sequence with gadolinium contrast showing Stage 3 AN tumor with the fundus of internal auditory meatus free from tumor

- Stage 3: Medium tumor, 11–25 mm, within CPA, touching and embedding the brainstem without distortion (Figs 7.10 to 7.13).
- Stage 4: Large tumor, 25–40 mm, with distortion of the brainstem and displacement of the IV ventricle (Fig. 7.14).
- Stage 5: Giant tumor, greater than 40 mm, extended over the middle line (Figs 7.15 and 7.16).

It is worth knowing that the distance between the porus acousticus and the midline is about 25–30 mm. Also, there are no radiological features to differentiate the AN from the facial schwannoma and the diagnosis is often made intraoperatively (Figs 7.17 to 7.19).

For each stage we used a further classification according to intracanalicular extension:

- *A (for absent)*: Tumor process absent in IAC.
- *B (for between)*: IAC fundus free of tumor process (Figs 7.2, 7.6, 7.10, 7.11 and 7.20).
- *C (for complete)*: IAC completely filled with tumor (Figs 7.1, 7.5, 7.15 and 7.21).

SURGICAL TECHNIQUE

Approach

The details of patient position, retrosigmoid exposure and craniotomy have already been discussed in Chapter 3 on MIRA. The key steps for MIRA as used for removal of Stage 1, 2 and 3 AN with grade A, B or C extension into the IAC by endoscope-guided retrosigmoid approach includes retrosigmoid craniotomy (Fig. 7.22), opening of cistern

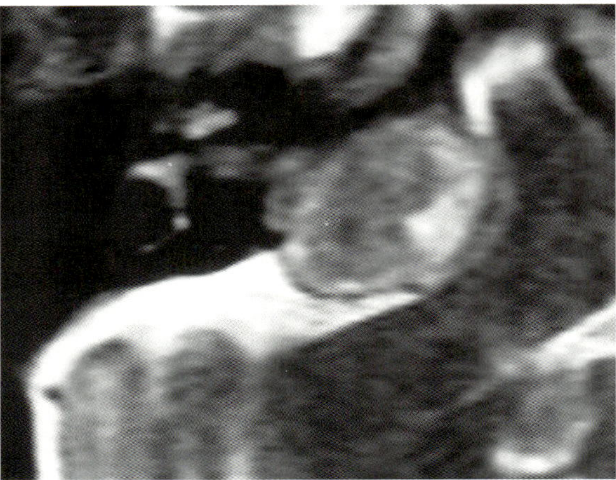

Fig. 7.11: Magnetic resonance imaging T2 sequence picture showing Stage 3 AN tumor with the fundus of internal auditory meatus free from tumor

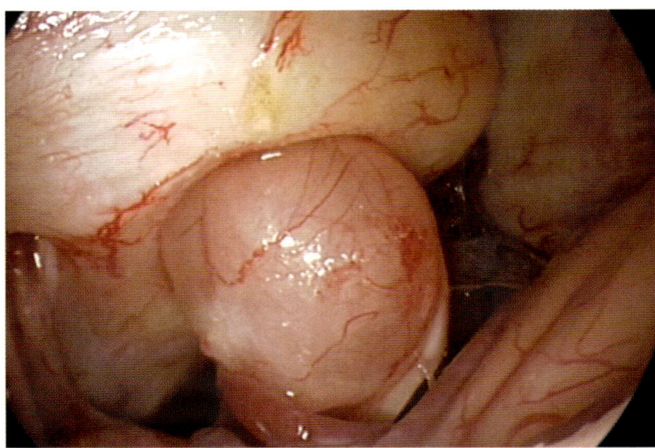

Fig. 7.12: Endoscopic view of Stage 3 AN tumor, within CPA, not touching the brainstem

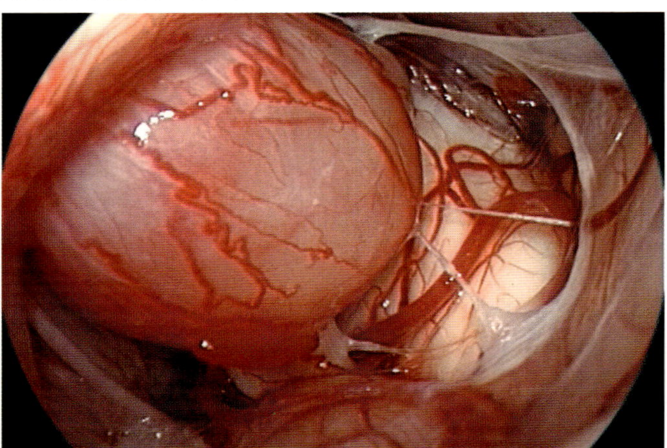

Fig. 7.13: Endoscopic view of Stage 3 AN tumor, just touching the brainstem without its distortion.

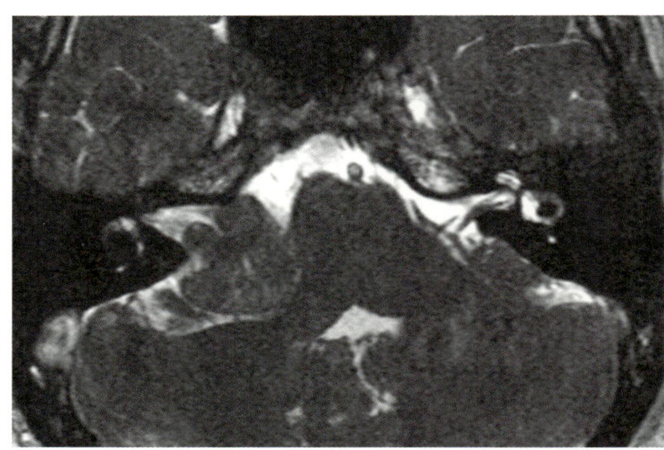

Fig. 7.14: Axial MRI in T2 sequence right Stage 3 AN tumor with brainstem distortion

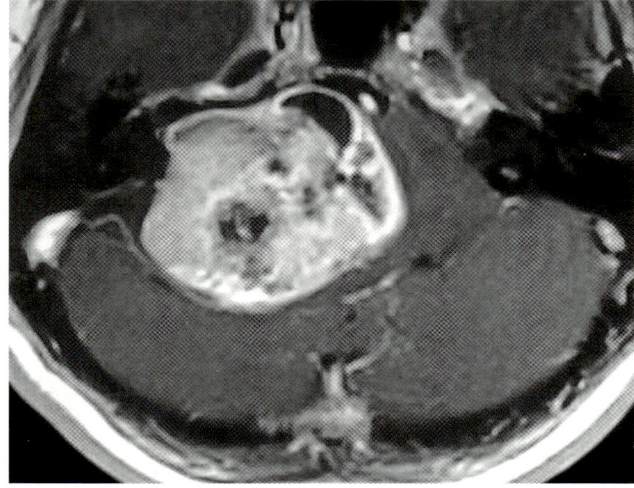

Fig. 7.15: Axial MRI with contrast showing giant Stage 5 AN tumor with distortion of the brainstem with midline shift

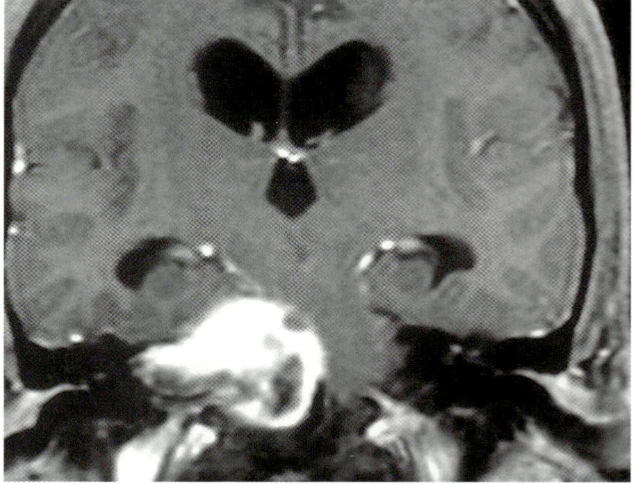

Fig. 7.16: Coronal MRI with contrast showing giant Stage 5 AN tumor with distortion of the brainstem and displacement of the IV ventricle

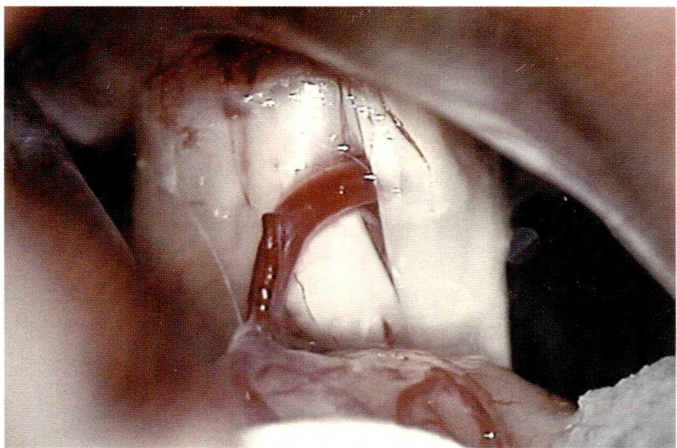

Fig. 7.17: Microscopic view of facial schwannoma with intact vestibulocochlear nerve fibers

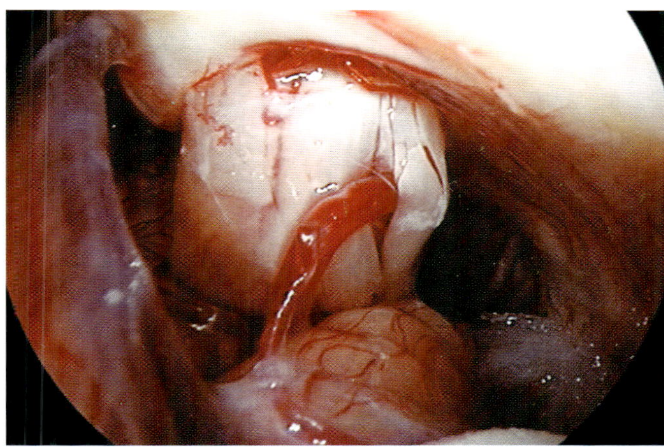

Fig. 7.18: Endoscopic view of facial schwannoma arising from anterosuperior part of porus with intact vestibulocochlear nerve fibers

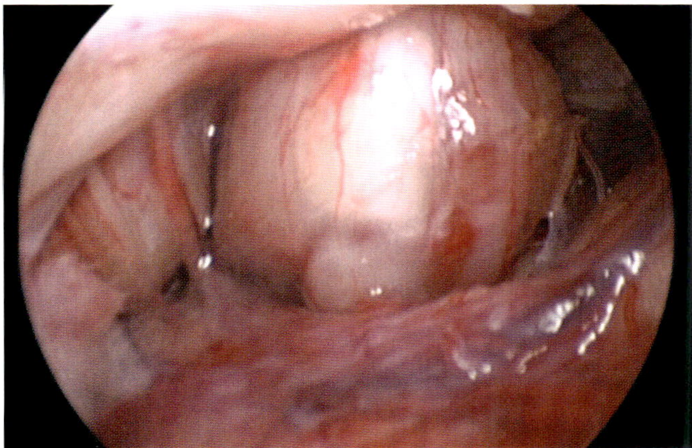

Fig. 7.19: Endoscopic view of Stage 3 facial schwannoma with intact but stretched vestibulocochlear nerve fibers with normal facial function preoperatively

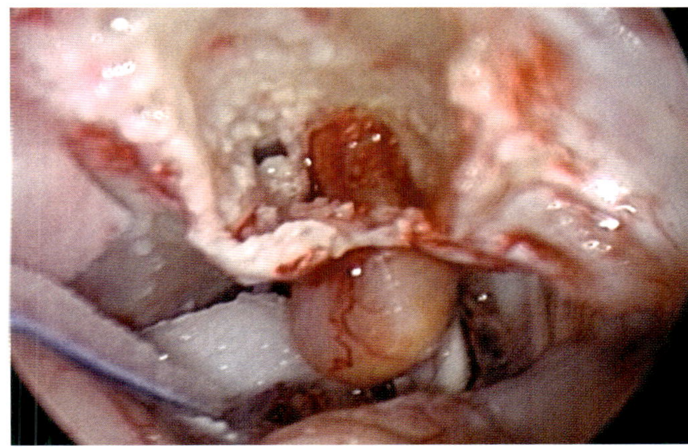

Fig. 7.20: Endoscopic view of Stage 2 AN tumor in CPA with grade B extension of tumor in IAC having fundus free of tumor process

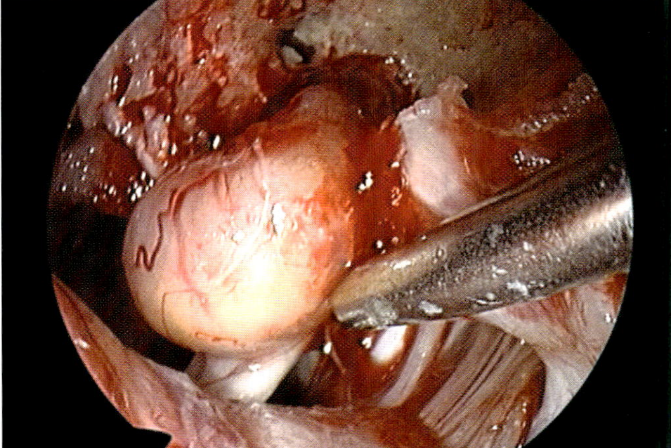

Fig. 7.21: Endoscopic view of Stage 2 AN tumor in CPA with grade C extension of tumor in IAC with involvement of fundus by tumor process

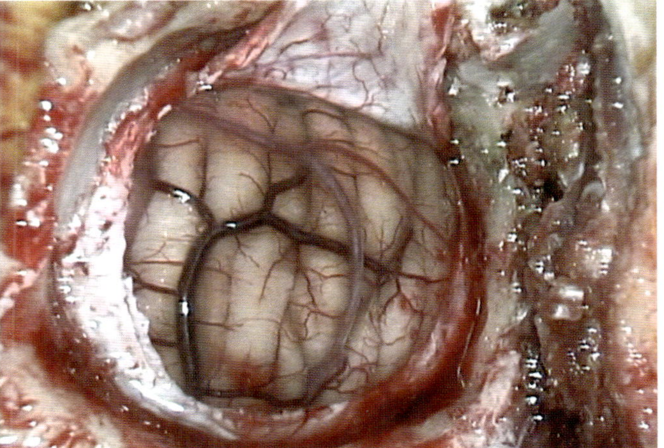

Fig. 7.22: Minimally invasive Retrosigmoid exposure for AN surgery

magna and drainage of CSF, exposure of AN (Fig. 7.23) and thorough dissection of arachnoid around AN (Figs 7.24 to 7.29).

"Mapping" of Contents of CPA with Endoscope

After exposure of CPA as mentioned in Chapter 4, the acoustic tumor can be undoubtedly visualized in the CPA abutting the porus part of the IAM (Fig. 7.23). The arachnoid draping the tumor (Figs 7.24 to 7.26) is swiftly pealed from the tumor to dissect the latter free from the anterior inferior cerebellar artery (AICA) and its branches (Figs 7.27 and 7.28). A 30°-angled endoscope with attached camera is introduced in the CPA to gain a panoramic view of the contents of the CPA. Endoscopy of CPA gives the surgeon a "mapping" of neurovascular structures adjacent to the tumor. Depending upon the stage of the tumor, the endoscopy gives information about various important structures like the medial pole of the neuroma, the cochlear nerve, the course of the AICA, the relation of the tumor to the facial nerve in CPA and at the porus and position of foramen of Luschka behind the protruding flocculus. We hereby illustrate the importance of endoscopic mapping in Stage 2, 3 and 4 AN by studying six different cases (Figs 7.30 to 7.50).

Cochlear and Facial Nerve Monitoring and Mapping for Acoustic Neuroma Surgery

Though discussed in the chapter on intraoperative nerve monitoring, we would like to highlight the role of nerve monitoring in modern acoustic neuroma surgery. Initially, we used only facial nerve monitoring by stimulation evoked measurement of facial muscles electromyography (EMG). We were not happy with the cochlear nerve monitoring

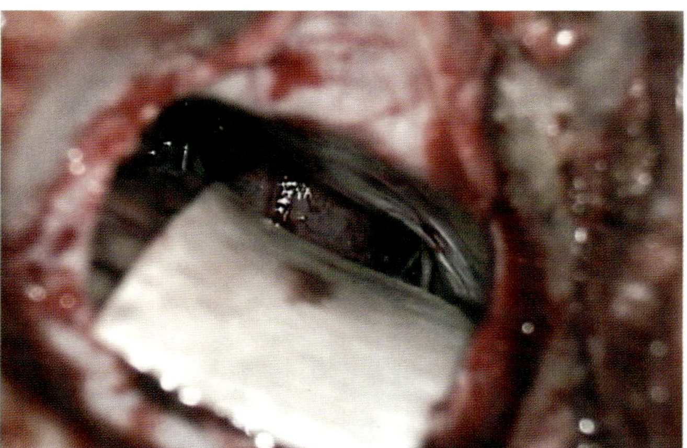

Fig. 7.23: The acoustic tumor visualized in the CPA abutting the porus part of IAM

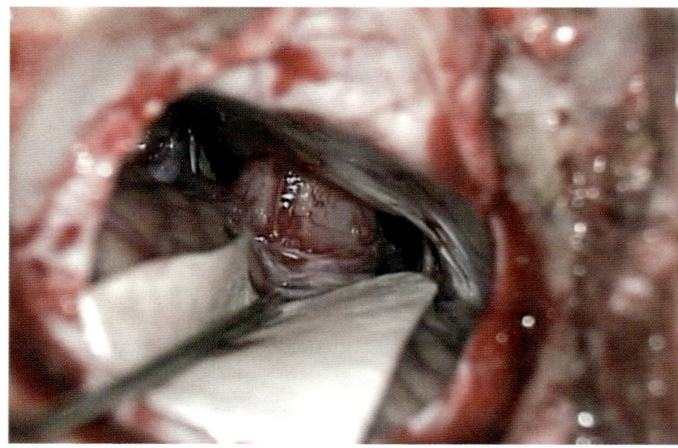

Fig. 7.24: The arachnoid draping the acoustic tumor in CPA

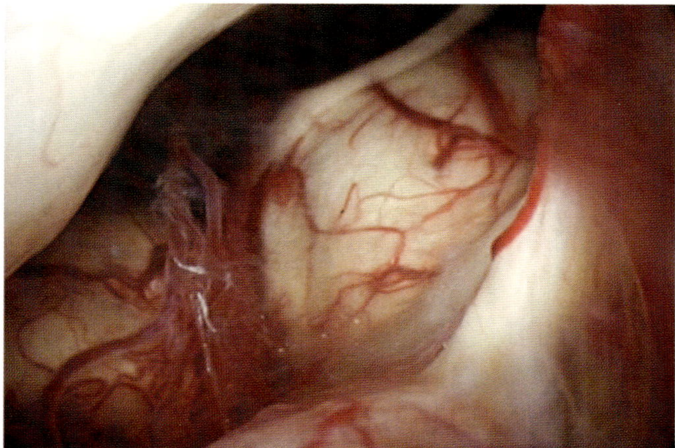

Fig. 7.25: Endoscopic examination of left CPA showing draping of arachnoid around the medial part of the acousticofacial nerve bundle

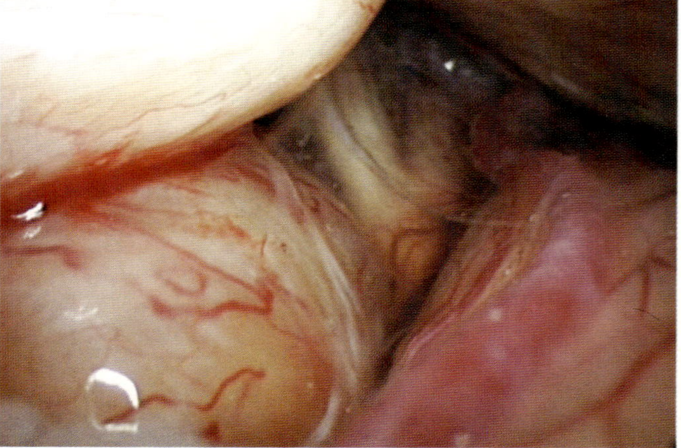

Fig. 7.26: Endoscopic examination of right CPA showing draping of arachnoid around the medial part of the AN and the auditory nerve

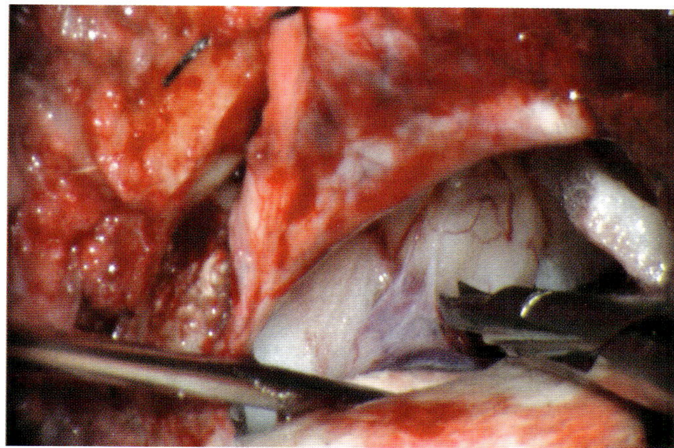

Fig. 7.27: The arachnoid draping the tumor and surrounding structures is thoroughly dissected away with sharp and blunt dissection

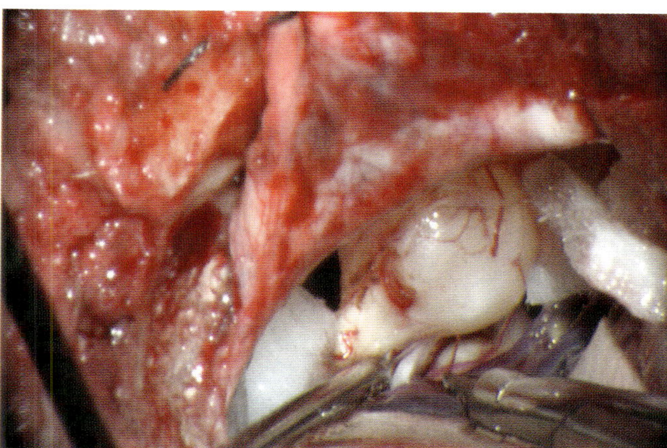

Fig. 7.28: The view of CPA and AN after dissection of the arachnoid draping the tumor

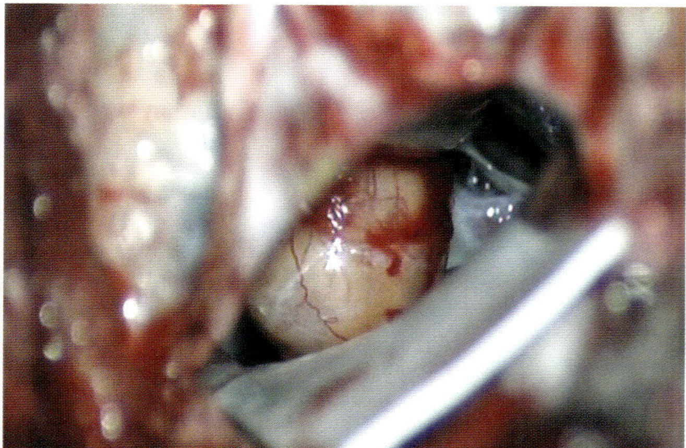

Fig. 7.29: The view of CPA and AN after dissection of the arachnoid draping the tumor

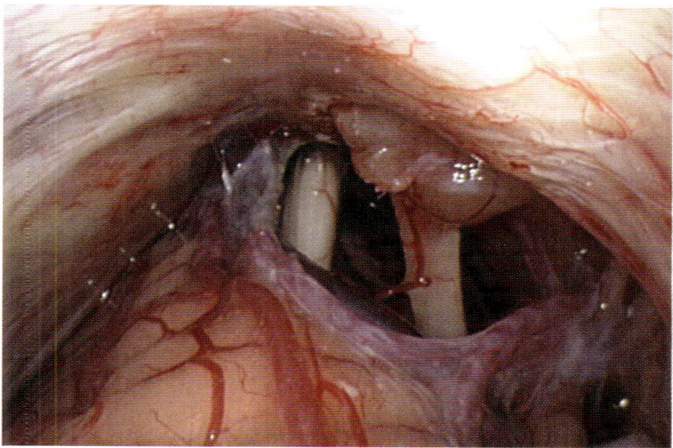

Fig. 7.30: Case 1 (Right CPA): Endoscopy of CPA showing the panoramic view of Stage 2 AN tumor in CPA

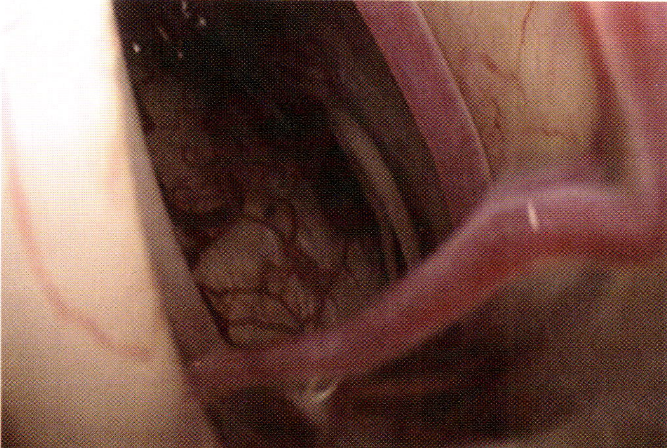

Fig. 7.31: Case 1: Endoscopic mapping of CPA showing the medial pole of the neuroma, the cochlear nerve, the course of the anterior inferior cerebellar artery and the relation of tumor to the facial nerve in CPA. Also seen in background is VIth nerve

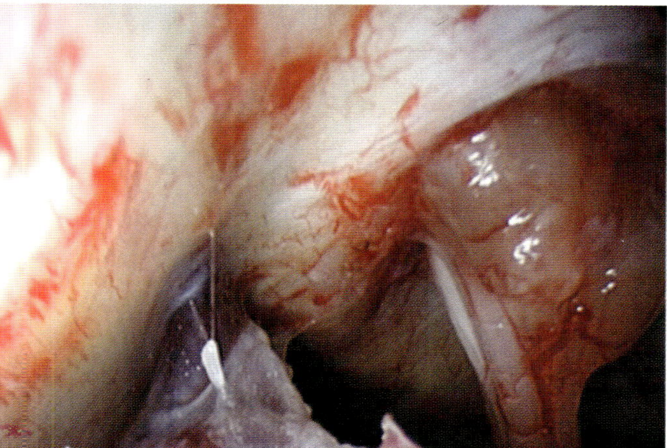

Fig. 7.32: Case 1: Endoscopic mapping of CPA showing the relation of facial nerve at the porus

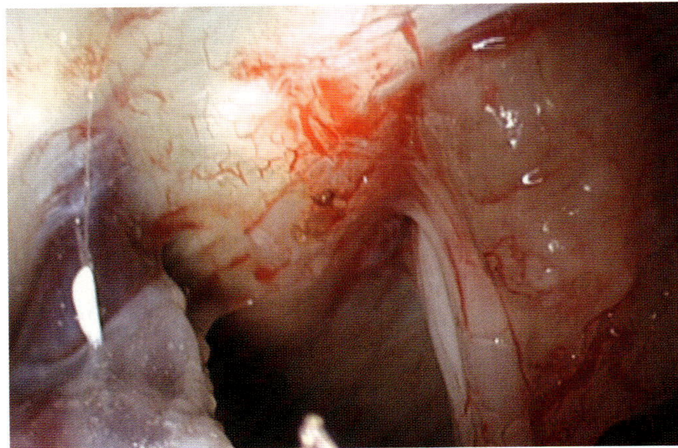

Fig. 7.33: Case 1: Endoscopic mapping of CPA showing the relation of facial nerve at the porus

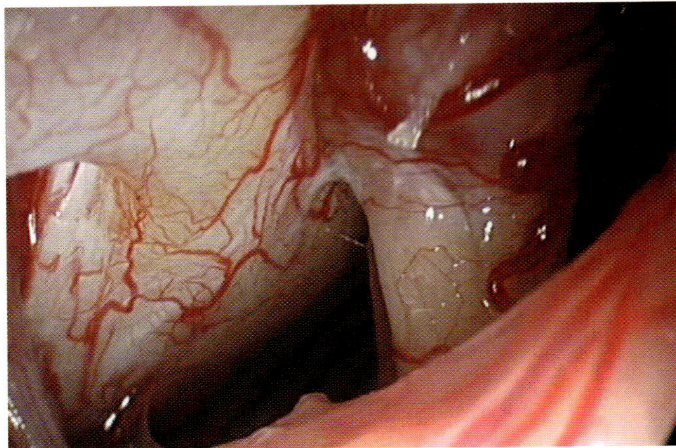

Fig. 7.34: Case 2 (Left CPA): Endoscopic mapping of CPA showing head on view of Stage 2 AN tumor arising from vestibular nerve

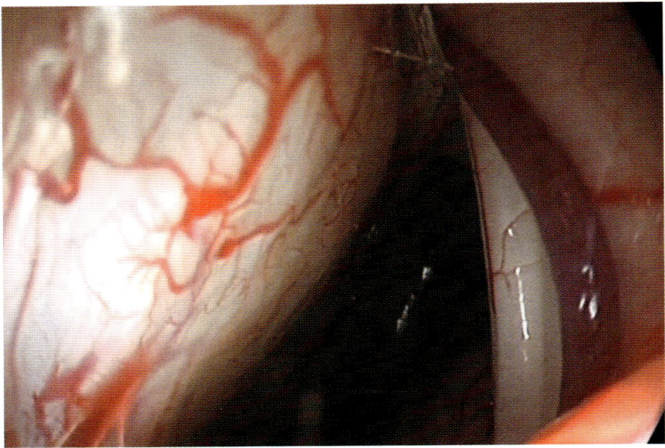

Fig. 7.35: Case 2: Endoscopic mapping of CPA showing relation of AN tumor to AICA and facial nerve in its cisternal course

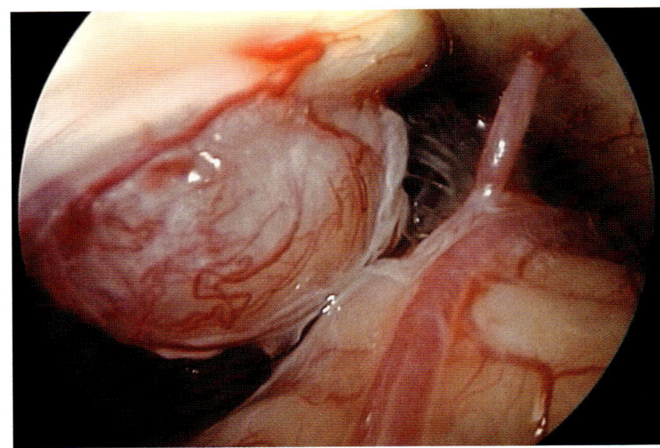

Fig. 7.36: Case 3 (Left CPA): Endoscopic mapping of CPA showing head on view of Stage 2 AN tumor

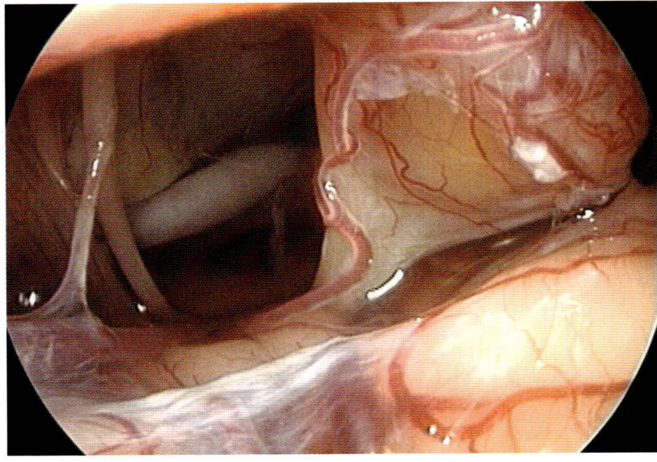

Fig. 7.37: Case 3: Endoscopic mapping showing medial end of tumor and its relation to lower cranial nerves

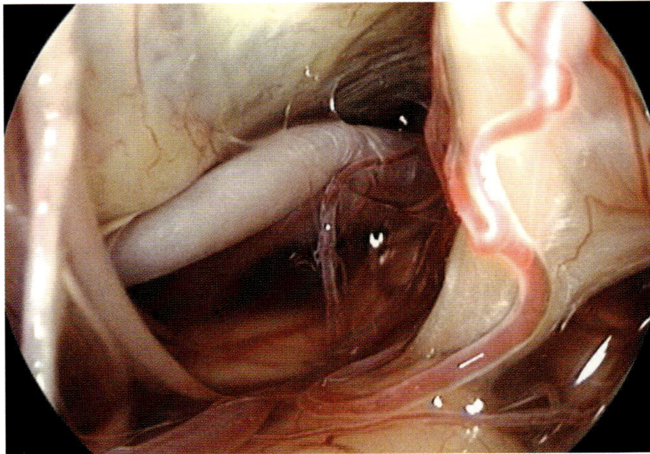

Fig. 7.38: Case 3: Endoscopic mapping showing medial end of tumor and its relations

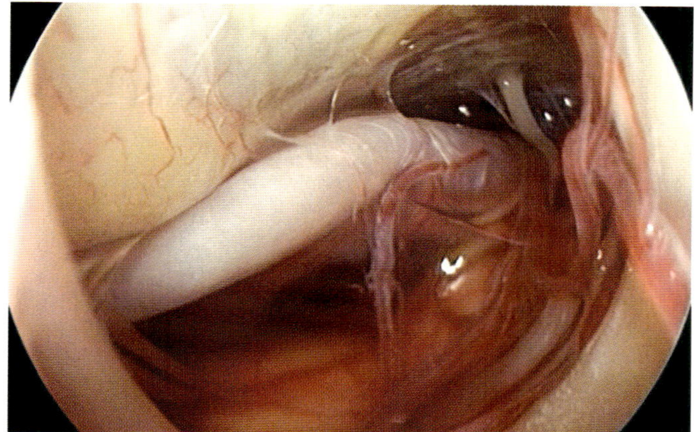

Fig. 7.39: Case 3: Endoscopic mapping showing medial end of tumor and its relations to AICA, facial nerve and lower cranial nerves. Also seen in background is vertebral arteries and VI nerve

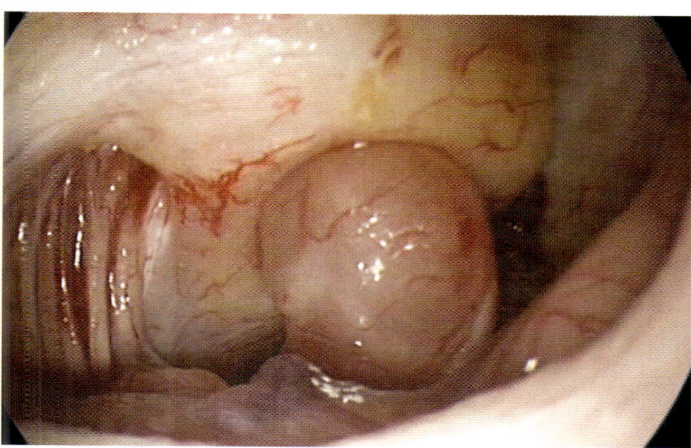

Fig. 7.40: Case 4 (Left CPA): Endoscopic mapping of CPA showing head on view of Stage 3 AN tumor

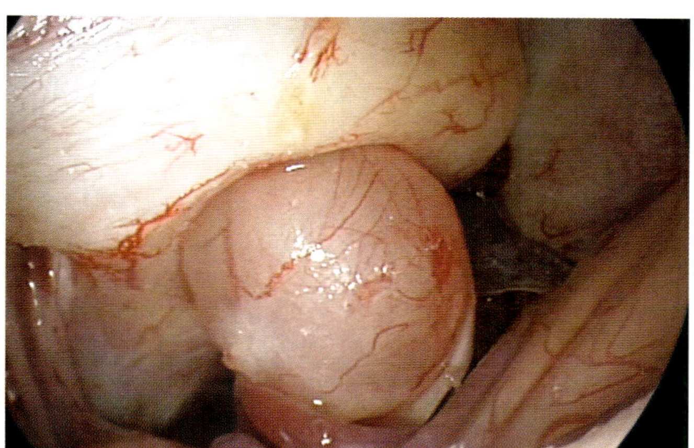

Fig. 7.41: Case 4: Endoscopic mapping of CPA showing closer view of Stage 3 AN tumor

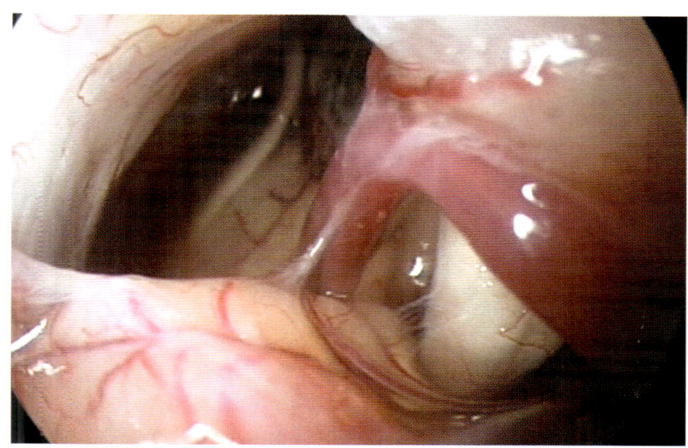

Fig. 7.42: Case 4: Endoscopic mapping showing closer view of medial end of Stage 3 AN tumor. Note the close relation to AICA and facial nerve in its background

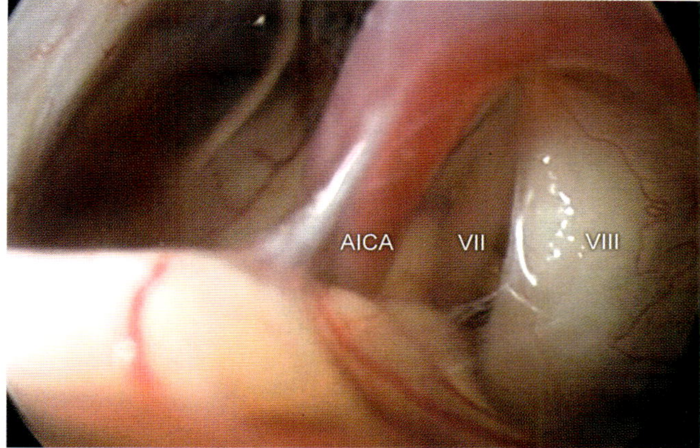

Fig. 7.43: Case 4: Endoscopic mapping showing closer view of medial end of Stage 3 AN tumor and its relation to AICA and facial nerve

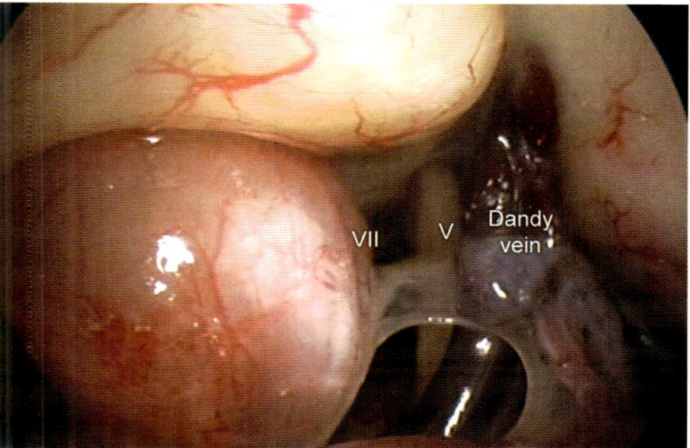

Fig. 7.44: Case 4: Endoscopic mapping showing closer view of lateral end of Stage 3 AN tumor and its relation to facial nerve and Dandy's vein. Note the relation of trigeminal nerve to superior pole of tumor

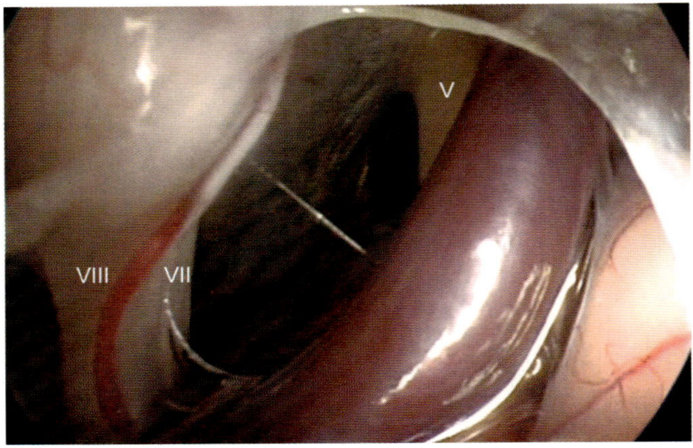

Fig. 7.45: Case 4: Endoscopic mapping showing closer view of lateral end of Stage 3 AN tumor and its relation to facial nerve and Dandy's vein. Note the relation of trigeminal nerve to superior pole of tumor

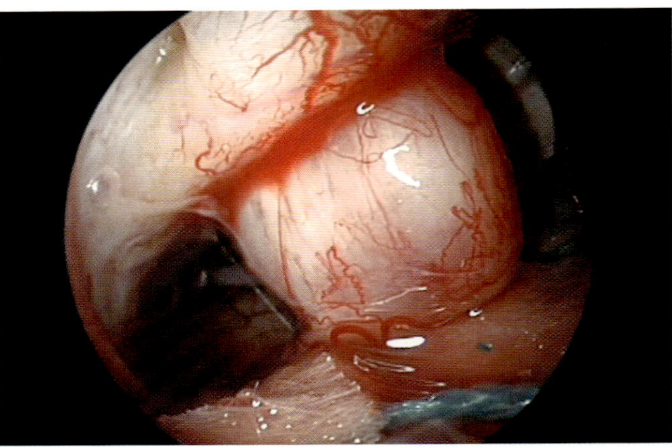

Fig. 7.46: Case 5 (Left CPA): Endoscopic mapping of CPA showing closer view of Stage 3 AN tumor

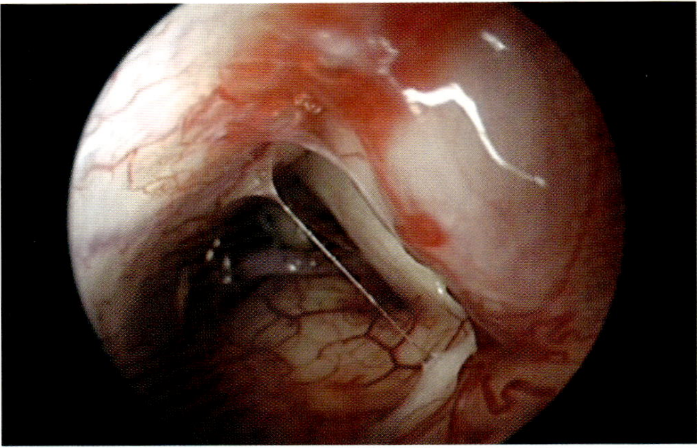

Fig. 7.47: Case 5: Endoscopic mapping of CPA showing relation of Stage 3 AN tumor to facial nerve at its medial end and at porus

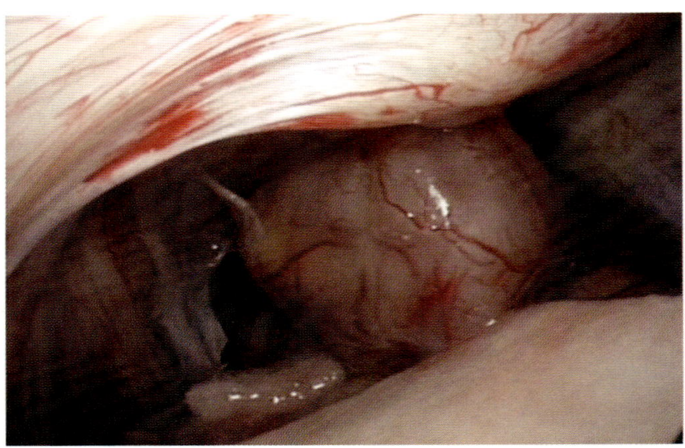

Fig. 7.48: Case 6 (Left CPA): Endoscopic mapping of CPA showing closer view of Stage 4 AN tumor

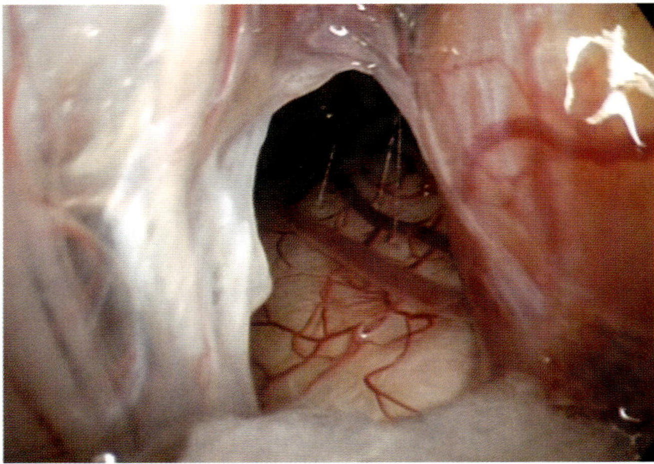

Fig. 7.49: Case 6: Endoscopic mapping of CPA showing medial relation of Stage 4 AN tumor to facial nerve

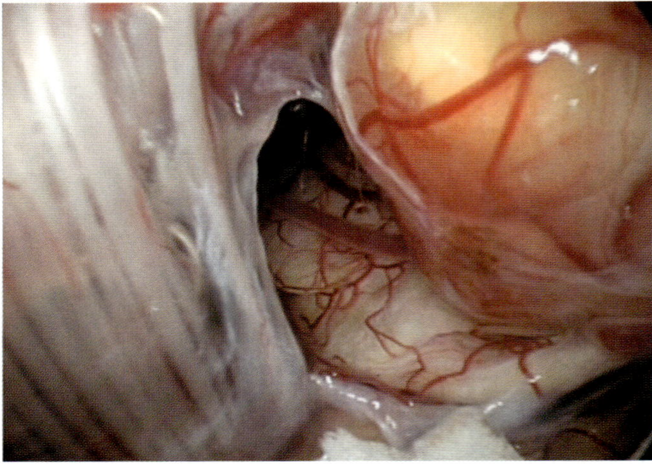

Fig. 7.50: Case 6: Endoscopic mapping of CPA showing medial relation of Stage 4 AN tumor to facial nerve

in 90s (as also experienced by many other centers) as measured by auditory brainstem responses (ABR) due to distraction caused by cumbersome techniques at that time, larger tumors and delayed responses of the ABR to surgical manipulation. However, lately with the advances in technology and advent of direct cochlear nerve and nucleus stimulated action potentials, the monitoring has become more real time and more reliable. So, we have been routinely using cochlear nerve monitoring in all the cases of AN by retrosigmoid approach for the past 2 years with better results in hearing preservation (unpublished data).

Once the mapping of CPA is complete with an endoscope, the cochlear nucleus electrode for free field monitoring of cochlear nucleus is inserted in the foramen of Luschka by guiding it along the superior border of the glossopharyngeal nerve, posteroinferior to the root exit zone (REZ) of nerve VIII and anterior to the flocculus. The choroid plexus coming out of the foramen of Luschka represents the most constant and valuable landmark. It is not necessary to visualize the foramen of Luschka as the electrodes measure free field potentials and need not be always accurately over the cochlear nucleus. Rather the electrophysiologist guides the surgeon to the best place where strong dorsal cochlear nucleus action potentials (DNAP) are obtained. The direct facial nerve stimulating electrode is next placed between the vestibulocochlear nerve and facial nerve such that it contacts the cisternal course of the facial nerve. The endoscope assists to acknowledge the position of electrodes for facial nerve monitoring in the CPA and for cochlear nerve monitoring in the foramen of Luschka for measurement of free field potentials from the dorsal cochlear nucleus (Figs 7.51 to 7.53). The ideal placements of both the electrodes

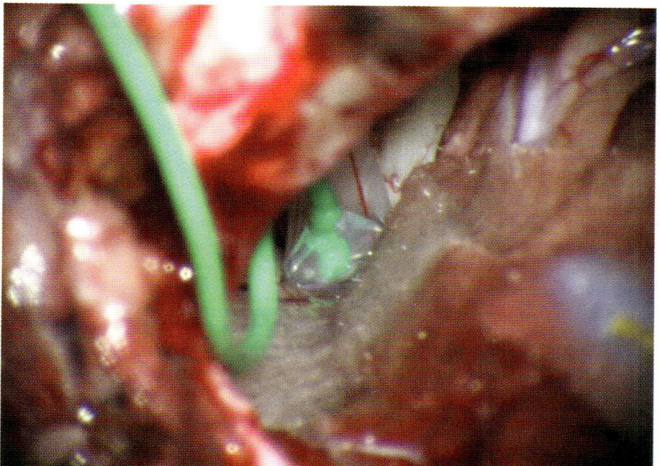

Fig. 7.51: Insertion of DNAP electrode along the plane of glossopharyngeal nerve close to the foramen of Luschka

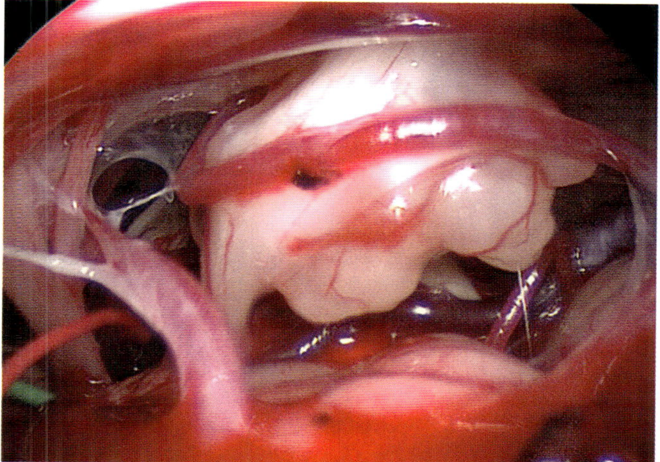

Fig. 7.52: 30°-angled endoscopic view of the setting of DNAP and FREMAP electrodes on the left side. FREMAP electrode is on top of the REZ of the facial nerve. The DNAP electrode is set on its caudal side in Foramen of Luschka and the green cord extending from DNAP electrode could be observed

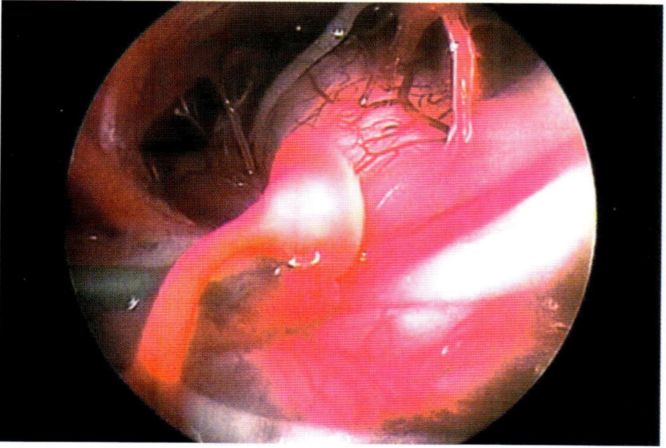

Fig. 7.53: Closer endoscopic view showing setting of DNAP and FREMAP electrodes on the left side. FREMAP electrode is on top of the REZ of the facial nerve. The DNAP electrode is set on its caudal side in Foramen of Luschka

are confirmed by evaluating nerve-stimulated EMG (FREMAP—facial nerve root evoked muscle action potential) and DNAP, and minor adjustments made so as to get the robust responses (Fig. 7.54). The origin of the tumor from the vestibular nerve is again confirmed to rule out cochlear or facial neuroma by confirming with nerve-stimulated potentials (Fig. 7.55). The plane of dissection between the vestibular and cochlear components of the nerve is similarly reconfirmed with nerve-stimulated potentials. Once the positions of the electrodes are confirmed, they are secured in the lower part of the CPA, so that they do not hinder the proceeding of subsequent steps.

When the tumors are large, there are cases where setting the DNAP and FREMAP electrodes become difficult and one would want to set the electrodes after reducing the size of the tumor. In such cases, the damage caused to the nerve during the surgical manipulation before setting the electrodes cannot be known. Although intraoperative continuous nerve monitoring could be performed even if the nerve is damaged, it is impossible to conduct an accurate nerve function preservation monitoring. Therefore, in acoustic tumor surgery for large tumor, special care is needed and it is important at an early stage of the surgery to decide the surgical field where an intraoperative continuous monitoring could be started.

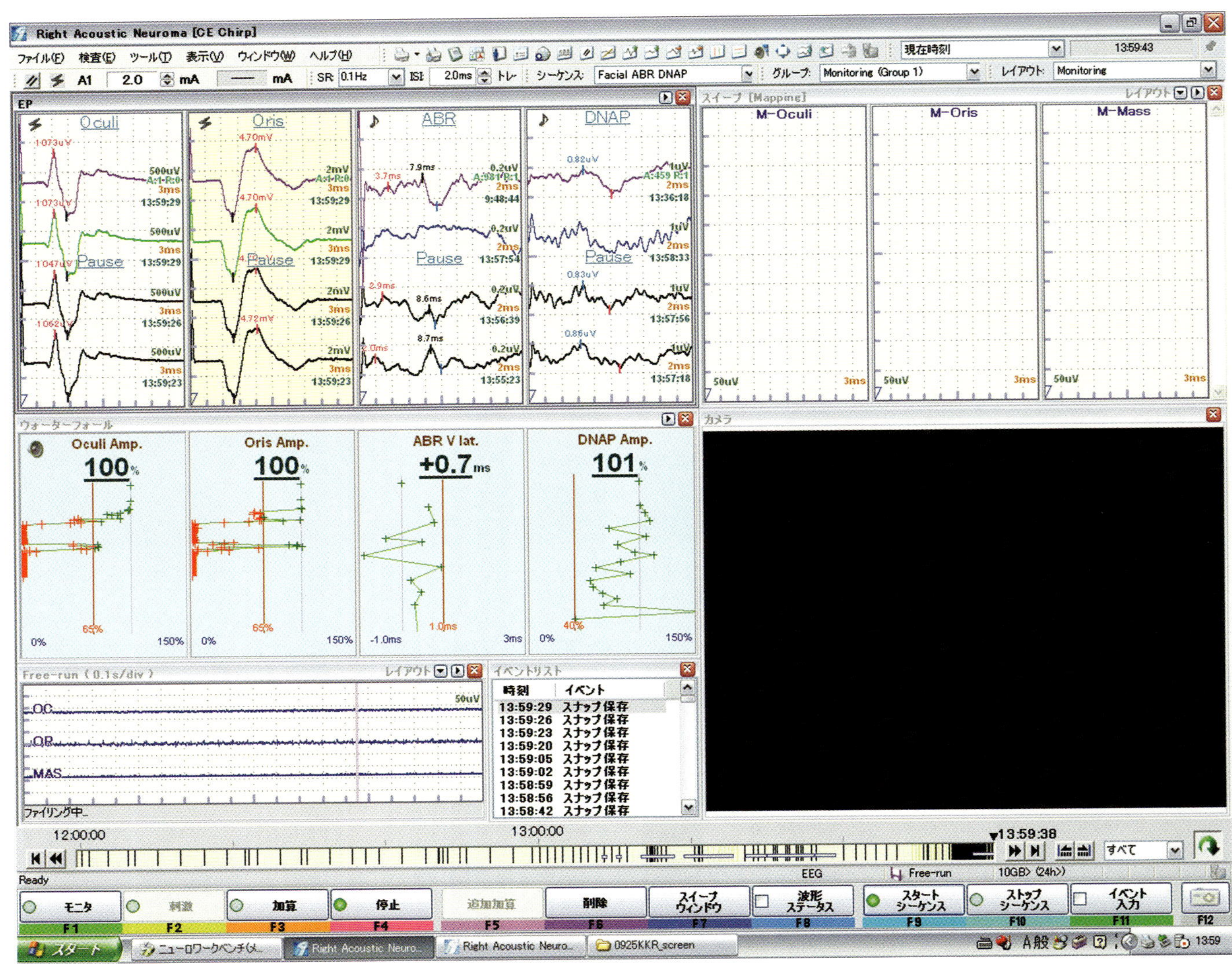

Fig. 7.54: The initial amplitude of the FREMAP is set at 100%, and the amplitude change in later steps is measured in this context

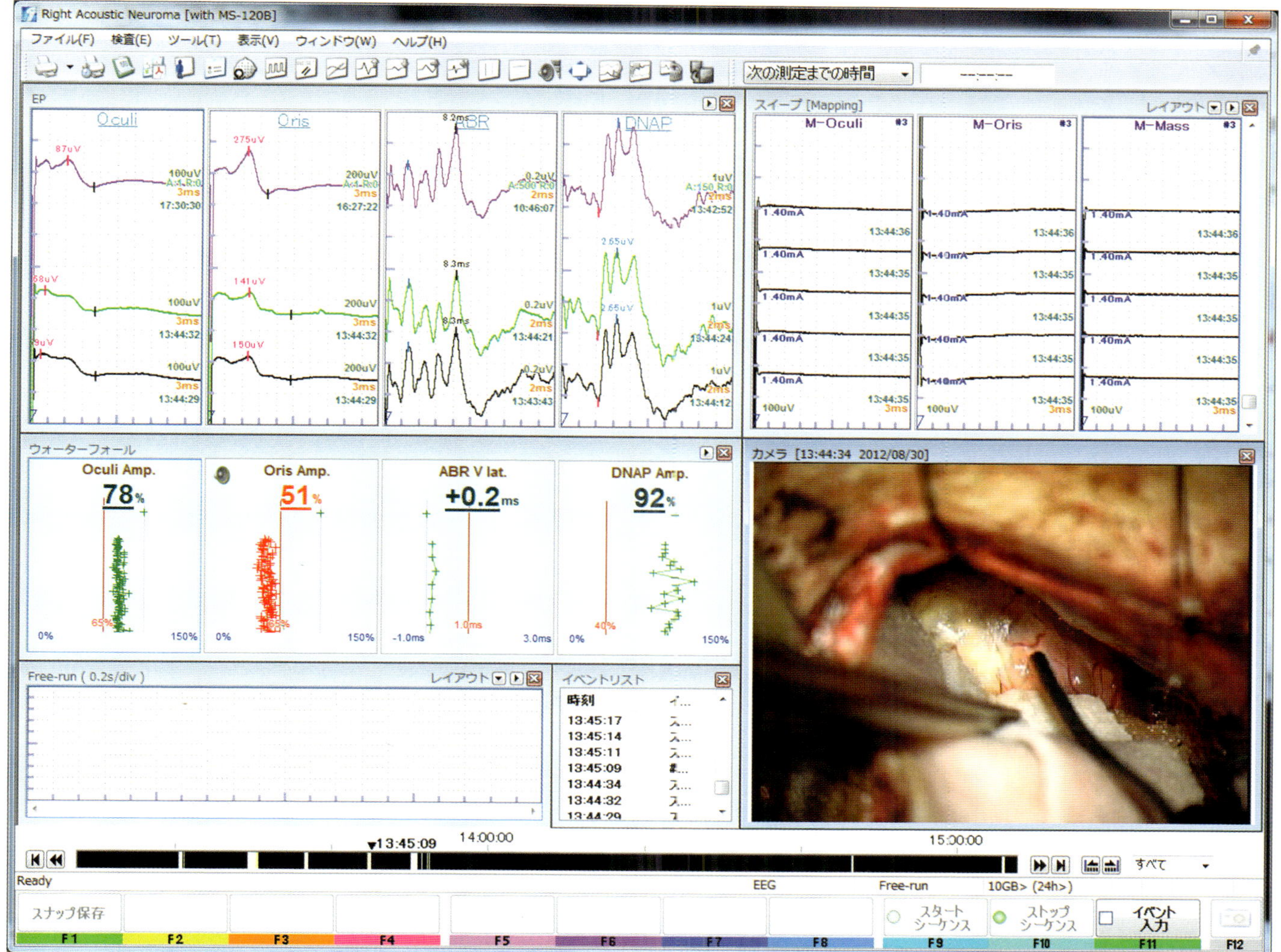

Fig. 7.55: Facial nerve mapping is conducted at 1.4 mA to rule out origin of tumor from facial nerve and confirm absence of facial nerve close to the tumor before initiating tumor debulking and bipolar coagulation. The initial DNAP can also be noted on the screen

If the lower cranial nerves could sufficiently be exposed by understanding their positions and their relation to tumor with the preoperative MRI, setting the electrodes are not necessarily difficult (Fig. 7.56).

To confirm the location of the nerve and to grasp the distance to the nerve, mapping is frequently conducted during the surgery. In acoustic tumor surgery, cochlear nerve and facial nerve mapping are conducted on the surface of the tumor. In cochlear nerve mapping, the tumor surface is stimulated from the rostal side toward the caudal side with an electrical current of 0.6 mA. Once there is a response at 0.6 mA, stimulation is repeated with a 0.2 mA current. If a response is obtained with a 0.2 mA current, it could be determined that it is right on top of the cochlear nerve and to distinguish it from a tumor it is marked with a crystal violet dye. Similarly for facial nerve mapping (Fig. 7.55), starting with an electrical current of 1.4 mA, the current is reduced sequentially and applied where response is obtained to 1, 0.6, 0.2 and 0.1 mA, which allows knowing the approximate distance, thereby making a mark with a crystal violet dye (Fig. 7.57). The relationship between the amount of the electrical current used for mapping and the distance of the considered nerve to the tumor differs depending upon the monitoring instrument and the stimulation probe.[44] If there is no response obtained at 1.4 mA (using intraoperative monitoring system MEE1200 made by NIHON KOHDEN), there could be a possibility of using a bipolar coagulation in the vicinity (Fig. 7.58).

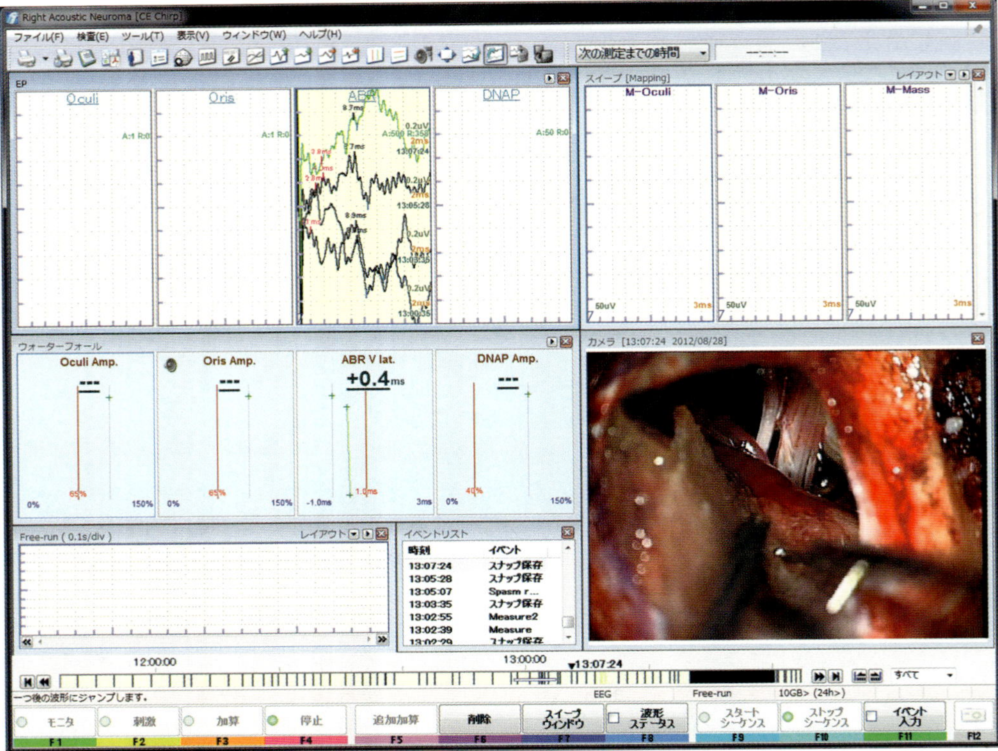

Fig. 7.56: In case of large tumor, lower cranial nerves are exposed initially by dissecting the arachnoid around them and they are used as a landmark to guide the DNAP electrode

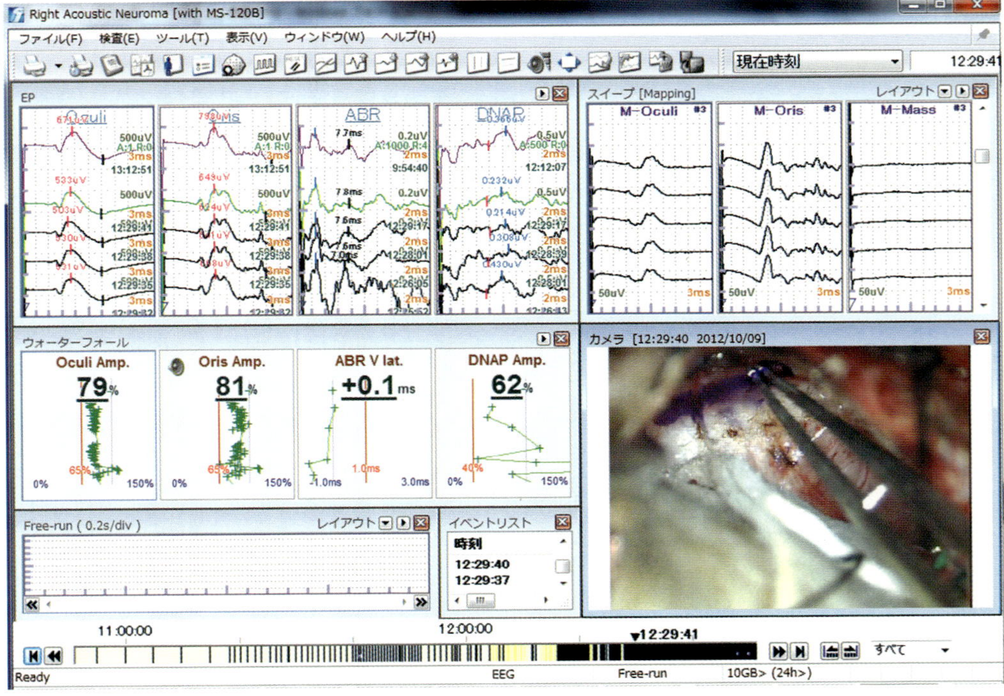

Fig. 7.57: After facial nerve mapping and cochlear nerve mapping, both facial and cochlear nerves are marked with a crystal violet dye

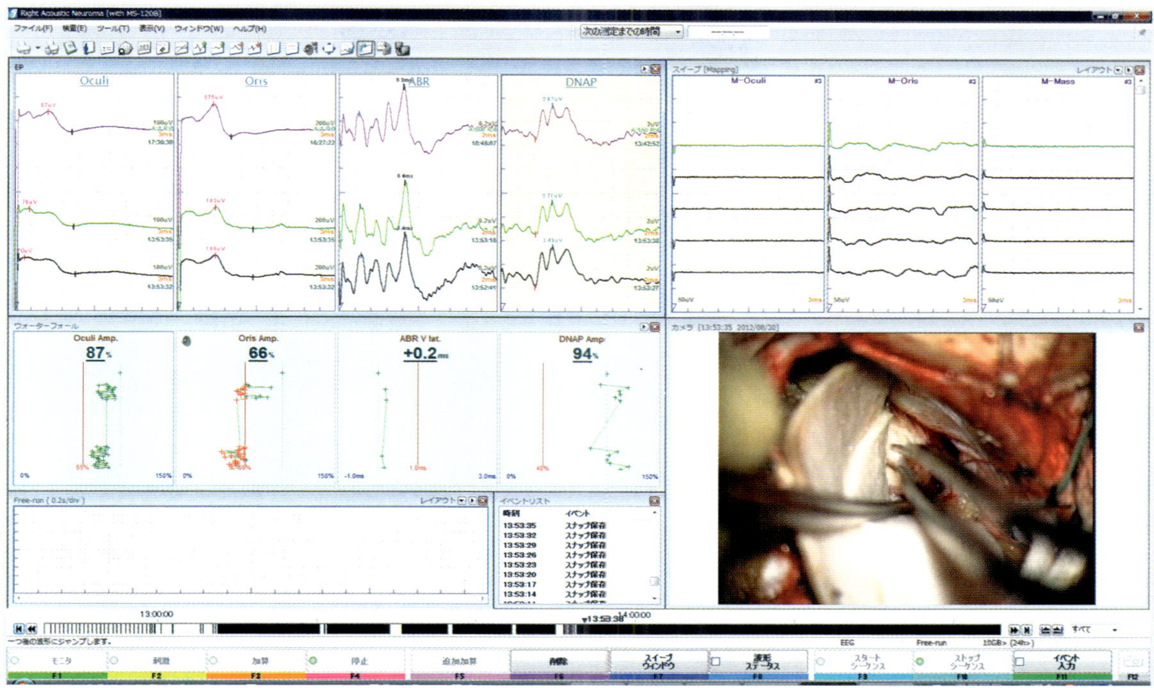

Fig. 7.58: After delineating the facial and cochlear nerves, it is safe to use bipolar coagulation over the tumor capsule to help debulk the tumor in avascular manner

Tumor debulking is started from places devoid of the cochlear nerve and the facial nerve fibers to reduce the inner pressure of the tumor. Debulking should not be conducted at just one place and the first step should be to reduce the total tumor volume while preserving the pseudo capsule. After the volume is reduced and the running of the cochlear nerve and the facial nerve becomes clear anatomically, the remaining tumor on the pseudo capsule is surgically removed. As small vessels running inside the pseudo capsule are important in preserving the functions of the cochlear nerve and facial nerve, in principle, the pseudo capsule is not removed surgically. During this debulking manipulation for reduction of the tumor size, one should carefully look for any change in the monitoring parameters that may occur and any event shown on the monitoring data should not be overlooked. Similarly, nerve mapping and monitoring are also useful after opening of the IAM for locating the facial nerve (Fig. 7.59) and dissecting the tumor from the fundus while doing hearing preservation surgery.

During the tumor removal, when either the amplitude of DNAP goes below 40% compared to that at the initial stage of the surgery or the amplitude of FREMAP goes below 65%, 15 or 30 min recuperating therapy should be conducted (Fig. 7.60). If the amplitude does not recover, wait for another 30 min and then conduct a recuperating therapy with a total maximum of 90 min. It is rare to see cases with further lowering after the recovery, but it could surely result in some kind of a loss in the nerve function if the surgical manipulation is continued in a case where the amplitude immediately gets low after restarting the surgery. We should talk to the patient prior to the surgery thoroughly on whether the patient wants the surgery continued or not, in case such a circumstance occurred during the surgery. One should understand firmly the will of the patient and the medical team that conducts the treatment should not make the decision unilaterally. However, there are cases where lowering and recovering of the amplitude take place more than twice during the surgery and a prolonged recuperation therapy is not possible. We should take the surgery duration time in consideration and decide upon the will of the patient as well as the goal of the surgery comprehensively.

To summarize, it is now possible to conduct a safe and accurate surgery based on monitoring; the rate of nerve preservation in AN surgery has improved dramatically.[45] Of the 46 cases who underwent AN surgery with recuperating therapy (including not so useful hearing cases) from May

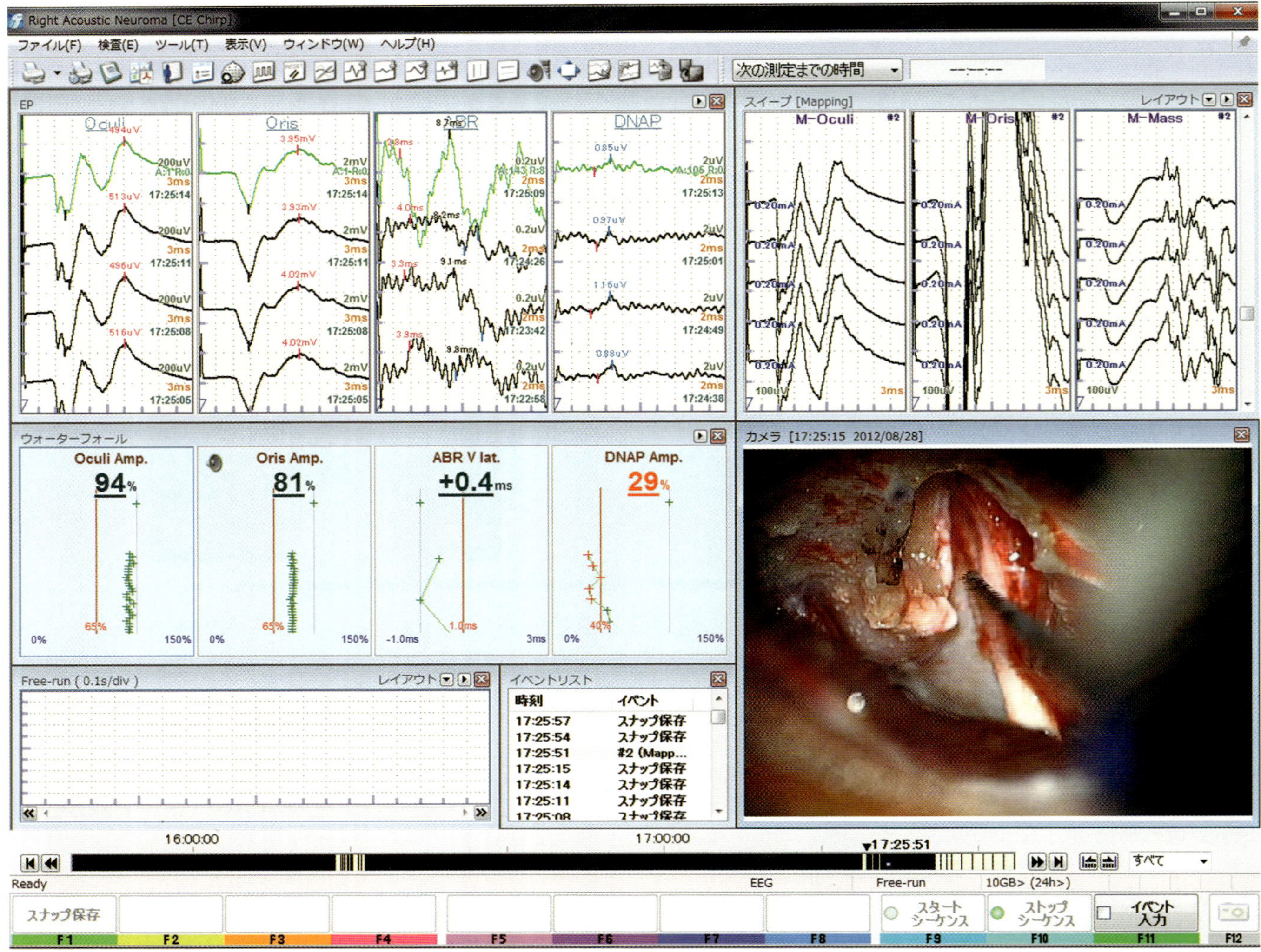

Fig. 7.59: The monitoring image shows facial nerve mapping at 0.1 mA being conducted in internal auditory canal and shows strong response even at 0.1 mA

2007 to Feb 2010, the rates of nerve preservation are 95% for normal facial nerve function and 80% for hearing (hearing class is same before and after surgery).[46]

Opening of Internal Auditory Meatus

The attachment of the tumor to the porus acousticus of the IAM identifies the location of the internal acoustic meatus (IAM). The next step is the opening of the IAM to expose the intrameatal part of tumor. It is not difficult to find the IAM via retrosigmoid approach, thus saving precious time. Hearing preservation surgery requires bone removal from the posterior wall of the IAM to be as conservative as possible, to prevent entering into the labyrinth. A rectangular dural flap is delineated over the IAM by cauterizing with bipolar forceps (Fig. 7.61) followed by incising it with a sharp micro-knife with its base toward the posterior lip of porus (Figs 7.62 to 7.64). The size of the flap is not based on some landmarks but an estimated one, with the width of the flap slightly larger than the IAM and the length is approximately twice its width. The dural flap is elevated from the bone that forms the posterior wall of the IAM with a straight elevator inward toward the neuroma and CPA (Figs 7.65 to 7.67). It is not necessary to preserve the dural flap and we often remove this dura as it impedes the drilling over the area (Figs 7.68 and 7.69).

The problem facing the surgeon is to obtain maximum exposure of the intrameatal tumor while at the same time minimizing the risk of inadvertent injury to the

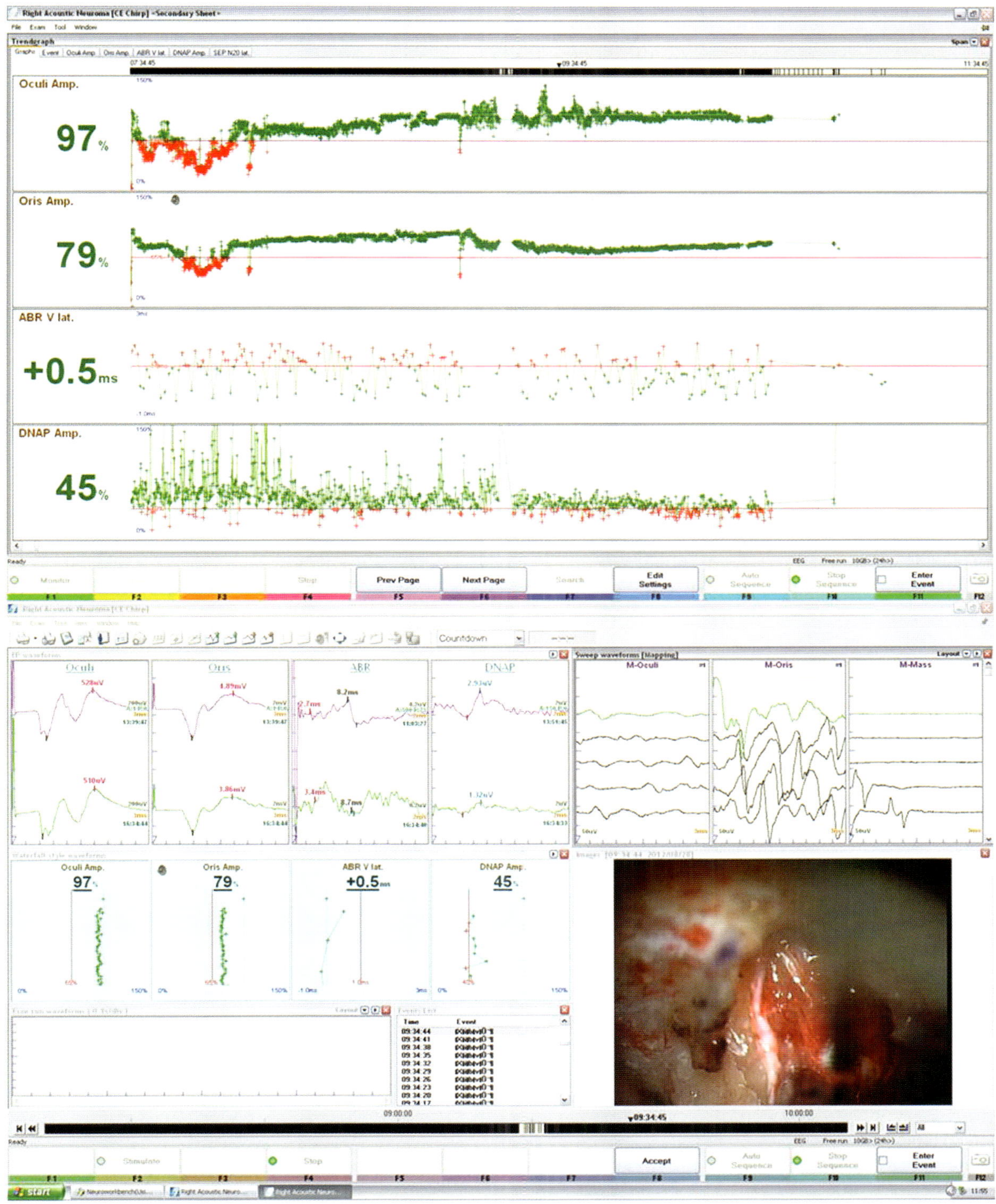

Fig. 7.60: Trend graph: DNAP amplitude percentage, orbicularis oculi muscle amplitude percentage, orbicularis oris muscle amplitude percentage and latency of ABR (I–V peak) are shown frcm the start to the end of monitoring with time. In this example, it could be understood that the DNAP amplitude became low and there was a 90-min standby in surgery and the surgery was resumed when its level recovered to above 40%. Neuromaster Intra-Operative Monitoring System MEE-1100 has dual screen, so we can see real-time monitoring and trend graph at the same time during the surgery

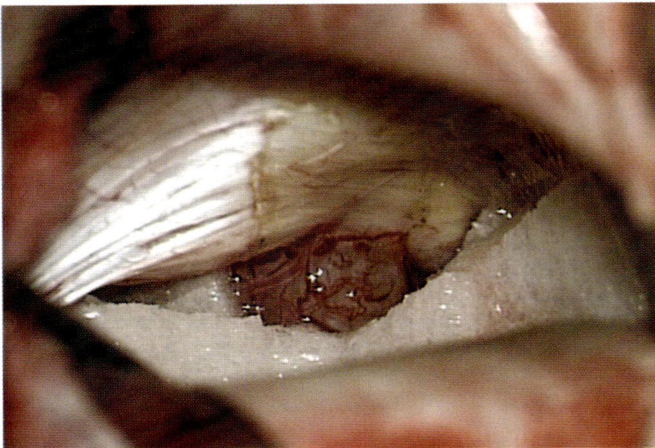

Fig. 7.61: A rectangular dural flap is delineated over the IAM by cauterizing the dural incision mark with bipolar cautery

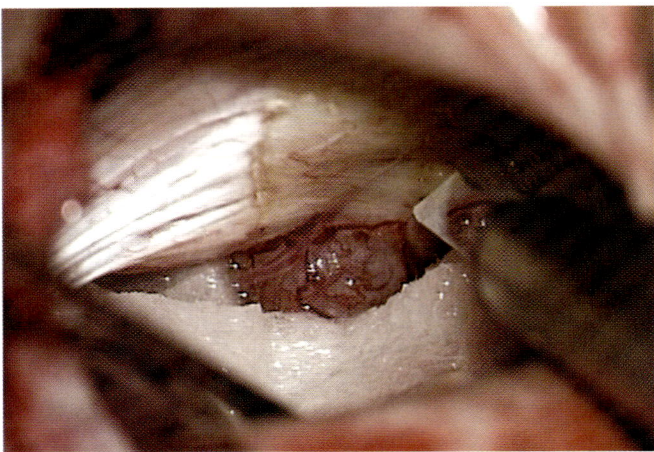

Fig. 7.62: An incision over the rectangular dural flap over the IAM is made by a sharp micro-beaver knife

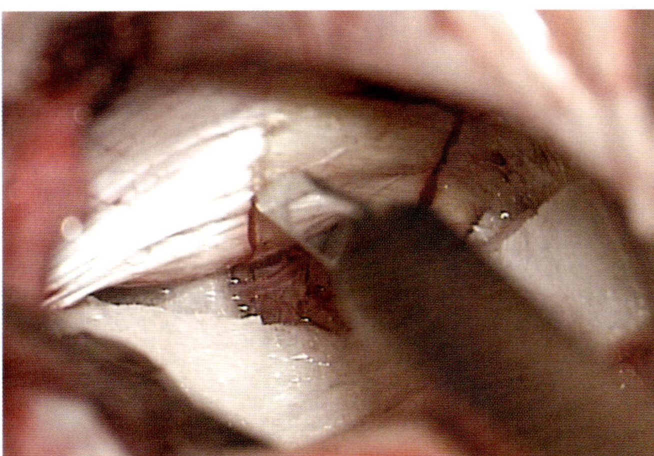

Fig. 7.63: A rectangular dural flap is delineated over the IAM with its base toward the posterior lip of porus

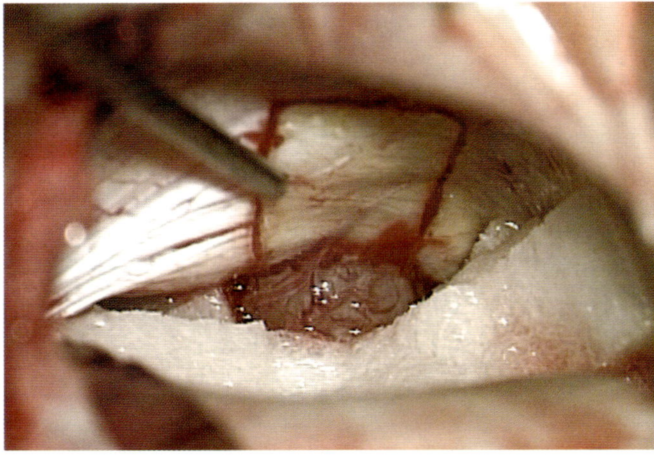

Fig. 7.64: A rectangular dural flap is delineated over the IAM with its base toward the posterior lip of porus

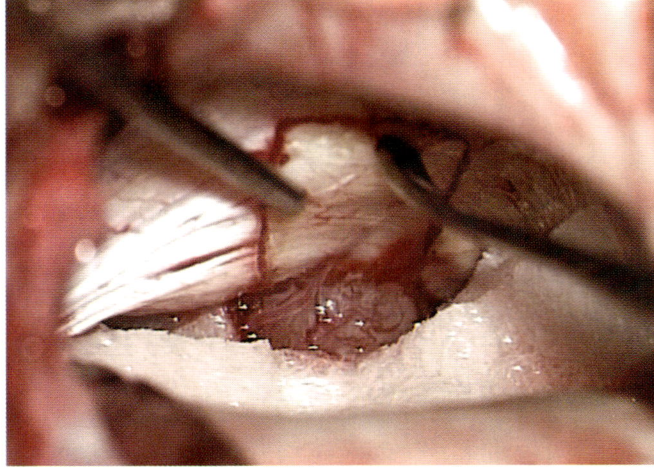

Fig. 7.65: The incised dural flap is elevated from the bone that forms the posterior wall of the IAM with a straight elevator

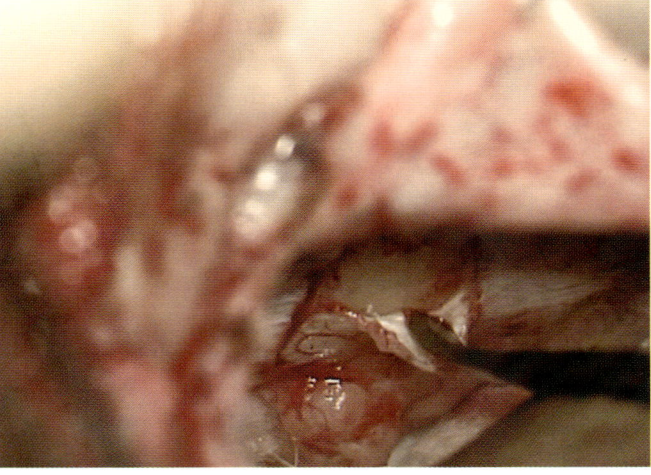

Fig. 7.66: The incised dural flap is elevated from the bone that forms the posterior wall of the IAM

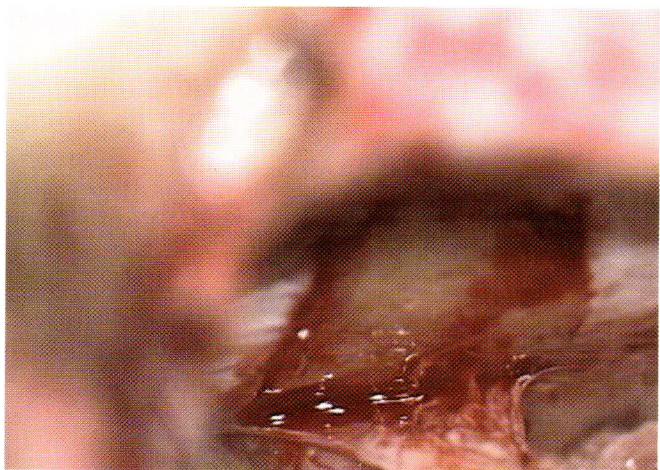

Fig. 7.67: The incised dural flap is elevated from the bone that forms the posterior wall of the IAM

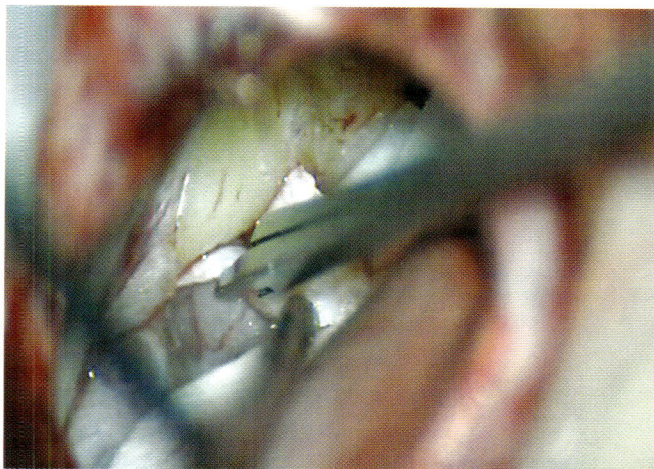

Fig. 7.68: The elevated dural flap is resected with sharp dissection by micro-scissors

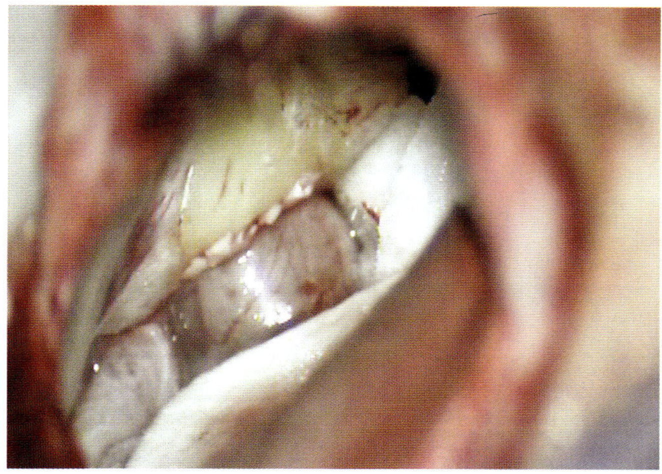

Fig. 7.69: The posterior wall of the IAM abutting the porus is now free of dural attachment. Two large strips of cottonoids are placed around the tumor in CPA to obliterate the subarachnoid space, so as to prevent the bone dust entering it on drilling the IAM to expose canalicular part of tumor

labyrinth. The most lateral part of the IAM leads to the labyrinth and therefore one should be precautious here. Unfortunately, there is no anatomical landmark to help identify the labyrinth. Neither the endolymphatic duct, transverse crest nor the singular foramen are consistently predictable landmarks.[47-50] Posteroinferiorly, the posterior semicircular canal and the common crus with the superior semicircular canal are at inadvertent risk for damage. The preoperative radiological data can give some idea about the distance of the labyrinth and posterior semicircular canal from the posterior meatal lip of the IAM and can be used during surgery by comparing the size of the head of bur with the distance drilled from the posterior lip.

Before drilling the posterior wall of the IAM, care should be taken to prevent bone dust created by drilling to enter the subarachnoid space of the CPA. Bone dust in the subarachnoid space is considered to be the reason for headache and postoperative hydrocephalus as observed in certain cases, especially in retrosigmoid approach. Two large strips of cottonoids are placed around the tumor near the IAM (Fig. 7.69) to obliterate the subarachnoid space temporarily. Initially, the drilling is performed along the expected direction of the IAM with a 4 mm diamond burr (Fig. 7.70) and later with a diamond one of smaller size (2 mm) when in proximity to the intracanalicular dura (Fig. 7.71). Drilling is performed parallel to the direction of IAM and from lateral to medial stopping just before the porus of IAM (Fig. 7.72). Occasional exposure of the common crus/posterior semicircular canal is immediately sealed with bone wax or periosteum and may not necessarily end up in profound hearing loss.[51] High jugular bulb (when close to inferior rim) is managed as in the translabyrinthine approach by using smooth dissection and compression by placing a large piece of Surgicel over the high jugular bulb followed by compressing it with bone wax to provide extra 2–3 mm of inferior exposure of IAM.

We believe in opening the medial two-third of the IAM, saving the labyrinth, but leaving around 2–3 mm of IAM hidden from microscope vision. The canal bottom may be the object of a particular dissection under endoscopic-assisted procedure. Once the intracanalicular dura is exposed partially, the exposure is widened to expose around

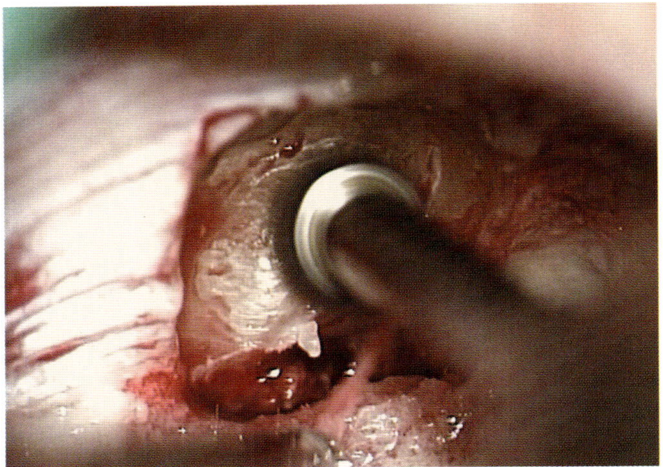

Fig. 7.70: The drilling of IAM is performed with a 4 mm diamond burr initially

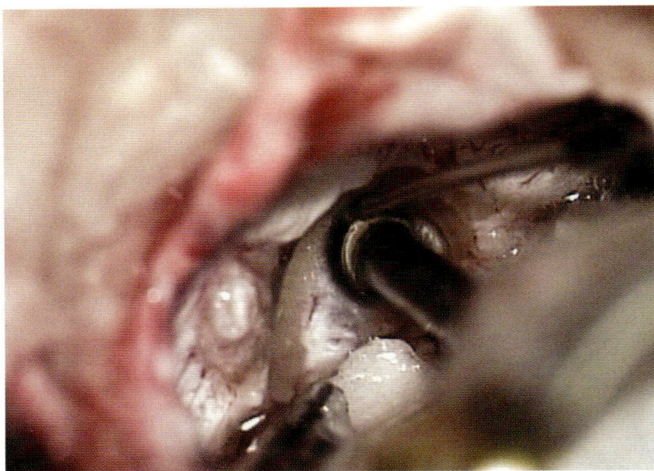

Fig. 7.71: Later as one proceeds toward the drilling of IAM roof, drilling is performed with a smaller 2 mm diamond burr

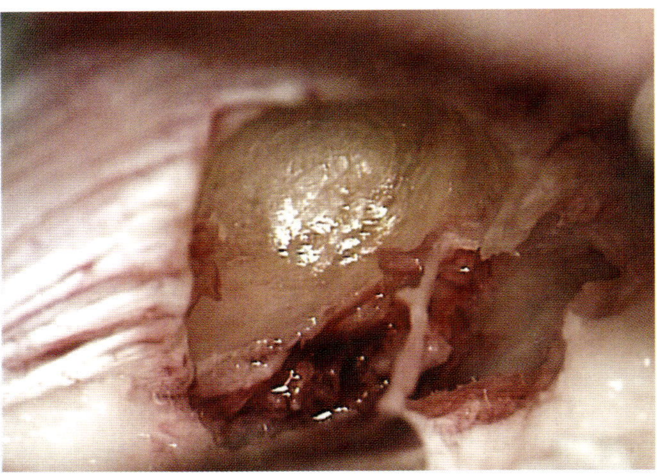

Fig. 7.72: Drilling is performed parallel to the direction of IAM and from lateral to medial stopping just before the porus of IAM

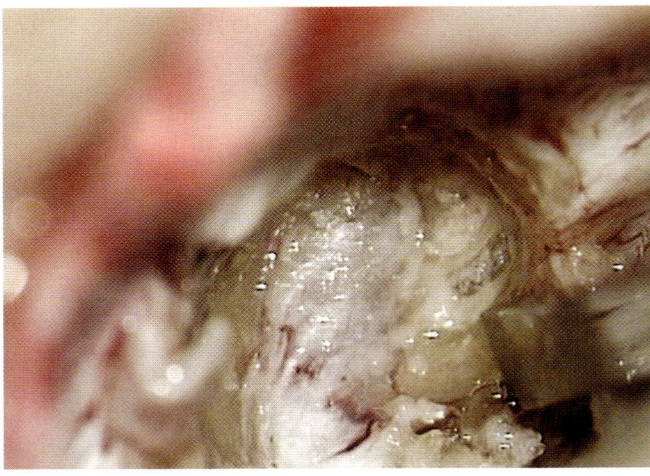

Fig. 7.73: The bone overlying canalicular dura is delineated by gradually drilling it with diamond burr. Overhang in the inferior part of posterior lip of IAM has to be often removed with 2 mm bayonet-shaped chisel and hammer

180° of the IAM (Fig. 7.73). Often there are overhangs both superiorly and inferiorly which are removed gently with 2 mm bayonet-shaped chisel (Figs 7.73 to 7.75), taking care to engage firmly in the bony lip before hitting with hammer. The intracanalicular component of the tumor is now visible in continuity with the cisternal component (Fig. 7.76). Strips of cottonoids placed around the tumor in the CPA to obliterate the subarachnoid space are now removed and saline wash given to clear the bone dust (Figs 7.77 and 7.78). Once the dura is completely exposed, it is opened with a sharp sickle knife. Any bleeding from the tumor is stopped with fine bipolar cautery on low power.

Debulking of Tumor

Once the tumor is completely delineated, blood vessels over the tumoral surface are coagulated with bipolar cautery forceps (Fig. 7.77). In smaller AN (intracanalicular stage I or stage II with less than 10 mm CPA component), there is hardly any debulking to be done. If the tumor is of larger size, the tumor surface is coagulated with bipolar forceps under constant irrigation and intracapsular debulking of tumor is done in its central region to reduce its size. The debulking can be done by bipolar coagulation and bayonet-shaped scissors or with the ultrasonic aspirator (which can induce intratumoral bleeding)

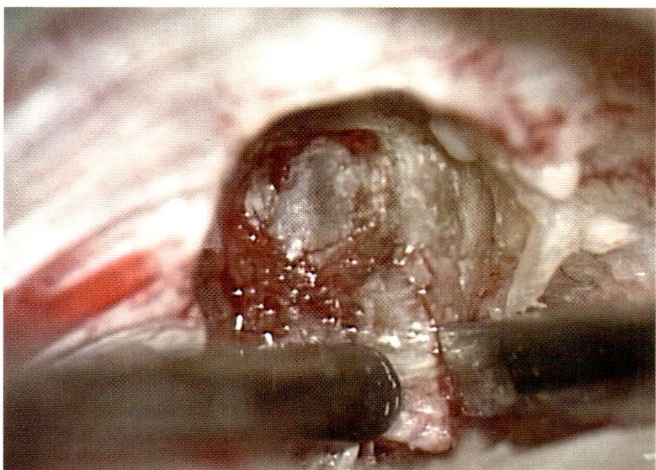

Fig. 7.74: Overhang over the IAM is removed with 2 mm bayonet-shaped chisel and hammer

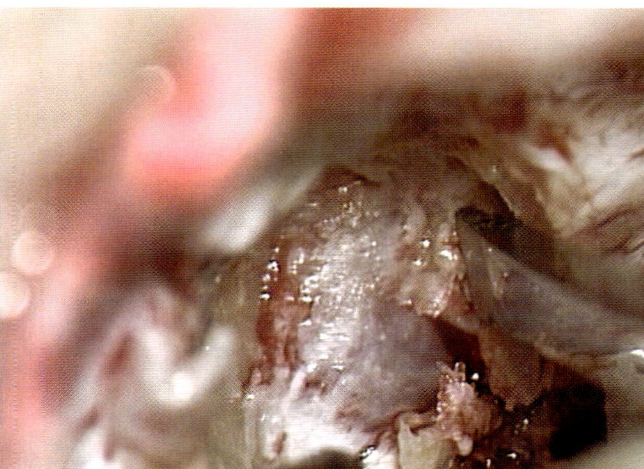

Fig. 7.75: Overhang over the IAM is removed with 2 mm bayonet-shaped chisel and hammer

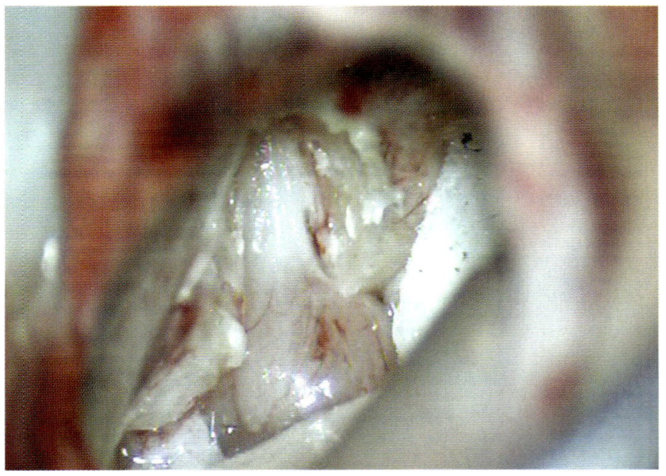

Fig. 7.76: Intracanalicular component of tumor is now visible in continuity with cisternal component

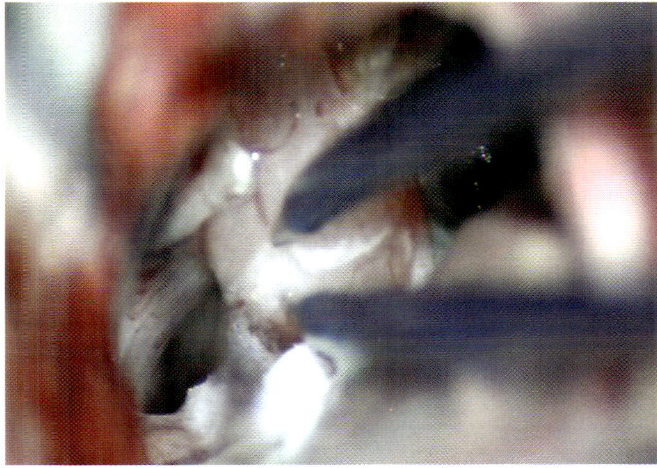

Fig. 7.77: Strips of cottonoids placed around the tumor in CPA to obliterate the subarachnoid space are now removed and saline wash given to clear the bone dust. Blood vessels over the tumoral surface are coagulated with bipolar cautery forceps

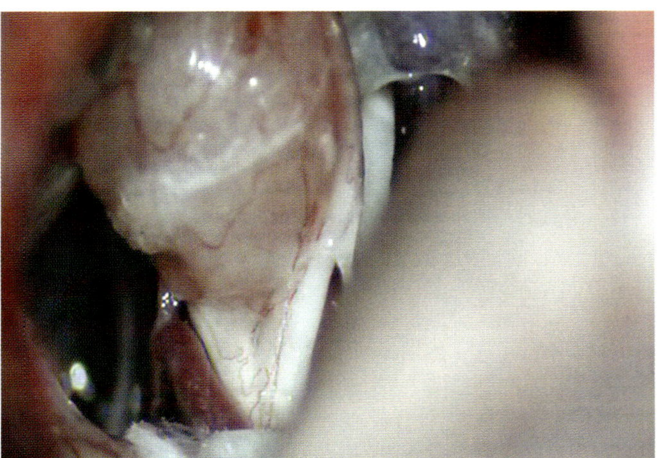

Fig. 7.78: Blood vessels over the tumoral surface are coagulated with bipolar cautery forceps. Arachnoid draping the tumoral surface is completely dissected. Medial end of vestibulocochlear nerve is delineated and the branch of AICA supplying tumor surface isolated

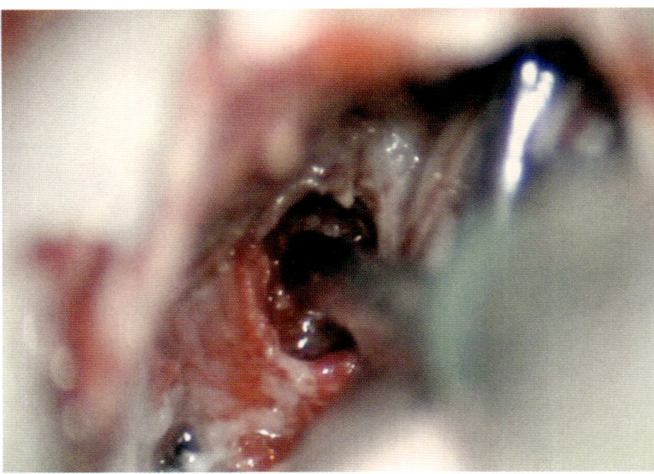

Fig. 7.79: Intracapsular debulking of tumor is done in its central region to reduce its size with ultrasound aspirator

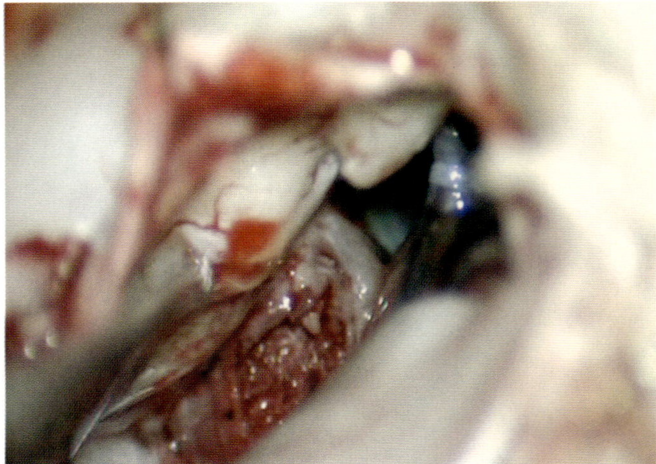

Fig. 7.80: Intracapsular debulking of tumor done with ultrasonic aspirator

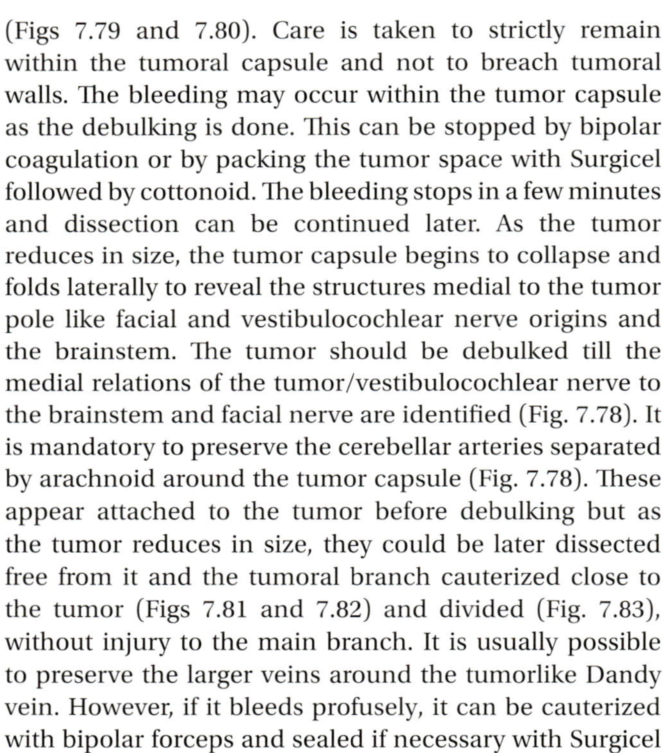

(Figs 7.79 and 7.80). Care is taken to strictly remain within the tumoral capsule and not to breach tumoral walls. The bleeding may occur within the tumor capsule as the debulking is done. This can be stopped by bipolar coagulation or by packing the tumor space with Surgicel followed by cottonoid. The bleeding stops in a few minutes and dissection can be continued later. As the tumor reduces in size, the tumor capsule begins to collapse and folds laterally to reveal the structures medial to the tumor pole like facial and vestibulocochlear nerve origins and the brainstem. The tumor should be debulked till the medial relations of the tumor/vestibulocochlear nerve to the brainstem and facial nerve are identified (Fig. 7.78). It is mandatory to preserve the cerebellar arteries separated by arachnoid around the tumor capsule (Fig. 7.78). These appear attached to the tumor before debulking but as the tumor reduces in size, they could be later dissected free from it and the tumoral branch cauterized close to the tumor (Figs 7.81 and 7.82) and divided (Fig. 7.83), without injury to the main branch. It is usually possible to preserve the larger veins around the tumorlike Dandy vein. However, if it bleeds profusely, it can be cauterized with bipolar forceps and sealed if necessary with Surgicel without any major sequelae.

Dissection from Medial to Lateral

Once the tumor is debulked (in very small tumors directly), the tumor along with the vestibular nerve to which it is attached is now dissected from the cochlear component of the vestibulocochlear nerve and the facial nerve. A plane of dissection is established between the tumor attached to the vestibular nerve, the cochlear and the facial nerve (Figs 7.84 to 7.87). The vestibular component of the acoustic nerve is located at the medial pole and is sectioned or dissected to keep the peritumoral capsular plane intact, to more efficiently preserve the facial nerve. Recently, we also add the information from cochlear nerve-stimulated DNAP responses to better guide us in differentiating the cochlear nerve fibers from the remnant vestibular nerve fibers.

The key to dissection is to preserve the peritumoral arachnoid curtain or capsule close to the cochlear and facial nerves. The facial nerve is well visualized at its REZ and at the medial end of the tumor. The tumor is gently lifted from lateral to medial direction from the cochlear and facial nerve bundles using alternatively small elevator and right-angled 2 mm blunt hook (Figs 7.84 to 7.87) while strictly protecting both the nerves by covering them with small cottonoid. The electrophysiologist is asked to give immediate feedback for the change in function in any of the two nerves. The strokes of the instruments used in removing the tumor should be directed along the vestibulocochlear nerve from medial to lateral rather than from lateral to medial, to prevent inadvertent damage to the cochlear nerve fibers arising from the modiolus of cochlea or facial nerve fibers that are often splayed and adherent to the porus. One should never pull the tumor capsule to dissect it free. Constant irrigation with warm saline and hydrotomy of capsular plane helps to improve the dissection of the cleavage plane between the tumor and the adjacent nerves. We use the Zini's procedure, combining irrigation-hydrotomy properties with mucolytic solution (MESNA) and blunt instruments, which greatly improve dissection and preservation of neural structures.

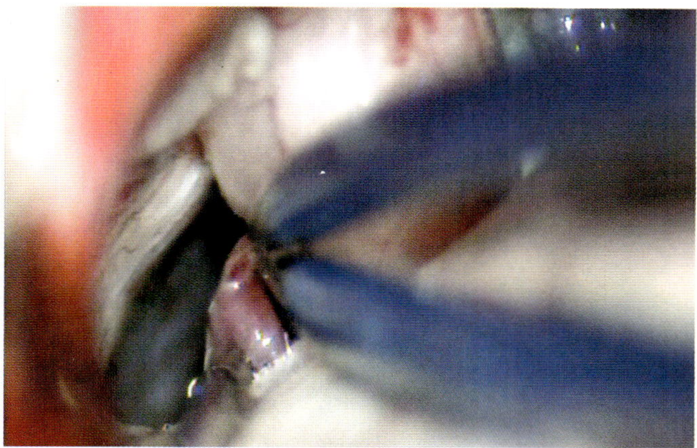

Fig. 7.81: The branch of AICA supplying tumor surface is isolated and coagulated with bipolar cautery close to tumoral surface

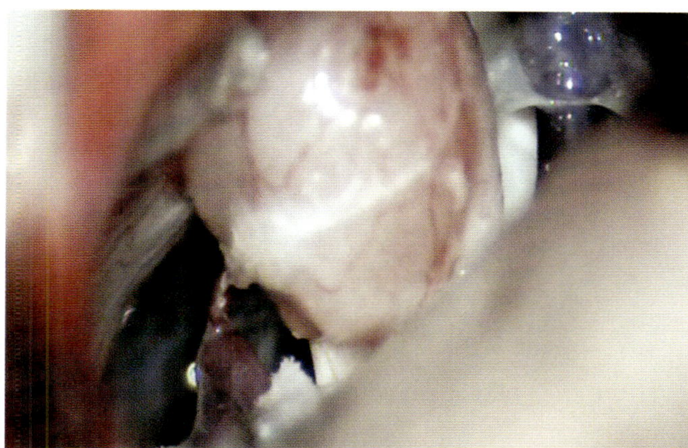

Fig. 7.82: The branch of AICA supplying tumor surface is coagulated close to tumoral surface

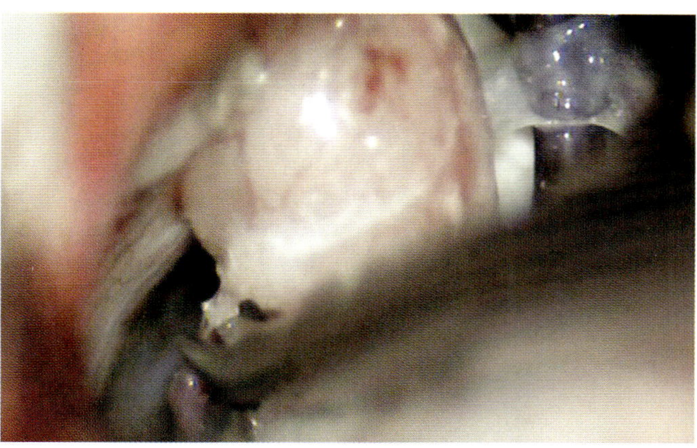

Fig. 7.83: The coagulated vascular branch supplying tumor surface is cut with bayonet scissors close to tumoral surface

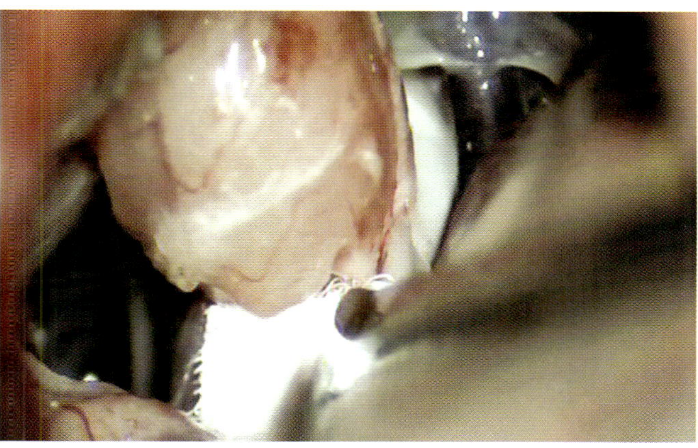

Fig. 7.84: Tumor is dissected from the underlying facial and cochlear nerve by blunt dissection while irrigating the tumor with warm saline

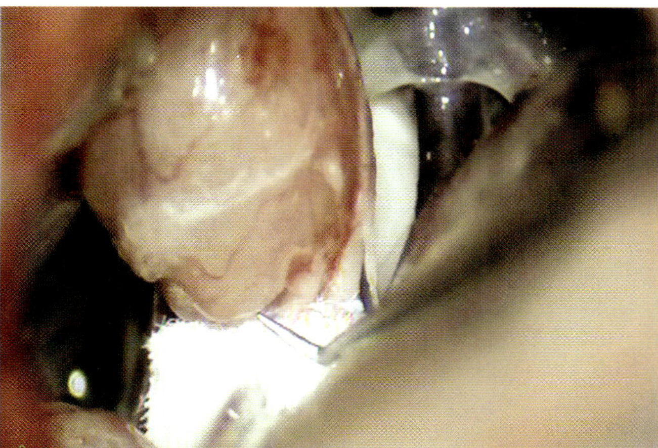

Fig. 7.85: The tumor is lifted from medial to lateral from the cochlear and facial nerve bundles using right-angled 2 mm blunt hook while protecting the two nerves with cottonoid between them and the tumor

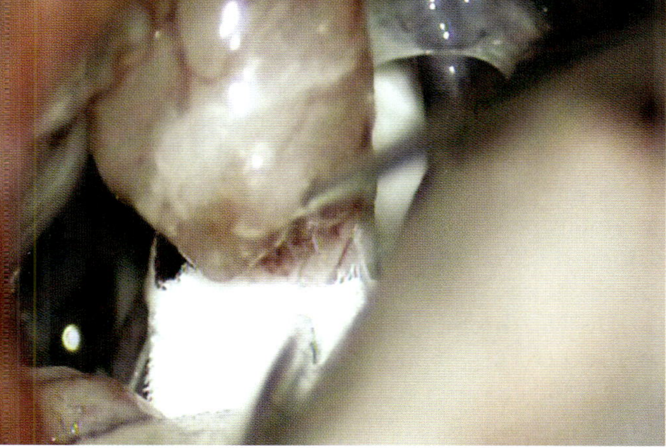

Fig. 7.86: The tumor is progressively dissected from medial to lateral from the underlying cochlear and facial nerve

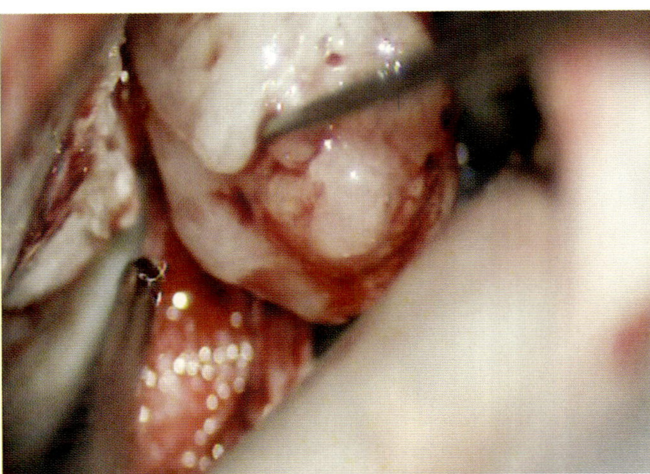

Fig. 7.87: The tumor is progressively dissected from medial to lateral from the underlying cochlear and facial nerve till the tumor extension into porus is reached. Facial nerve has variable adherence to tumor close to the porus of internal auditory meatus depending upon the size of tumor

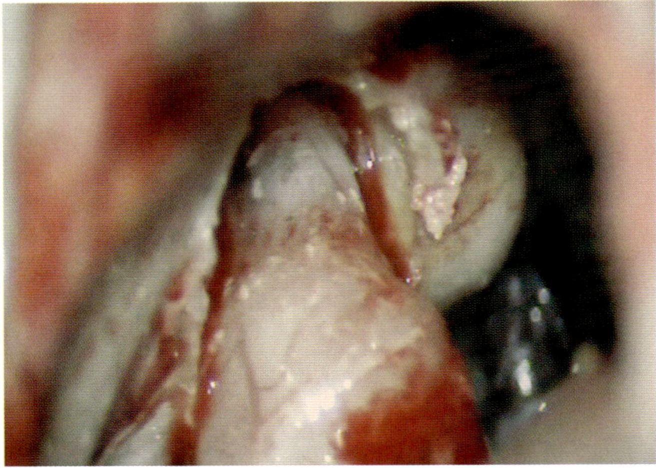

Fig. 7.88: The dissection is now shifted to lateral fundal end of IAM

Removal of Intracanalicular Part and Endoscopic Inspection of Fundus

The intracanalicular extension of neuroma is fortunately enucleated en bloc from the bottom of the IAM in majority of cases by establishing a plane of dissection between the tumor and the facial and cochlear nerve (Figs 7.88 to 7.92) without injury to the inner ear structures.

The facial nerve gains variable contact and adherence to the tumor when getting closer to the porus of the IAM (Fig. 7.93). The intermedius nerve is a good landmark to perform dissection where the facial nerve changes direction around the tumor approaching the meatal porus. The dissection is continued till we are well beyond the porus into the IAM (Figs 7.94 and 7.95). The cleavage plane becomes better again in its intracanalicular part.

Toward the end of the dissection exercise, the lateral most part of the IAM must be checked for residual tumor using a 30° endoscope (Fig. 7.96). Residual tumor is cleared by endoscope-assisted dissection, using bayonet-shaped ring curette (Figs 7.97 and 7.98) or right-angled curved elevator (Fig. 7.99), both of them being specially designed for this purpose. The 30° endoscope is held in the left hand and is stabilized keeping its tip against the walls of the drilled bone of the IAM (Fig. 7.96). The bayonet ring curette instrument is held in the right hand and is glided parallel to the endoscope under external vision till the tip of the instrument is seen by the endoscopic picture (Fig. 7.97). The diameter of the ring of the curette is 2 mm and the length of the shaft of the curette is 1 cm. The ring is angled at 120° from the shaft and is not straight. This instrument allows an accurate dissection of the remnant tumoral fragment from the fundus laterally and cochlear and facial nerves anteriorly (Fig. 7.98). A free canal allows insight to the transverse crest and penetration of cochlear and facial nerves in the petrous bone (Figs 7.100 and 7.101). Needless to say, the entire dissection of the cisternal and intracanalicular component of the tumor should be done in an extremely delicate manner taking care not to injure the blood supply of the cochlear nerve and cochlea (Figs 7.102 and 7.103). Though it is not possible to preserve the hearing at present in all the cases, the effort is worth the result that is received in majority of the patients while we are striving for improvement in our results. The causes for loss of hearing in such hearing preservation techniques are many. The direct injury to the vestibule or semicircular canal, cochlear nerve fibers, injury to the blood vessels supplying the cochlear nerve and more commonly cochlea and postoperative fibrosis leading to further worsening in the blood supply are some of the factors we guess we know at present. But we believe there are various other reasons that are not conceived as the cause for such loss and further advances in basic research and electrophysiological advances may help us to understand this better.

Final Evaluation

Final assessment of the fundus and CPA is performed with 30° endoscope (Figs 7.102 and 7.103).

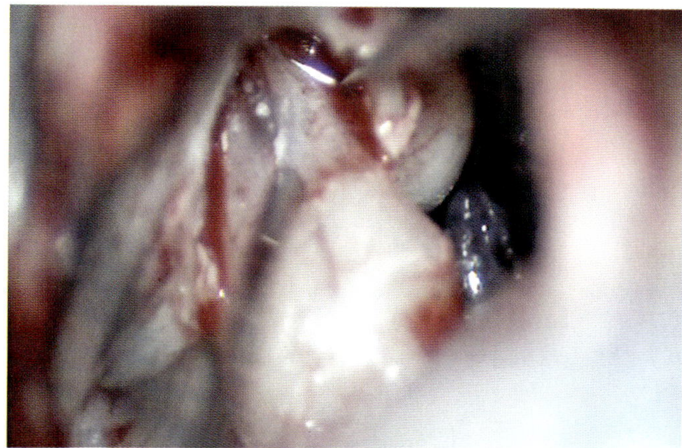

Fig. 7.89: The tumor is lifted from lateral to medial from the cochlear and facial nerve bundles using right-angled 2 mm blunt hook by finding the plane between tumor and the nerves

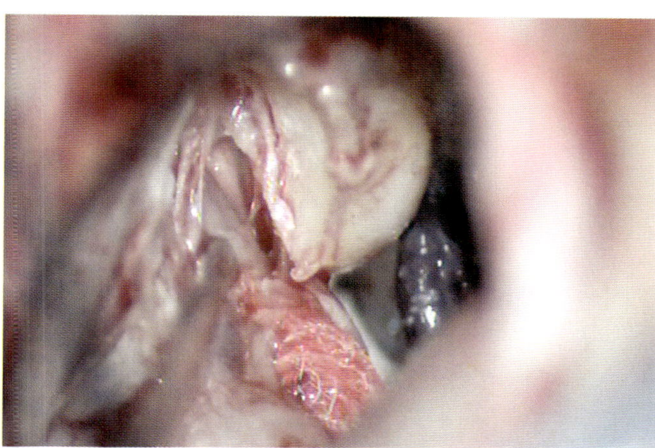

Fig. 7.90: Facial nerve is identified in anterosuperior quadrant of IAM after dissecting the tumor capsule from it

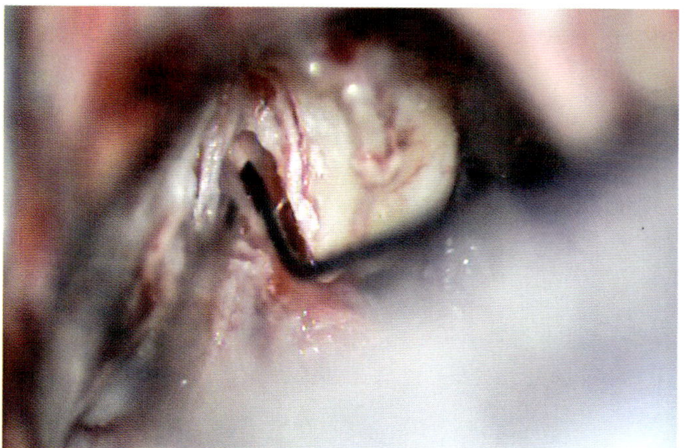

Fig. 7.91: Facial nerve identification is reinforced by stimulating it with low power (less than 0.5 mA current) facial nerve stimulation

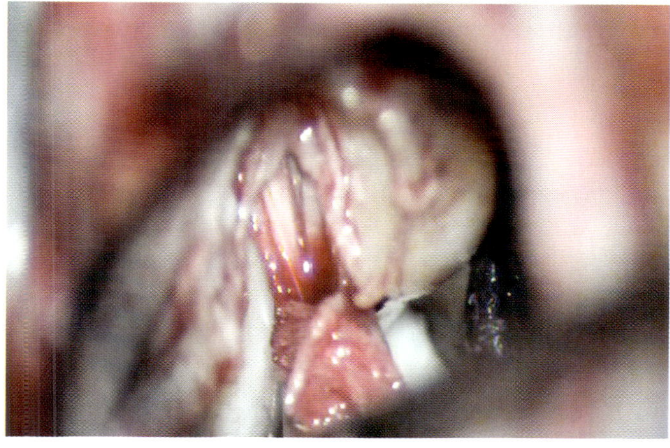

Fig. 7.92: The tumor is lifted from lateral to medial from the cochlear and facial nerve bundles up to porus attachment using right-angled 2 mm blunt hook while protecting the two nerves with cottonoid between them and the tumor

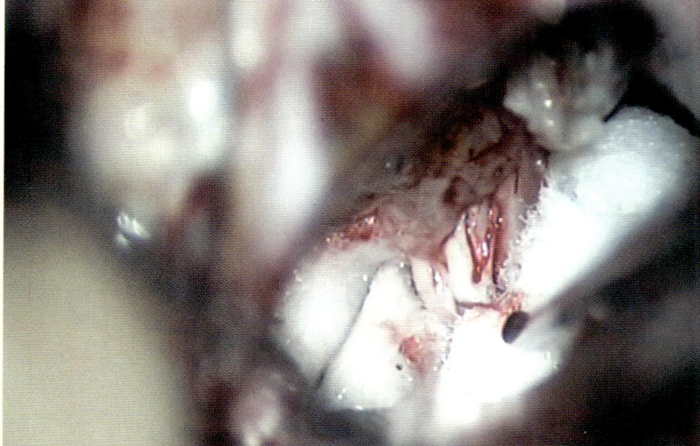

Fig. 7.93: Final dissection is carried out at the porus to dissect the firm tumor attachments to the underlying nerve and dura

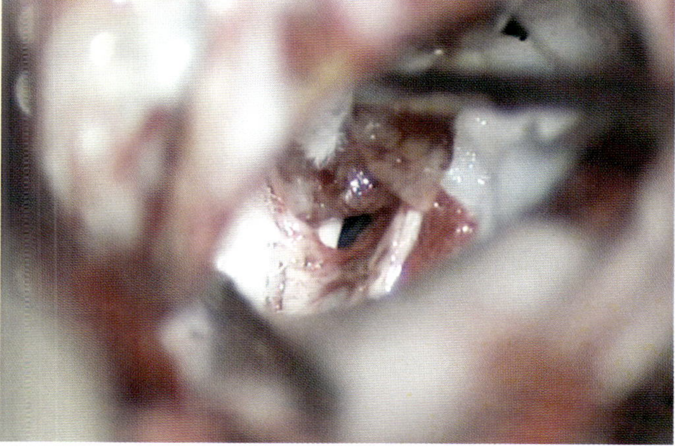

Fig. 7.94: The facial and cochlear nerve are maximally splayed at the porus due to firm adhesions between tumor and facial nerve

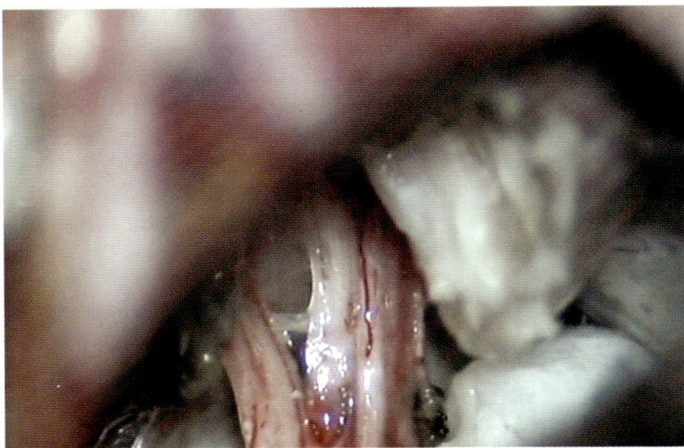

Fig. 7.95: The facial and cochlear nerve are maximally splayed at the porus. Facial nerve has variable adherence to tumor close to the porus of internal auditory meatus depending upon the size of tumor

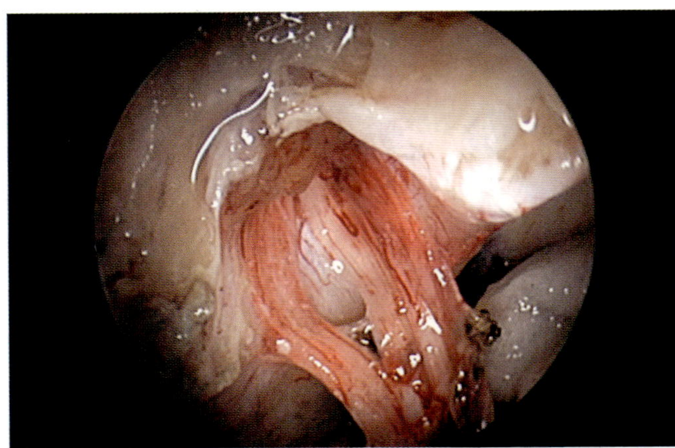

Fig. 7.96: Lateral most fundal part of IAM is checked for residual tumor using a 30° endoscope

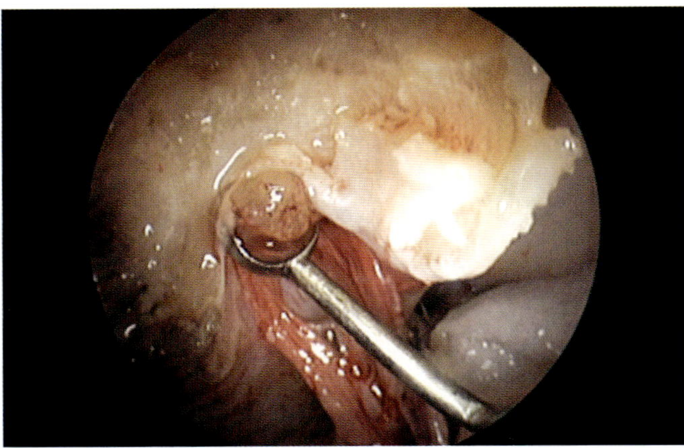

Fig. 7.97: The 30° endoscope is held in the left hand and is stabilized against the bone of the IAM and bayonet-shaped ring curette specially designed for endoscopic dissection of tumor from lateral most part of IAM is inserted under guidance

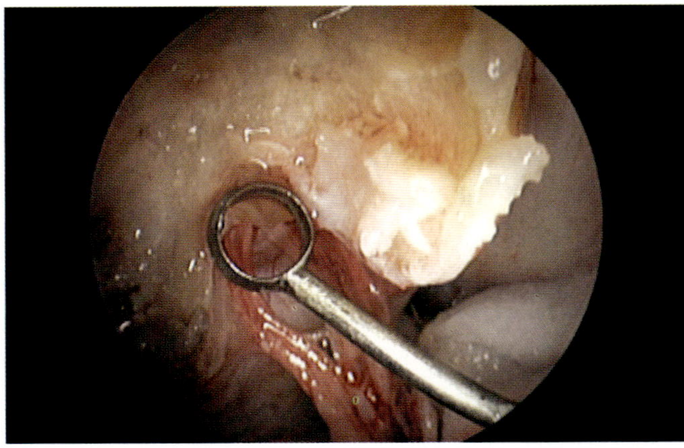

Fig. 7.98: Tumor from fundus of IAM is removed using bayonet-shaped ring curette specially designed for endoscopic dissection of tumor from lateral most part of IAM

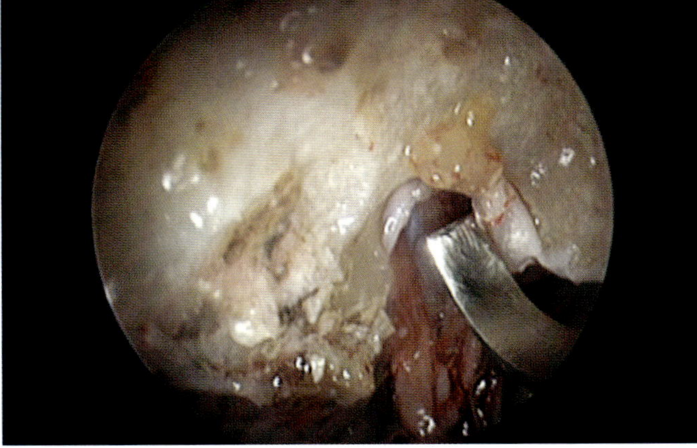

Fig. 7.99: Sometimes other instruments like curved elevator is used for this terminal dissection of tumor from fundus

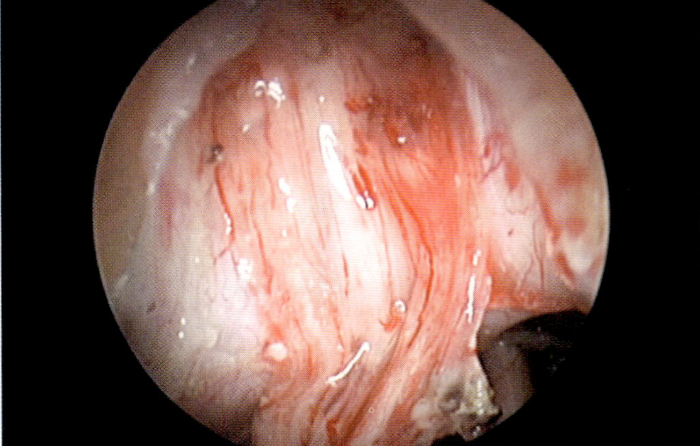

Fig. 7.100: Endoscopic picture of the lateral end of IAM after the tumor is removed

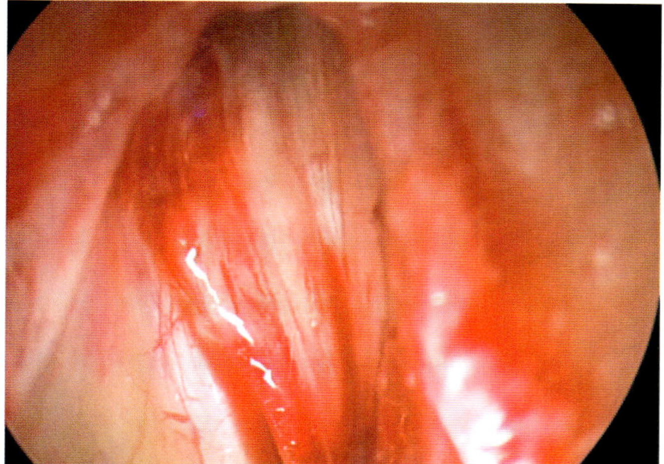

Fig. 7.101: Close up endoscopic view of the lateral end of IAM after the tumor is removed

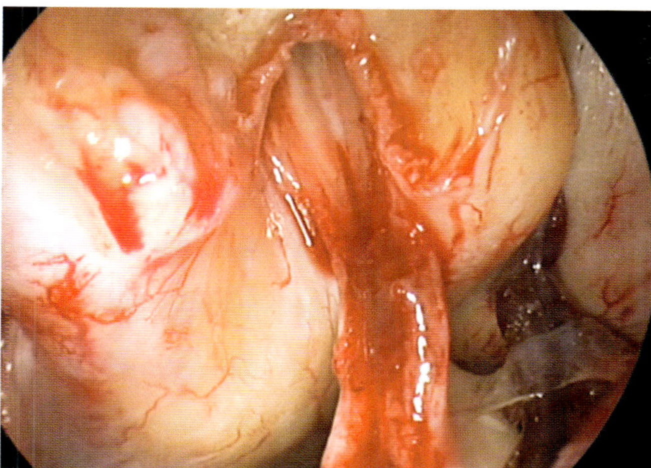

Fig. 7.102: Endoscopic picture showing removal of the entire cisternal and intracanalicular component of the tumor with preservation of the cochlear and facial nerve with the blood supply

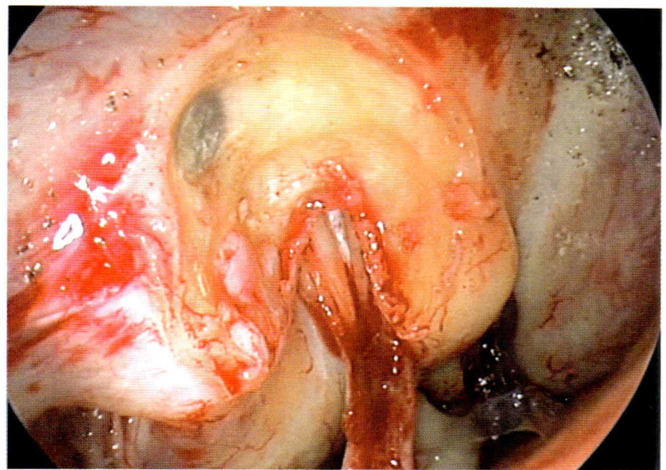

Fig. 7.103: Final endoscopic picture showing removal of the entire cisternal and intracanalicular component of the tumor with preservation of the cochlear and facial nerve. The top of jugular bulb is seen exposed during the drilling of the IAM

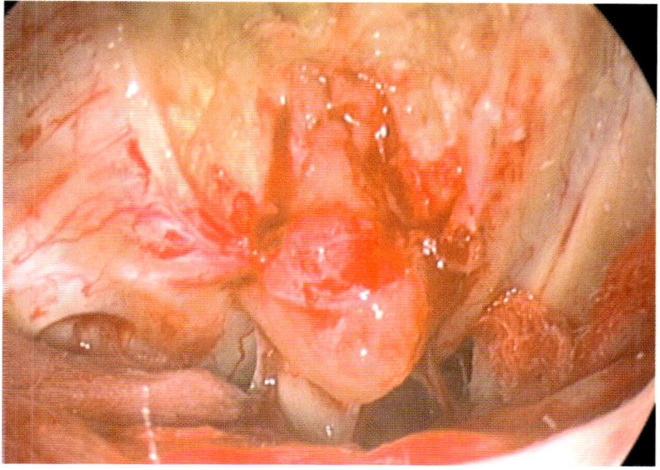

Fig. 7.104: Case 2: In tumors with small cisternal extension like this, no debulking is required. After drilling of IAM, intracanalicular component of tumor is now visible in continuity with cisternal component

We would like to reinforce the importance of dissection of cisternal and intracanalicular tumor along with endoscopic clearance from the fundus with illustrations from various other cases (Figs 7.104 to 7.131).

The electrophysiological nerve integrity (or lack of it) of both the facial and the cochlear nerves are evaluated by direct nerve stimulation (Fig. 7.131). The ABR alone (especially its absence at the end of dissection) is not a reliable indication for hearing results postoperatively, as they may be disturbed temporarily by multiple parameters.

Closure

Protective cottonoids are removed from the CPA. The posterior fossa is washed with physiological solution at 37°C to clear residual bone dust and blood clots and to ensure small vessel hemostasis. The mastoid air cells accidentally opened around the IAM are meticulously sealed with bone wax. The opening of IAC is closed with free subcutaneous fat and fortified by Surgicel and fibrin glue (Figs 7.132 to 7.135) preferred to a muscle tissue, whose

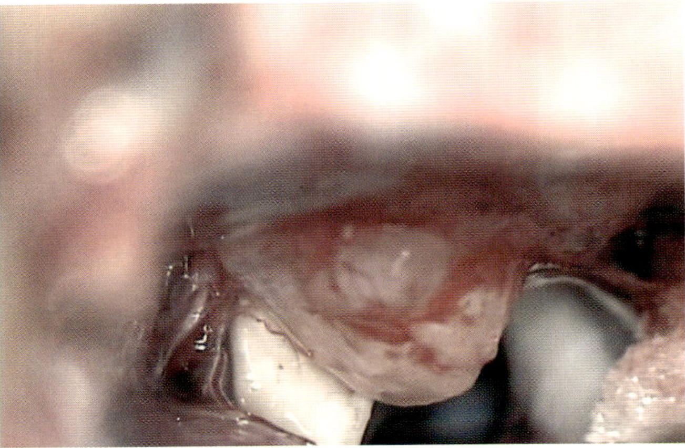

Fig. 7.105: Case 2: The vestibulocochlear nerve is delineated at the medial end of tumor

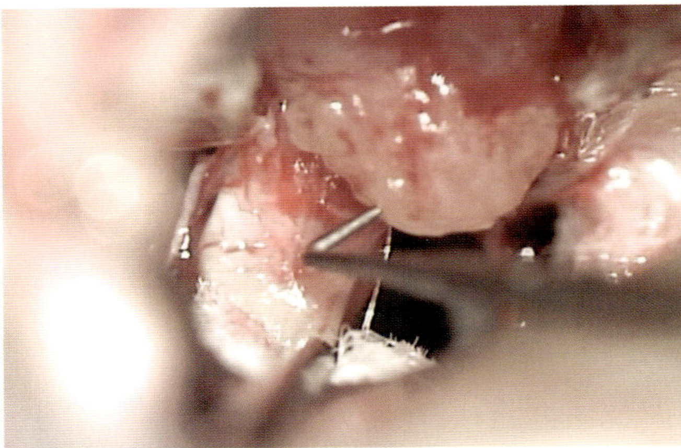

Fig. 7.106: Case 2: The tumor is lifted from medial to lateral from the cochlear and facial nerve bundles using right-angled 2 mm blunt hook while protecting the two nerves with cottonoid between them and the tumor

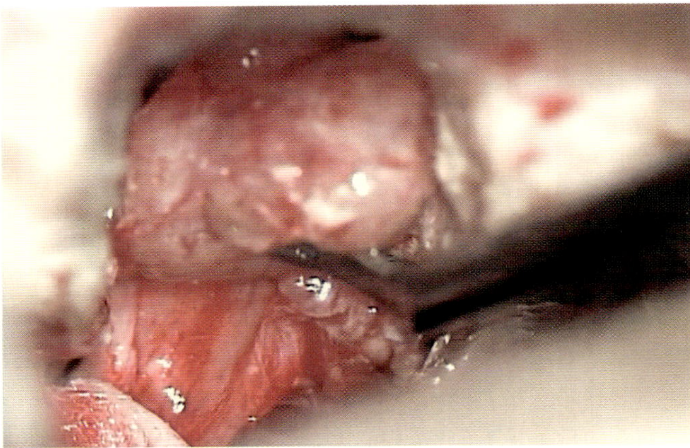

Fig. 7.107: Case 2: The tumor is progressively dissected from medial to lateral from the underlying cochlear and facial nerve till the tumor extension into porus is reached

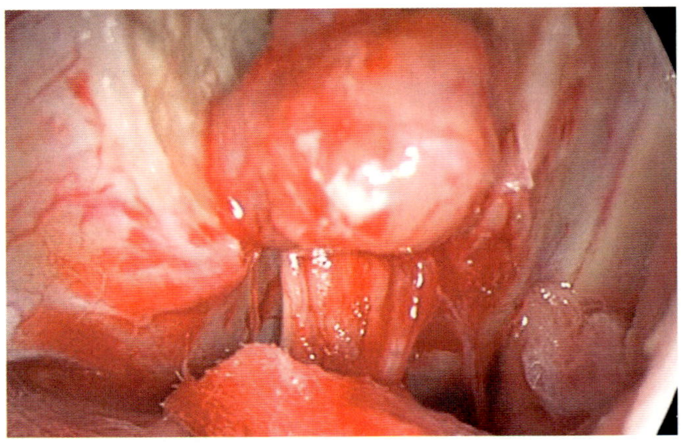

Fig. 7.108: Case 2: Endoscopic view of tumor dissected from underlying facial and cochlear nerve up to porus

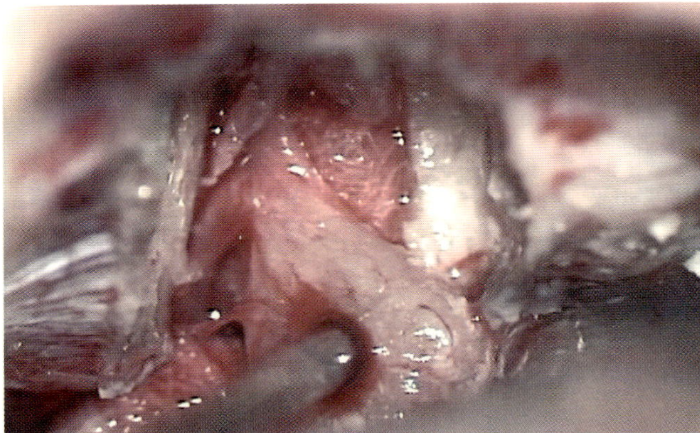

Fig. 7.109: Case 2: The dissection is now shifted to lateral fundal end of IAM. The tumor is lifted from lateral to medial from the cochlear and facial nerve bundles using right-angled 2 mm blunt hook by finding the plane between tumor and the nerves

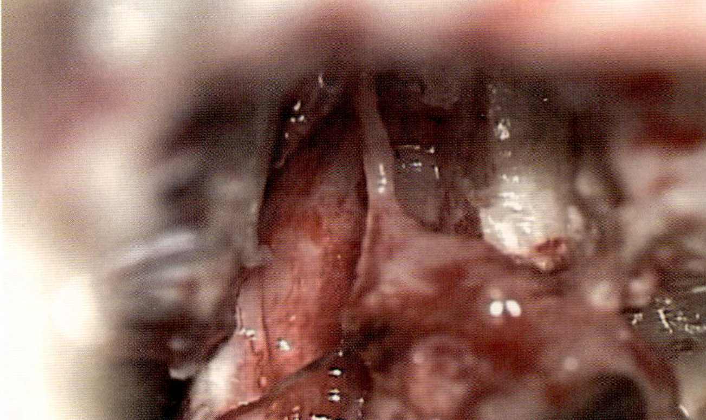

Fig. 7.110: Case 2: The tumor dissected from lateral fundal part with attachment with the lateral end of inferior vestibular nerve

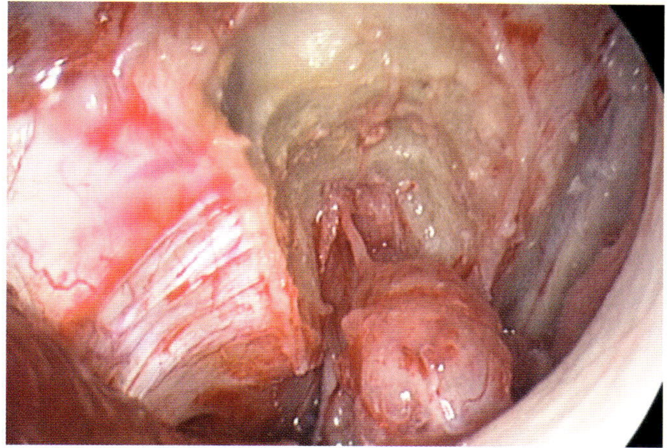

Fig. 7.111: Case 2: Endoscopic view showing the tumor dissected from lateral fundal part with attachment with the lateral end of inferior vestibular nerve

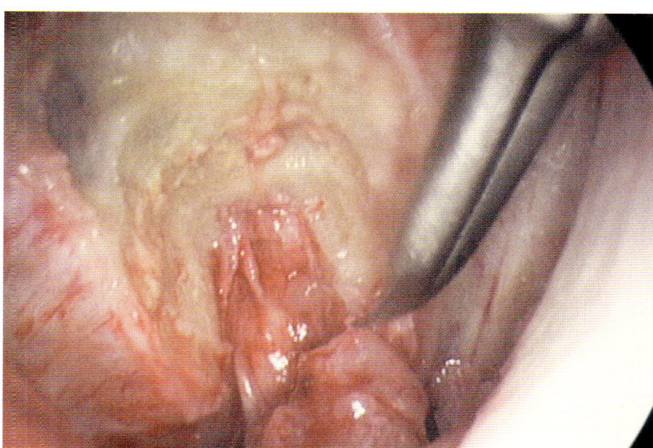

Fig. 7.112: Case 2: The lateral attachment of the tumor is cut with scissors

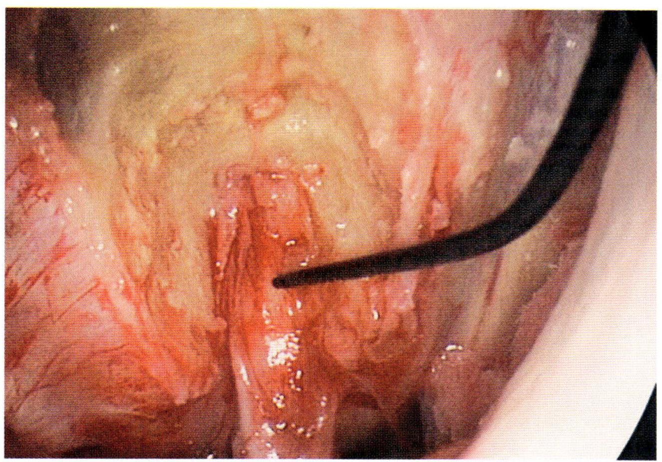

Fig. 7.113: Case 2: Final endoscopic view after tumor removal with stimulation of facial nerve

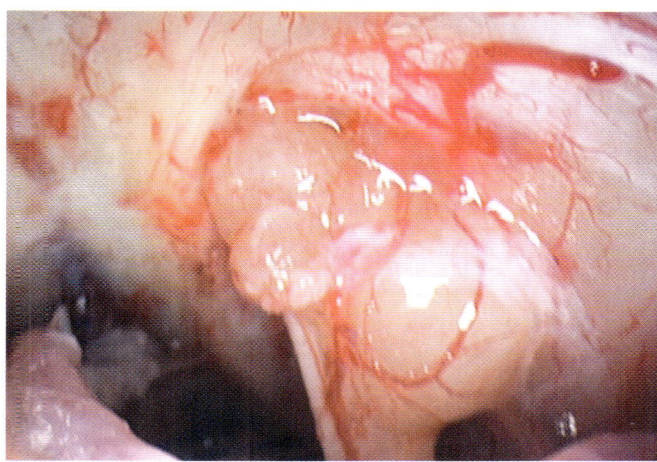

Fig. 7.114: Case 3: Stage 2 tumor with small cisternal extension

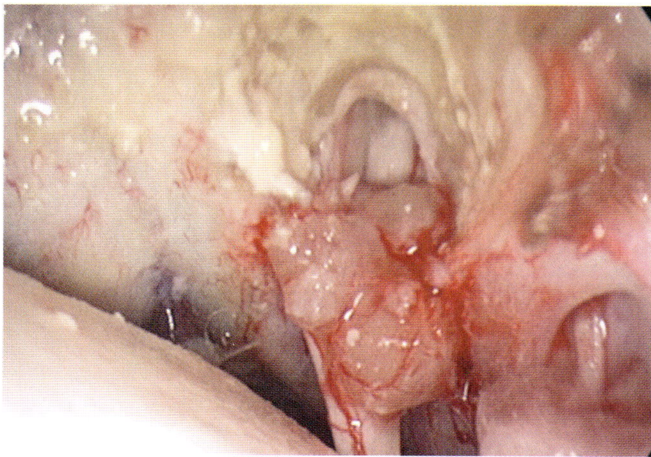

Fig. 7.115: Case 3: The IAM is drilled open and intracanalicular extension dissected from underlying facial and cochlear nerves

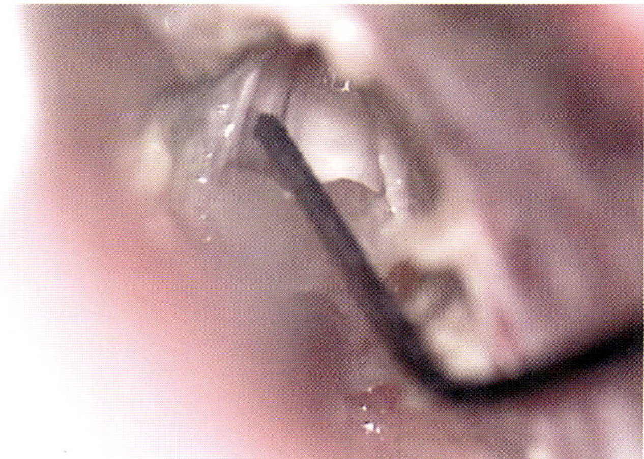

Fig. 7.116: Case 3: Facial nerve reconfirmed with stimulation

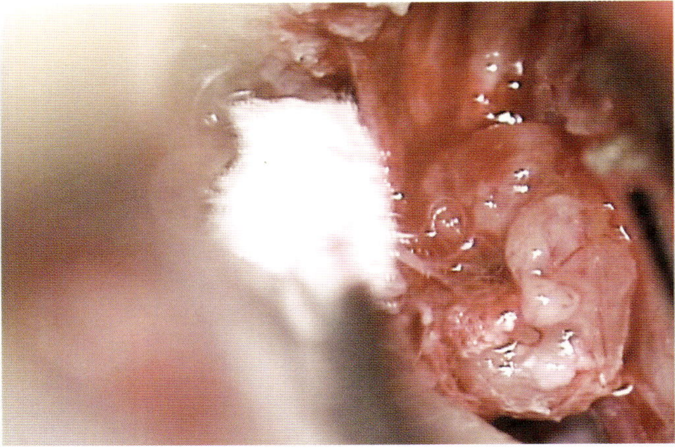

Fig. 7.117: Case 3: Dissection of tumor from underlying facial and cochlear nerves

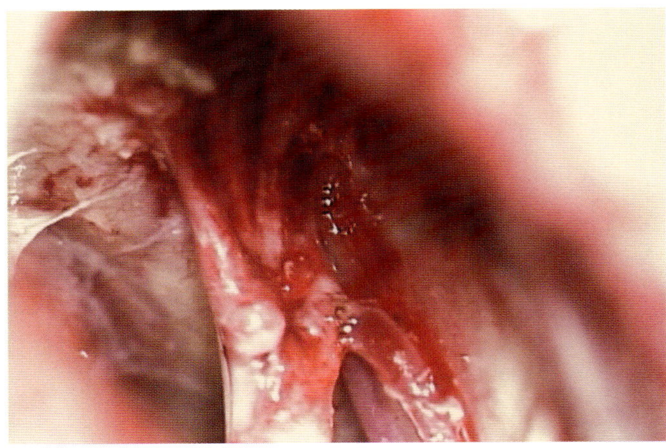

Fig. 7.118: Case 3: Final microscopic view after tumor removal

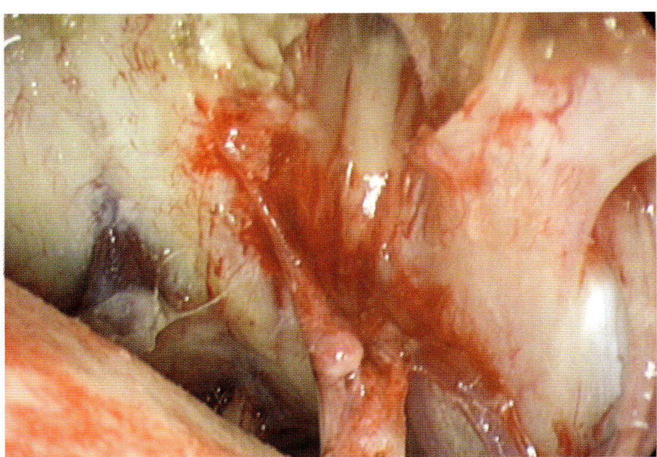

Fig. 7.119: Case 3: Final endoscopic view after tumor removal

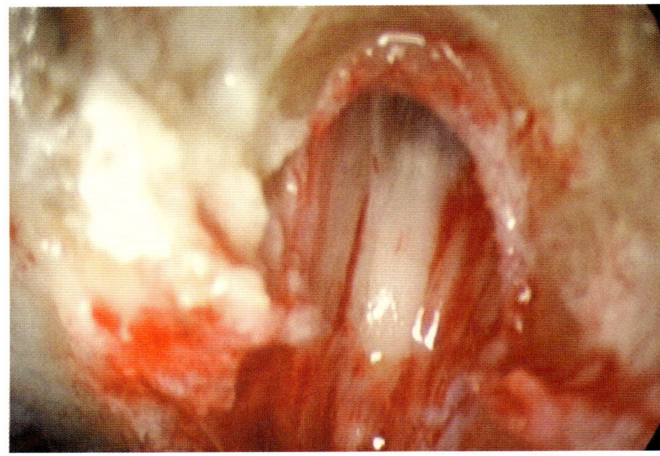

Fig. 7.120: Case 3: Final endoscopic view of fundus of IAM after tumor removal

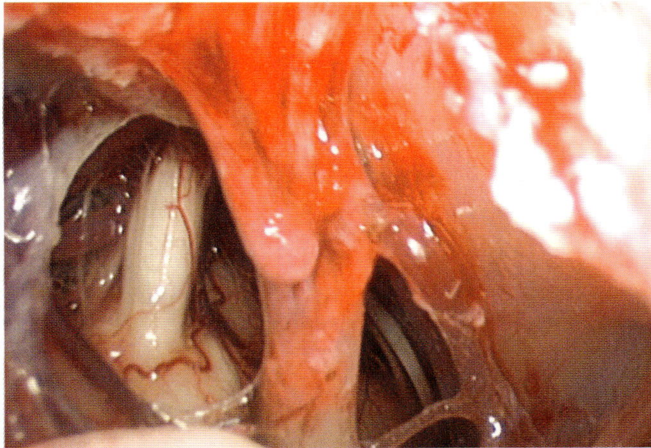

Fig. 7.121: Case 3: Final endoscopic view of CPA after tumor removal

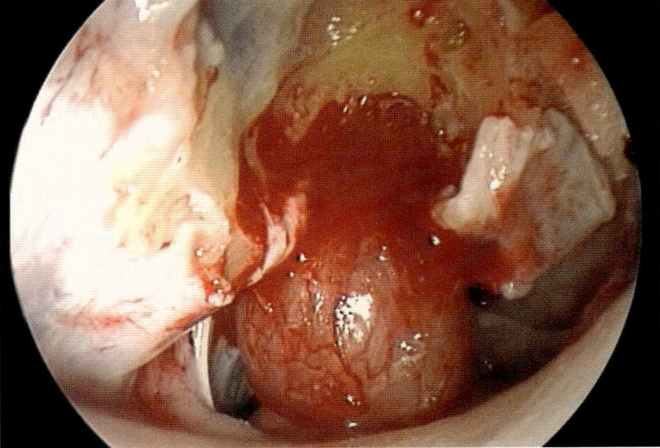

Fig. 7.122: Case 4: Stage 3 AN tumor touching the pons surface without its distortion. The IAM is drilled open showing grade C extension up to fundus

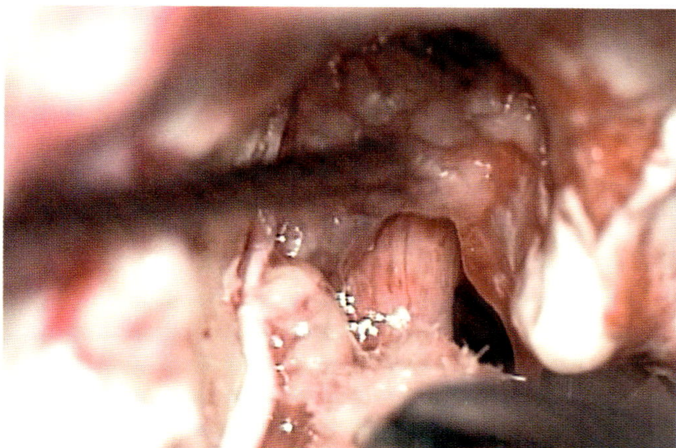

Fig. 7.123: Case 4: After debulking of tumor the medial end is dissected from underlying facial and cochlear nerves up to porus

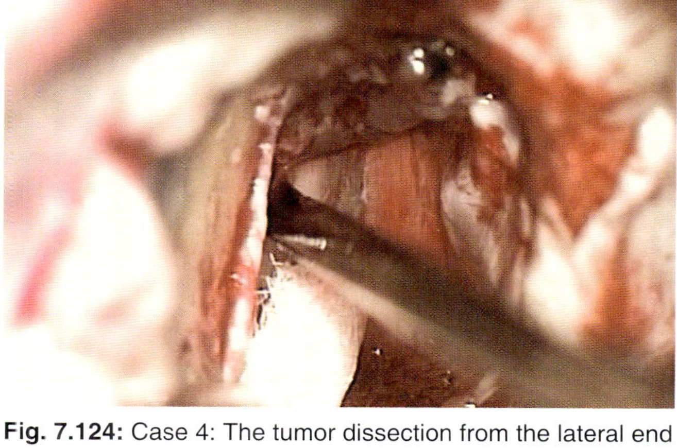

Fig. 7.124: Case 4: The tumor dissection from the lateral end of IAM is complete with remnant in the fundus

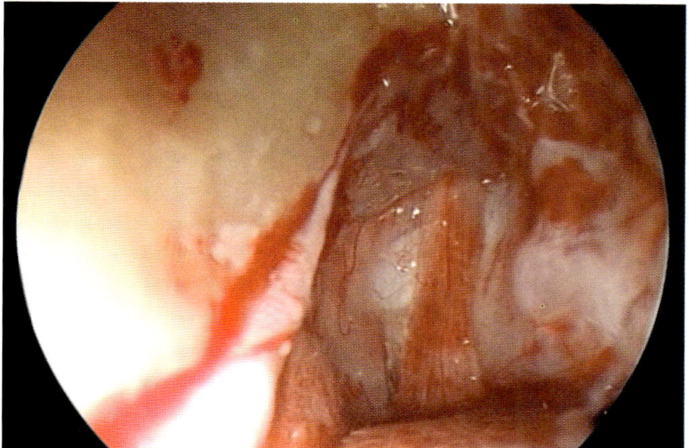

Fig. 7.125: Case 4: Endoscopic view showing the remnant tumor in the lateral fundal end of IAM

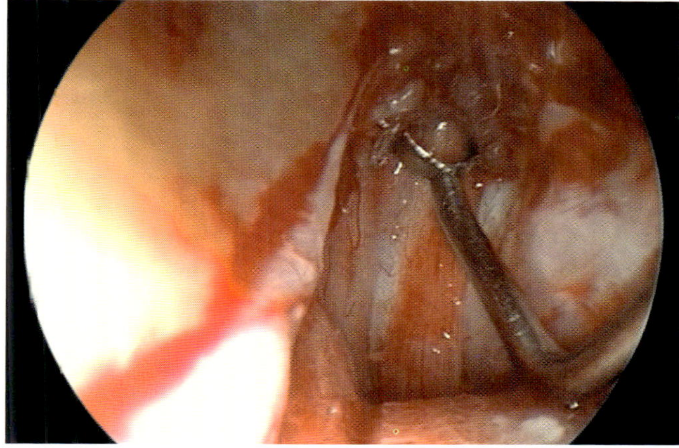

Fig. 7.126: Case 4: Endoscopic dissection of remnant tumor in fundus using specially designed bayonet-shaped ring curette. The 30° endoscope is held in the left hand and is stabilized against the bone of the IAM and bayonet-shaped ring curette specially designed for endoscopic dissection of tumor from lateral most part of IAM is inserted under guidance

MRI signal can be confusing in the postoperative period as residual tumor. Before assuring closure of the dura, the posterior fossa must be completely filled with saline solution to avoid pneumocephalus. The closure of the craniotomy defect and subcutaneous tissue is discussed in detail in Chapter 4. The dura mater is sutured using 5-0 silk sutures over the Durapatch. The dural opening does not always allow a waterproof stitch suture, so it may be sealed with periosteal muscular fragments fixed with biological glue. Craniotomy defect is obliterated with bone paste. Periosteal incision is closed with 2-0 Prolene. Skin incision is closed with 3-0 Nylon.

POSTOPERATIVE CARE

The average time for operation is 4 h. Then the patient is taken to step down unit and is back to his hospital room on the same day. Antibiotic and analgesic coverage is started. The mean hospitalization time is 8 days.

RESULTS

From a study of 171 patients[6] with CPA tumors that underwent surgery in our unit from October 93 to December 98, 119 patients had an AN stage I, II or III with preoperative hearing threshold preserved. The 52 patients

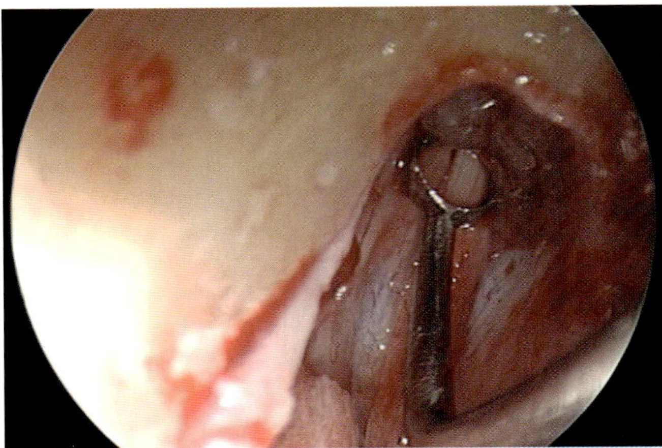

Fig. 7.127: Case 4: Endoscopic dissection of remnant tumor in fundus using specially designed bayonet-shaped ring curette. Endoscopic dissection of the remnant tumor from the fundus laterally and cochlear and facial nerves anteriorly with ring curette

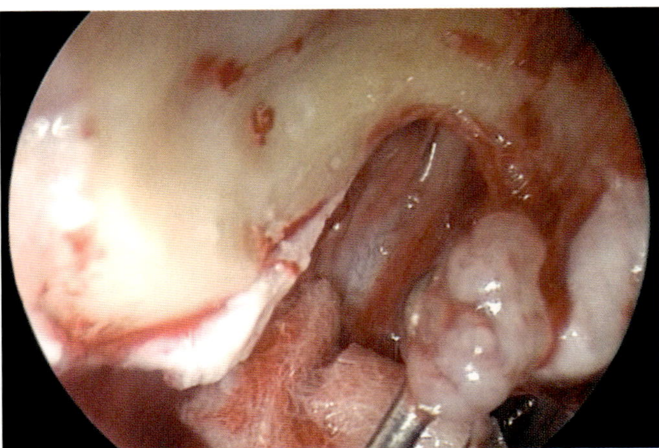

Fig. 7.128: Case 4: Endoscopic dissection of remnant tumor in fundus completed using specially designed bayonet-shaped ring curette

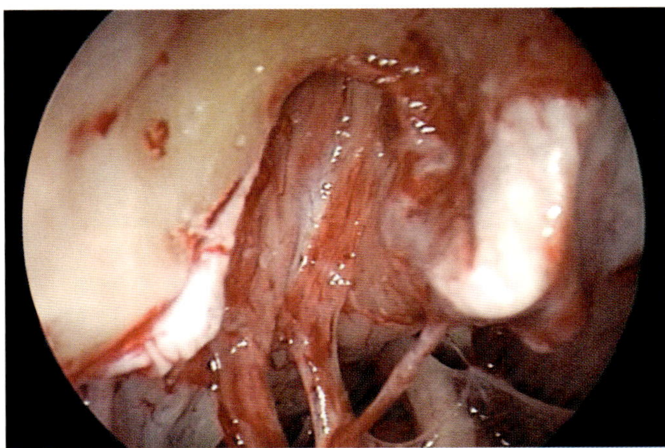

Fig. 7.129: Case 4: Final endoscopic view after tumor removal

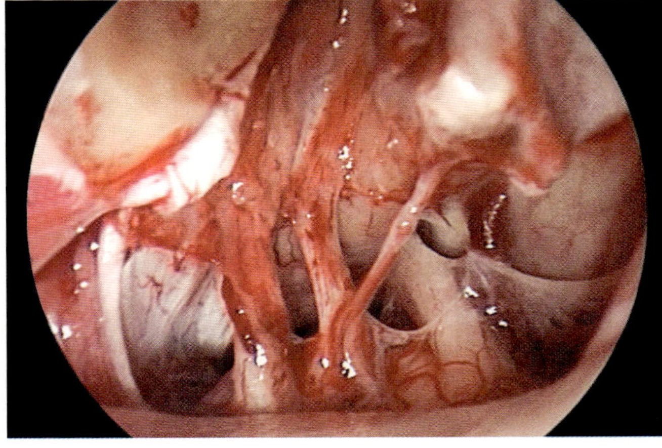

Fig. 7.130: Case 4: Final endoscopic view after tumor removal. Removal of the entire cisternal and intracanalicular component of the tumor with preservation of the cochlear and facial nerve

excluded from analysis had 2 facial nerve neuromas, 8 cochlear nerve neuromas, 42 tumors greater than 25 mm in CPA or with bad or miserable hearing threshold (Shelton's type D).

Survival in AN surgery is now granted; there was no mortality in 171 CPA tumors operated on in the above period. Morbidity is low with 10 cases of CSF leak, 5 of which required revision surgery. Out of 119 retrosigmoid approaches performed, two cases had persistent headache and one had unexplained paralysis of abducent nerve. The 119 patients' functional results were analyzed.

Classification according to tumor stages and facial nerve function after 1-year follow-up is shown in Table 7.1.

The two grade IV patients had tumors abnormally adherent to facial nerve and in one case the facial nerve was situated behind the tumor.

The overall hearing results showed 58 patients with hearing preserved out of a series of 119 patients. The classification of patients according to Shelton's is shown in Table 7.2.

Besides the tumor stage and difficulty of tumor dissection, the predictive factors for hearing preservation in AN removal are, as far as we observed, the presence of synchronized ABRs or preoperative otoacoustic emission (OAE), as well as the preoperative hearing level.

Actually, in the group with preserved hearing postoperatively, synchronized ABR and spontaneous

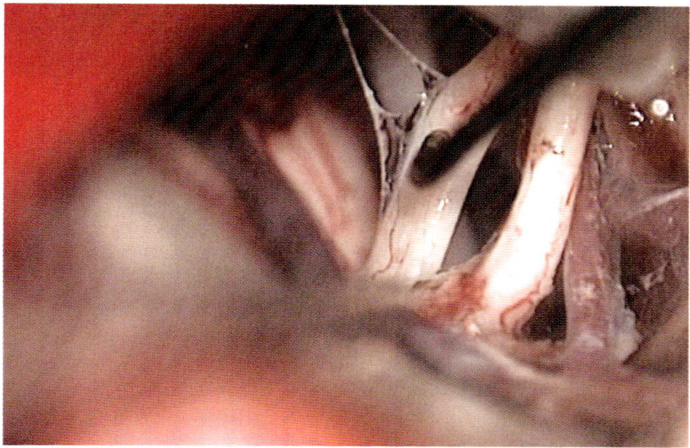

Fig. 7.131: Functional integrity of both the facial and cochlear nerve are reconfirmed at the end of the procedure

Fig. 7.132: The mastoid air cells opened accidentally around the IAM are meticulously sealed with bone wax. IAM is obliterated with subcutaneous fat

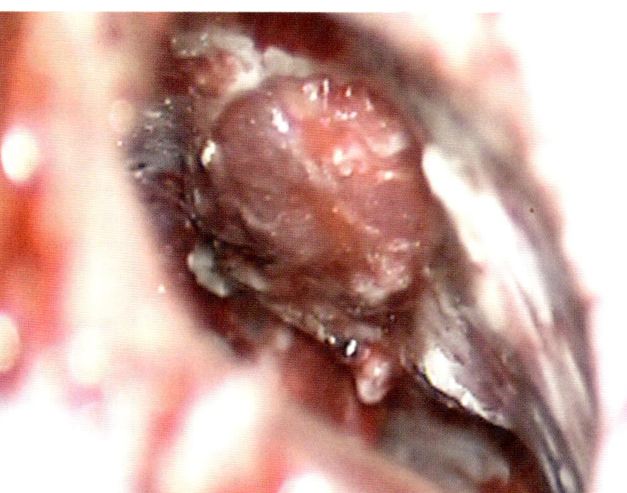

Fig. 7.133: Internal auditory meatus obliteration with subcutaneous fat is reinforced with fibrin glue

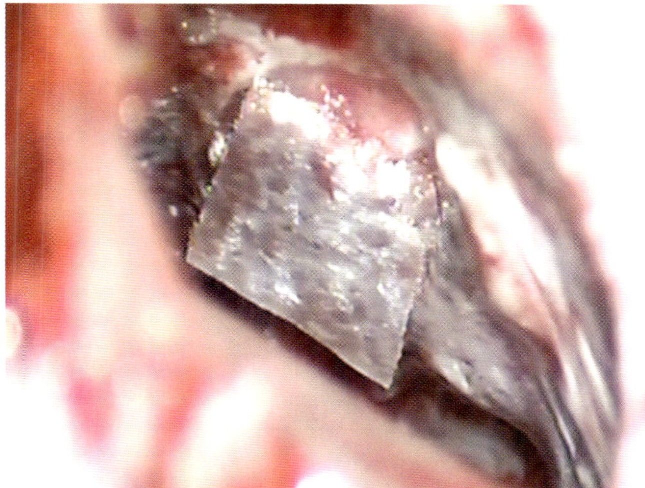

Fig. 7.134: Internal auditory meatus obliteration is further fortified with a piece of Surgicel

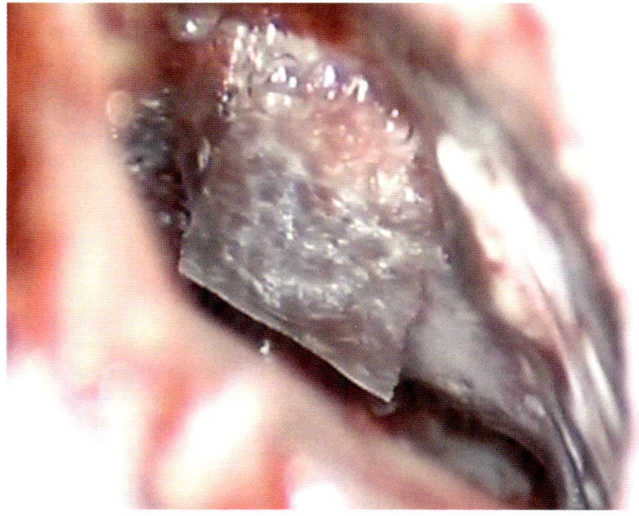

Fig. 7.135: Internal auditory meatus obliteration with subcutaneous fat and Surgicel are glued to each other with fibrin glue

Table 7.1: Retrosigmoid acoustic neurinomas according to the Brackmann House facial nerve classification*

Tumor	*Grade I (91%)*	*Grade II (96%)*	*Grade III*	*Grade IV*
Intracanal	19	1		
< 10 mm	66	2	2	1
< 25 mm	25	2		1

*n=119

Source: Otology & Neurotology, Vol. 23, No. 2, 2000

Table 7.2: Hearing function before and after surgery according to Shelton classification

Classification	*Before*	*After*
Type A (0–30 dB)	37 (31%)	17 (14.5%)
Type B (30–50 dB)	50 (42%)	18 (15.5%)
Type C (+ 50 dB)	32 (27%)	23 (19%)
Type D (deafness)		61 (51%)

OAE were detected in greater percentage than the group with hearing lost. Equally, as for the preoperative hearing level studied in the "hearing preserved" group and "postoperative deafness" group, it is higher in the "hearing preserved" group with an average 34.8 dB loss, for 48.9 dB loss in the "postoperative deafness" group.

Preoperative hearing level is thus an indirect predictive sign for cochlear nerve–tumor surgical cleavage. Imaging monitoring is done at 2 and 5 years.

CONCLUSION

Acoustic neuroma surgery for small or medium size tumors is completely different from the techniques used for neuromas greater than 20 mm in CPA: while the latter is an intracranial tumor, the former is a tumor of acoustico-facial nerve bundle where functional prognosis is of primary importance. The goal for this surgery should be to preserve the facial nerve function in 100% of cases and hearing function in 50% of cases. The keyhole retrosigmoid approach allows one to obtain results not far from this ideal. Long-term experiences in neurotologic surgery with sincere postoperative follow-up and critical analysis of failures, and appropriate modifications have simplified and standardized the surgical procedure to get facial nerve preservation (House Brackman Grade I/II) in more than 97% and hearing preservation for small and medium tumors (less than 2 cm) in 54% of our cases.[52]

REFERENCES

1. Douglas D. Backous, Huong T. Pham. Guiding patients through the choices for treating vestibular schwannomas: balancing options and ensuring informed consent. Neurosurg Clin N Am. 2008;19:379–92.
2. Friedman WA, Bradshaw P, Myers A, et al. Linear accelerator radiosurgery for vestibular schwannomas. J Neurosurg. 2006;105:657–61.
3. Lunsford LD, Niranjan A, Flickinger JC, et al. Radiosurgery of vestibular schwannomas: summary of experience in 829 cases. J Neurosurg. 2005;102(Suppl):195–9.
4. Hasegawa T, Fujutani S, Katsumata S, et al. Stereotactic radiosurgery for vestibular schwannomas: analysis of 317 patients followed more than 5 years. Neurosurgery. 2005;57:257–65.
5. Shokek O, Terezakis S, Hughes MA, et al. Hypofractionated stereotactic radiotherapy as primary treatment of acoustic neuroma: interim results of the Johns Hopkins experience. Int J Radiat Oncol Biol Phys. 2004;60(Suppl 1):314.
6. Magnan J, Barbieri M, Mora R, et al. Retrosigmoid approach for small and medium sized acoustic neuromas. Otol Neurotol. 2002;23:141–5.
7. Lassaletta L, Fontes L, Mecon E, et al. Hearing preservation with the retrosigmoid approach for vestibular schwannoma: myth or reality? Otolaryngol Head and Neck Surg. 2003;129:397–401.
8. Brackmann D, Owens R, Friedman R, et al. Prognostic factors for hearing preservation in vestibular schwannoma surgery. Am J Otolaryngol. 2000;21(3):417–24.
9. Weber P, Gantz B. Results and complications from acoustic neuromas excision via middle cranial fossa approach. Am J Otolaryngol. 1996;17:669–75.
10. Satar B, Jackler R, Oghalai J, et al. Risk-benefit analysis of using the middle fossa approach for acoustic neuromas with less than 10 mm cerebello-pontine angle component. Laryngoscope. 2002;112:1500–6.
11. Ito K, Kurita H, Sugasawa K, Okuno T, Mizuno M, Sasaki T. Neuro-otological findings after radiosurgery for acoustic neuromas. Arch Otolaryngol Head Neck Surg. 1996;122:1229–33.
12. Wiet R, Micco A, Bauer G. Complications of the gamma knife. Arch Otolaryngol Head Neck Surg. 1996;122:414–6.
13. Sekhar L, Gormlex W, Wright J. The best treatment for vestibular schwannoma (Acoustic Neuroma): microsurgery or radiosurgery? Am J Otol. 1996;17:676–82.
14. Hanabusa K, Morikawa A, Murata T, et al. Acoustic neuroma with malignant transformation: case report. J Neurosurg. 2001;95:518–21.

15. Shin M, Ueki K, Kurita H, et al. Malignant transformation of a vestibular schwannoma after gamma knife radiosurgery. Lancet. 2002;360:309–10.
16. Yoshimoto Y. Systematic review of the natural history of vestibular schwannoma. J Neurosurg. 2005;103(1):59–63.
17. Raut V, Walsh R, Bath A, et al. Conservative management of vestibular schwannomas: second review of a prospective longitudinal study. Clin Otolaryngol Allied Sci. 2004;29(5):505–14.
18. Brémond G, Garcin M, Magnan J. Preservation of hearing in the removal of acoustic neuroma (minima posterior approach by retrosigmoid route). J Laryngol. 1980;94: 1199–204.
19. Rand R, Kurze T. Preservation of vestibular, cochlear and facial nerves during microsurgical removal of acoustic tumor. Report of two cases. J Neurol Surg. 1968;28:158–61.
20. Smith M, Miller R, Coxe D. Suboccipital microsurgical removal of acoustic neuroma of all sizes. Ann Otol Rhinol Laryngol. 1973;82:407–14.
21. Smith M, Laqger R. Hearing conservation in acoustic neurilemmoma surgery via retrosigmoid approach. Otolaryngol Head Neck Surg. 1984;92:168–75.
22. Sterkers J. Préservation de l'audition dans la chirurgie des neurinomes de l'acoustique par la voie d'abord rétrosigmoide (80 cas). Rev Laryngol Otol Rhinol. 1982;103:21–4.
23. Magnan J, Deveze A, Miyazaki H, Canani FB. Cerebellopontine angle surgery by the retrosigmoid approach: our experience in elderly patients. Mediterr J Otol. 2005;1:1–7.
24. Harner S, Beatty C, Ebersole M. Retrosigmoid approach of acoustic neuroma. Exper Otolaryngol Head Neck Surg. 1990;103:40–5.
25. Nadol J, Chong C,Ojemann R. Preservation of hearing and facial nerve function in resection of acoustic neuroma. Laryngoscope. 1992;102:1153–8.
26. Cohen N, Lewis W, Ramsohoff J. Hearing preservation in cerebellopontine angle tumor surgery, the NYU experience 1974–1991. Am J Otol. 1993;14:423–33.
27. Sterkers J, Morrison G, Sterkers O, Badre El-Dine. Preservation of facial, cochlear, and other nerve functions in acoustic neuroma treatment. Otolaryngol Head Neck Surg. 1994;110:146–55.
28. Silverstein H, Rosenberg P, Flanzer J. An algorithm for the management of acoustic neuromas regarding age, hearing, tumor size and symptoms. Otolaryngol Head Neck Surg. 1993;108:1–10.
29. Shelton C, Alavi S, Li J, Hitselberger W. Modified retrosigmoid approach: use for selected acoustic tumor removal. Am J Otol. 1995;16:664–8.
30. Colleaux B, Chays A, Dubreuil C, Magnan J, Boulud B. Neurinome de l'acoustique et conservation de l'audition par voie retrosigmoide. JF ORL 1994;43:101–5.
31. Arriaga M, Chen D, Fukushima T. Individualizing hearing preservation in acoustic neuroma surgery. Laryngoscope. 1997;107:1043–8.
32. Hetch C, Honrubia V, Wiet R, Sims S. Hearing preservation after acoustic neuroma resection with tumor size used as clinical prognosticator. Laryngoscope. 1997;107:1122–6.
33. Moffat D, De Cruz M, Baguley D. Hearing preservation in solitary vestibular schwannoma surgery using retrosigmoid approach. Otolaryngol Head Neck Surg. 1999;121:781–8.
34. Bruzzo M, Broder L, Chays A, Magnan J. Nos résultats actuels de la chirurgie du neurinome de l'acoustique. Ann d'Otolaryngol (Paris). 2000;117:110–7.
35. Bruzzo M, Broder L, Laurent, El Garem H, Chays A, Magnan J. Retrosigmoid for hearing preservation in unselected patients with small and medium acoustic neuroma. In: Sanna M (Ed.). Acoustic neurinoma and other CPA tumors. Roma: Monduzzi edit.; 2000; 629–35.
36. Jaisinghani V, Levine S, Nussbaum E, et al. Hearing preservation after acoustic neuroma surgery. Skull Base Surg. 2000;10:141–7.
37. Holsinger C, Coker N, Jenkins H. Hearing preservation in conservation surgery for vestibular schwannoma. Am J Otol. 2000;21:695–700.
38. Schessel D, Nedzelski J, Kand E, Rowed D. Recurrence rate of acoustic neuroma in hearing preservation surgery. Am J Otol. 1992;13:231–4.
39. Mazzoni A, Calabrese V, Moschini L. Residual and recurrent: acoustic neuroma in hearing: preservation procedures: neuroradiologic and surgical findings. Skull Base Surg. 1996;6:105–12.
40. Magnan J, Chays A, Lepetre C, Pencroffi E, Locatelli P. Surgical perspectives of endoscopy of the cerebellopontine angle. Am J Otol. 1994;15:366–70.
41. Miyazaki H, Deveze A, Magnan J. Neuro-otologic surgery through minimally invasive retrosigmoid approach. Endoscope-assisted microvascular decompression, vestibular neurotomy, and tumor removal. Laryngoscope. 2005;115(9);1612–7.
42. Zini C, Magnan J, Piazza F, Chays A, Passanisi E, Girard N. New radio-surgical classification of acoustic neuromas. In: Sanna M (Ed.). Acoustic neurinoma and other cpa tumors. Roma: Monduzzi edit.; 2000; 117–20.
43. Tos M, Thomsen J. Acoustic neuroma. Amsterdam: Kugler Publications; 1992.
44. Sasaki T. Acoustic neuroma. Tokyo: Igaku-Shoin; 2009.
45. Nakatomi H, Miyazaki H, Tanaka M, Kin T, Yoshino M, Oyama H, Usui M, Sano H, Okada M, Moriyama H, Kaga K, Saito N. Visualizing, tracking neural function with continuous direct brainstem evoked potentials and

discriminating reversible injury by intraoperative extended recuperating treatment improved functional preservation in acoustic neuroma surgery (Submitted to J Neurosurg).

46. Miyazaki H, Nakatomi H. Developing of the new intraoperative cochlear monitoring and hearing preservation surgery for acoustic neuroma: keyhole retrosigmoid approach and extended retrosigmoid approach. Kyosai-ihou, Jpn. 2011;60(2):196–8.
47. Tran Ba Huy P, Lot G, Herman P. La dissection aquatique du nerf facial dans la chirurgie du neurinome de l'acoustique. À propos de 212 cas. Ann Otolaryngol Chir Cervicofac. 1998;115:42–4.
48. Domb G, Chole R. Anatomical studies of the posterior petrous apex with regard to hearing preservation in acoustic neuroma removal. Laryngoscope. 1980;90: 1769–76.
49. Kartusch J, Telian S, Graham M, Kennink J. Anatomic basis for labyrinthine preservation during posterior fossa acoustic tumor surgery. Laryngoscope. 1986;96:1024–8.
50. Roland P, Meyerhoff W, Wright C, Michey B. Anatomic considerations in the posterior approach to the internal auditory canal. Ann Otol Rhinol Laryngol. 1988;97:621–5.
51. Smouha E, Inouye M. Partial labyrinthectomy with hearing preservation: frequency-specific data using tone-burst auditory brainstem response. Otolaryngol Head Neck Surg. 1999;120:146.
52. Magnan J. Surgical classification and predictive factors in acoustic neuromas. In acoustic neuroma: consensus on systems for reporting results series: Keio University International Symposia for Life Sciences and Medicine. Kanzaki J, Tos M, Sanna M, Moffat D, Kunihiro T, Inoue Y (Eds). Springer Japan. 2003;10:39-43.

Auditory Brainstem Implants

8

INTRODUCTION

The ideal goal in the management of acoustic neuroma (AN) patients should be early detection and hearing preservation surgery. However, lack of residual hearing is a common sequelae after removal of acoustic neuroma, not only in transmastoid approaches but also in substantial portion of hearing preservation procedures, especially for larger tumors and patients with neurofibromatosis type 2 (NF2). When this happens in patients with bilateral acoustic tumors as in NF2, it leaves the patients without any means for auditory verbal communication. The auditory brainstem implant (ABI) was developed after the success of cochlear implant technology to address the problem of these profoundly deaf individuals who do not have residual functional cochlear nerves and so are not suitable for cochlear implants (CIs). The implant bypasses the cochlear nerve and stimulates the auditory pathway through the cochlear nucleus.

To better understand the probable mode of action and the outcomes of ABI, it is necessary to understand the evolution and mechanism of action of the cochlear implant technology. Cochlear implantation is now an established procedure for rehabilitation of bilateral severe to profound hearing loss due to cochlear pathologies of varied etiology in both prelingual children and postlingual adults. The common end point of all these cochlear pathologies is severe damage to the hair cells of Organ of Corti with an intact functioning cochlear nerve. The implanted prosthesis stimulates the spiral ganglion cells and the functioning cochlear nerve transmits the electric signals to the central auditory pathways. The cochlear implantation is probably more effective due to anatomically accessible and highly tonotopic organization of the cochlea (with high-frequency tones at the basal end of the cochlea and low-frequency sounds at the apical end). This tonotopic information of sounds is replicable by having frequency-specific electrodes being placed at similar frequency-specific locations in cochlea. This is made possible by a microphone that picks up the sound, sound processor that converts the sound into electrical signal, transmitter that transmits this signal through the skin into the receiver coil, which then transmits it to the electrodes into the cochlea. The mechanism of course is not that simple and has involved various modifications and advances in technology to bring the cochlear implant technology at present stage. There was a perceived gap in the application of this technology in patients with malfunctioning or no cochlear nerve.

First attempts to overcome this handicap were made by House and Hitselberger as early as 1979[1] by placing a single ball electrode implant (that they called cochlear nucleus implant) to directly stimulate the cochlear nucleus in the lateral recess of the fourth ventricle after removal of acoustic neuroma in the NF2 patient. The mode of action and the principle behind the modern ABI is similar but has undergone tremendous evolution in the hardware and the sound-processing technology. However, the understanding of the central auditory pathway has till date remained elusive. Although useful auditory sensation is provided by the ABI, the results with this device usually do not match the exceptional results seen with cochlear stimulation. Because of variations in brainstem anatomy, electrode placement and stimulation patterns seen in patients with ABI, the complexity of their programming is increased significantly relative to CIs.

INDICATION AND PATIENT SELECTION

Auditory brainstem implants (ABIs) have been shown to partially restore the auditory pathway function for the majority of patients implanted. The original candidate group was patients with neurofibromatosis type 2 (NF2) who had lost their hearing as a result of bilateral vestibular schwannomas or due to the surgery to remove them. While ABIs have represented a significant advance in the management of NF2 patients, hearing rehabilitation is far from ideal. After the results of ABI in NF2 patients, newer candidate groups viable for ABI have been suggested by Colletti et al.[2-5] including bilaterally deaf postlingual adults, who are not suitable for CIs (by etiologies like meningitis with complete cochlear ossification, temporal bone fractures with cochlear nerve avulsion trauma and for treating congenitally deaf children born with bilateral severe cochlear dysplasia and cochlear nerve aplasia).

Despite limited audiological benefit with ABI, it is common to observe that most of the NF2 patients implanted with ABI preferred to use their ABI throughout the day. Though it is unusual for ABI candidates to have significant open speech, the role of ABI is to work best in conjunction with lip reading. Nevertheless, the patients with poor vision can have surprising benefits thanks to the brain plasticity.

After ascertaining the levels of expectations, the potential benefits and associated limitations, the NF2 patients are prepared for the loss of hearing that the surgery may incur and the present technological options available. The candidates receiving ABI must be managed by a multidisciplinary team including otologist, audiologist, neurologist, psychotherapist and speech therapist. The family should be educated about the limited benefit from the device and possible nonauditory stimulation of other cranial nerves in the early postoperative period and reassured that the causative electrode can be switched off after its identification. Occasionally the choice to go for cochlear implant or ABI has to be made intraoperatively, stressing the importance of high quality of intraoperative cochlear monitoring in the decision making. Hearing preservation in the intraoperative period after tumor removal is indicated by preservation of brainstem-evoked response auditory (BERA), cochlear nerve action potential (CNAP) and dorsal cochlear nucleus action potential (DNAP), and these cases are implanted with cochlear implant. Absence of hearing preservation with absence of BERA and CNAP but anatomical integrity of the cochlear nerve with positive cochlear mapping with DNAP response again represents an indication of cochlear implant. The ABI represents the unique procedure for hearing rehabilitation when there is absence of anatomical cochlear nerve integrity after acoustic tumor removal in NF2 patients with bilateral tumors.

APPLIED ANATOMY FOR THE AUDITORY BRAINSTEM IMPLANT

The surgical procedure for ABI requires a perfect understanding of the related anatomy of dorsal and ventral cochlear nuclei, the lateral recess of fourth ventricle and the foramen of Luschka. The cochlear nucleus complex, comprising of ventral and dorsal cochlear nuclei, is the optimal target site to place the electrode. The ventral cochlear nucleus is the principal nucleus for transmission of neural impulses from the eighth pair and form the main ascending route of the cochlear nerve. Neither the ventral nor the dorsal nuclei are visible during surgery and their location depends on the identification of adjacent anatomical structures. The cochlear nuclei are located on the dorsolateral aspect of the brainstem at the level of the rostral medulla. They are superficially situated on the dorsal and lateral aspects of the inferior cerebellar peduncle and form part of the floor of the lateral recess of the fourth ventricle (Fig. 8.1), which opens into the CPA through the foramen of Luschka (Figs 8.1 to 8.3). Apart

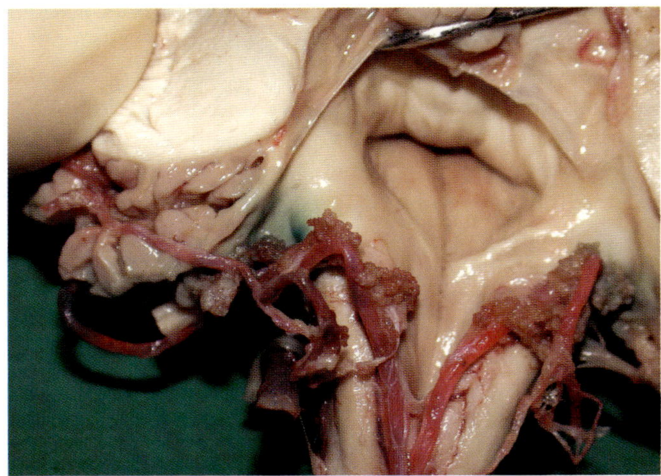

Fig. 8.1: Posterior view of the floor of fourth ventricle cavity located between the cerebellum posteriorly (removed here) and the brainstem. It is connected rostrally through the aqueduct with the third ventricle, caudally through the foramen of Magendie with the cisterna magna and laterally through the foramina of Luschka with the cerebellopontine angles. It has a roof, a floor and two lateral recesses. Most of the cranial nerves arise near its floor

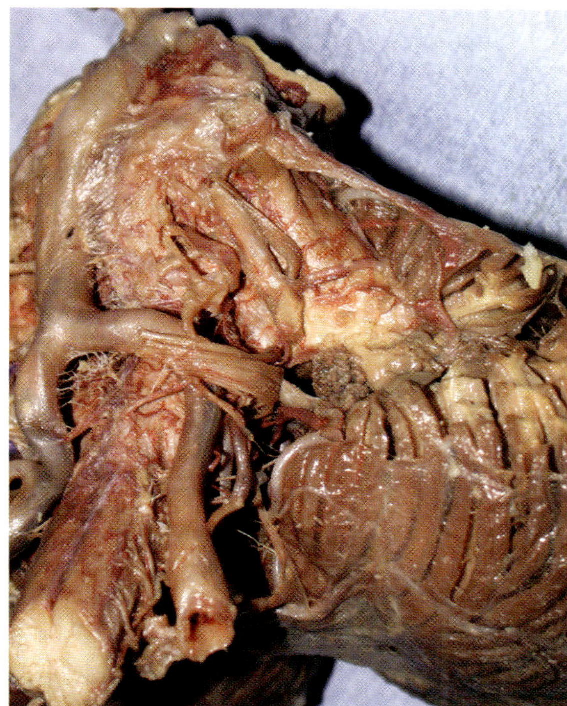

Fig. 8.2: Cadaveric specimen showing foramen of Luschka (left side) located at the lateral most part of pontomedullary junction between the brainstem entries of facial (VII), vestibulocochlear (VIII), glossopharyngeal (IX) and vagal (X) nerves. Foramen of Luschka is the lateral opening of the fourth ventricle through which the CSF formed in the ventricle by choroid plexus communicates with the subarachnoid space. Also visible are the upper spinal cord, medulla, pons and the left cerebellar hemisphere. Bilateral vertebral arteries anastomose to form the basilar artery at the pontomedullary junction. Anterior inferior cerebellar artery (AICA) is seen arising from the basilar artery and supplying the petrosal surface of the cerebellum. The posterior inferior cerebellar artery (PICA) is seen arising from the vertebral artery and supplying the occipital surface of the cerebellum

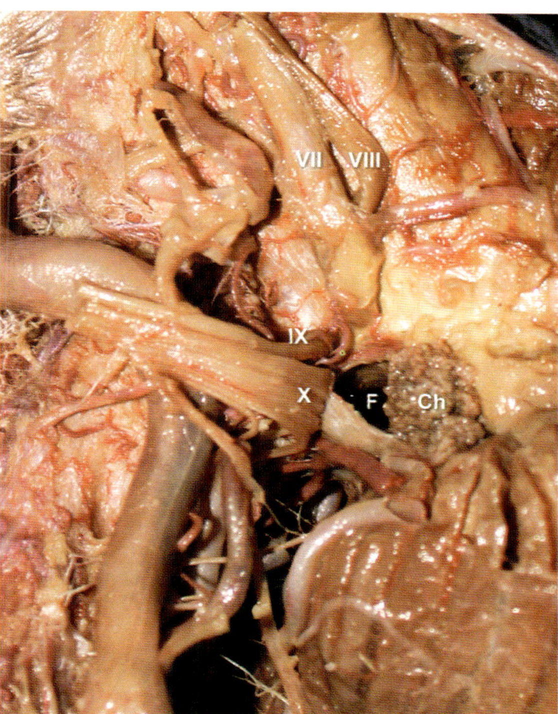

Fig. 8.3: The close-up view of foramen of Luschka (F) with choroid plexus (Ch) within it. It is closely related to the brainstem entries of facial (VII), vestibulocochlear (VIII), glossopharyngeal (IX) and vagal (X) nerves. The topographical anatomy of foramen of Luschka has recently gained more importance as it is the site of placement of auditory brainstem implant.

from cochlear nuclei, the floor of fourth ventricle contains sensory and motor nuclei of other cranial nerves like facial, hypoglossal, trigeminal and vagal nerve. Therefore, the precise placement of the ABI is essential to avoid side effects on adjacent cranial nerve nuclei and pathways. The ideal position for the electrode placement is completely within the lateral recess, adjacent to the dorsal nucleus and the inferior aspect of the ventral nucleus. This position results in optimal auditory stimulation and the least stimulation of adjacent cranial nerve nuclei.

Foramen of Luschka is the most important anatomical landmark for placement of the ABI over the cochlear nuclei. The view to foramen of Luschka is blocked by cerebellar flocculus. The choroid plexus marks the entrance to lateral recess (at foramen of Luschka) (Figs 8.2 to 8.8). Foramen of Luschka is located at the lateral most part of pontomedullary junction (Figs 8.2 and 8.3) just superior to the glossopharyngeal nerve root and inferior to the vestibulocochlear nerve root (Figs 8.2 to 8.8). Foramen of Luschka leads to lateral recess of fourth ventricle and the dorsal and ventral cochlear nuclei are located on the superior aspect of lateral recess. Thus, the electrode array has to be inserted through the foramen of Luschka, well within the superior aspect of lateral recess to prevent instability. Stimulation of the ventral nucleus is considered to be the primary source of auditory sensations in ABI.

SURGICAL TECHNIQUE

Preoperative Decision Making for Neurofibromatosis Type 2 Patients with Bilateral Acoustic Neuroma

The decision making in management of the acoustic neuroma in the NF2 patient (Fig. 8.9), or in the patient with AN tumor in only the hearing ear is a difficult task.

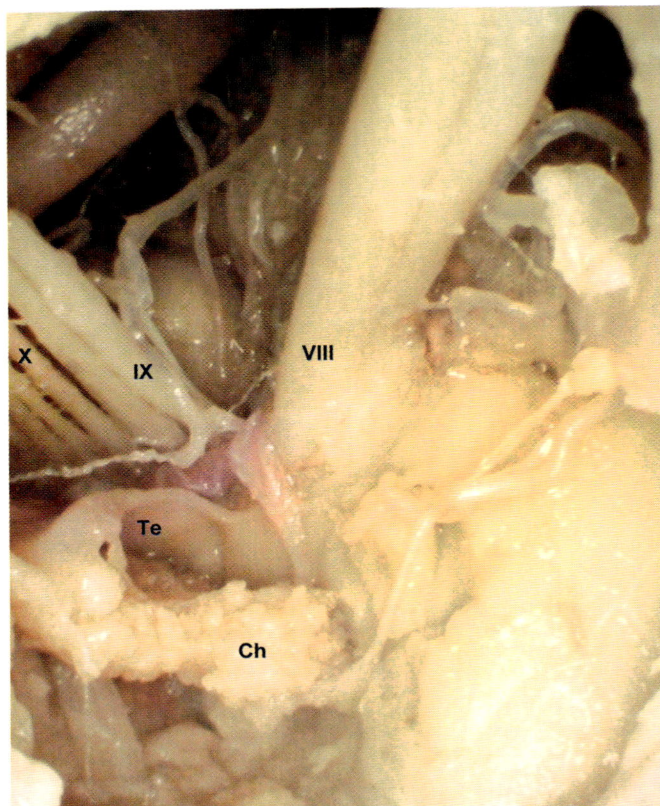

Fig. 8.4: View of left foramen of Luschka with VIIIth nerve anterosuperiorly and IXth nerve inferior to it. It is partially covered by choroid plexus (Ch). The PICA is closely related to foramen of Luschka. Te: Tenia covering the foramen of Luschka

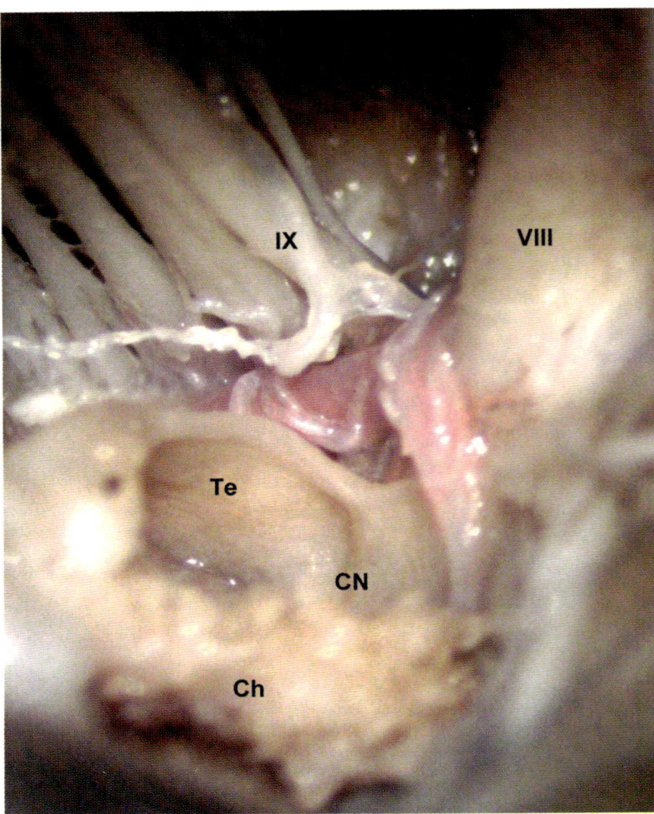

Fig. 8.5: Close-up view of foramen of Luschka with VIIIth nerve anterosuperiorly and IXth nerve inferior to it. CN: Dorsal cochlear nerve nucleus

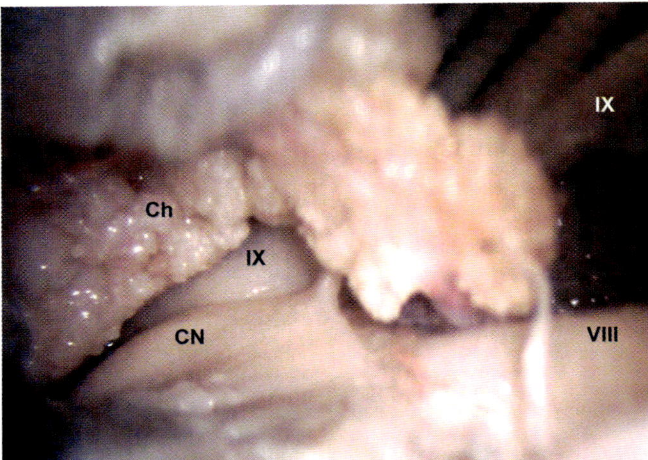

Fig. 8.6: Close-up view of foramen of Luschka leading into lateral recess with cochlear nucleus (CN) bulge visualized

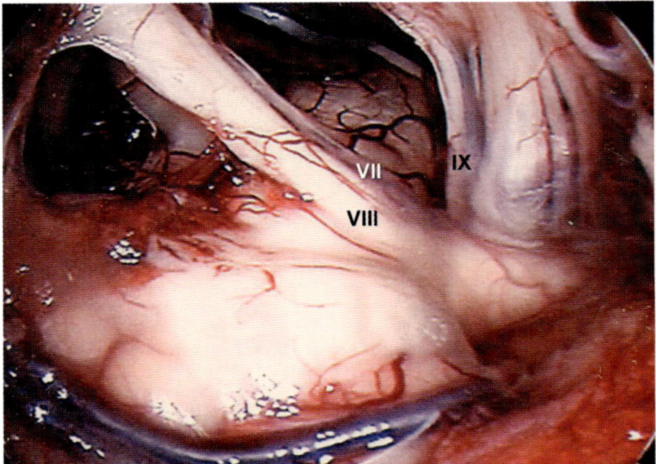

Fig. 8.7: Intraoperative endoscopic picture of right foramen of Luschka. The glossopharyngeal nerve is related just inferiorly and the vestibulocochlear nerve (VIII) forms the superior relation. The facial nerve (VII) is related anterosuperiorly

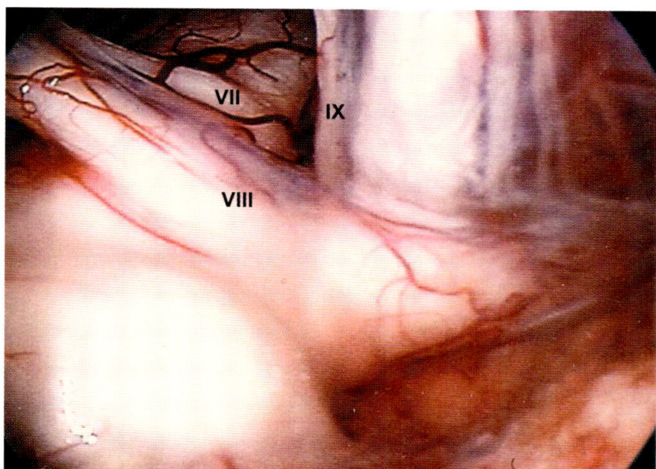

Fig. 8.8: Closer endoscopic picture of foramen of Luschka with the glossopharyngeal nerve (IX) located just inferiorly and the vestibulocochlear nerve (VIII) forms the superior relation. The facial nerve (VII) is related anterosuperiorly

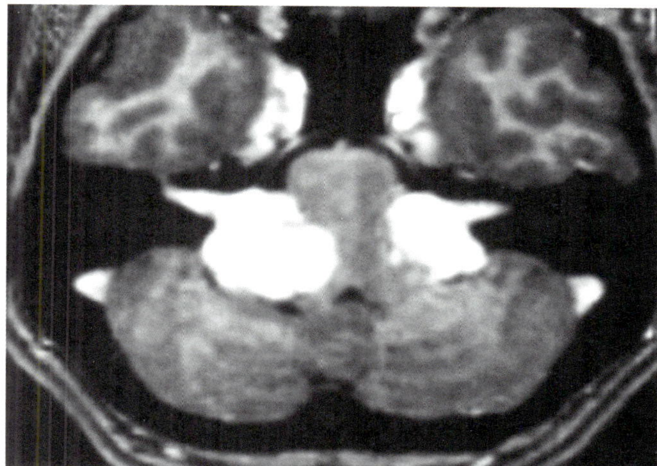

Fig. 8.9: Magnetic resonance imaging with contrast in a patient of NF2 with bilateral acoustic neuromas

The treatment for AN patients (unilateral and bilateral) is diverse, including observation, surgery and radiotherapy.[6] Treatment of the worst hearing ear in NF2 patients could leave an only hearing ear with tumor and the risk of further hearing loss. Moreover, treatment of AN in an only hearing ear can also lead to deafness. Both situations represent a therapeutic dilemma.[7] The ideal management of bilateral acoustic neuromas involves complete tumor resection with preservation of hearing in at least one ear (Fig. 8.9).

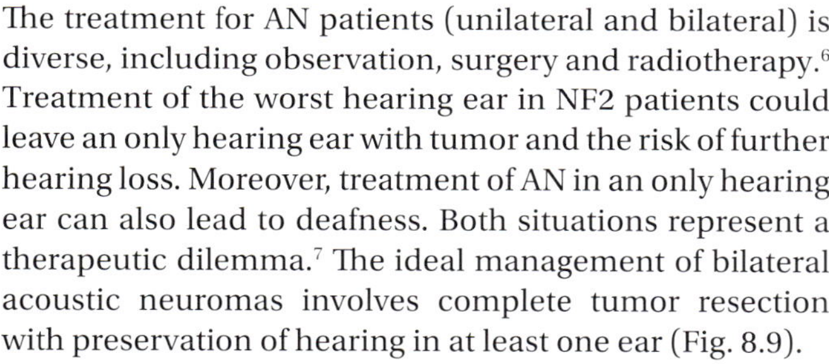

Interventional surgery should now be done at earlier ages to preserve hearing. According to us, NF2 patients with small to medium size AN with 2 cm maximal diameter, and speech discrimination scores of ≥ 50% in both ears, are good candidates for cochlear preservation surgery by retrosigmoid approach. Generally, when bilateral small growing AN is present, the more "favorable" tumor for hearing preservation is removed first. If hearing is preserved following surgery, the second AN will be carefully removed later attempting to preserve the cochlear nerve. If, however, hearing is not preserved following surgery on the first tumor, a sleeping cochlear or brainstem implant could be performed in the same stage. The unoperated ear retains preoperative level of serviceable hearing. Careful observation is then required of the nonoperated side (increase in size or impairment of audiometric tests) before decision making for the second side (Gamma Knife or surgery).

Unfortunately, the advanced size of tumors at presentation often precludes attempted hearing preservation and cochlear nerve preservation. Cochlear nerve function is not always preserved in spite of anatomic preservation of the cochlear nerve. In spite of preservation of the cochlear nerve during surgery, several patients lose hearing in the postoperative period. Although patients with NF2 are often not the candidates for cochlear implantation (CI) because of the cochlear nerve disruption or trauma, CI has given superior results to ABI when indicated. Cochlear implantation has been used in selected cases of NF2 following tumor removal[8-12] by both translabyrinthine (TL) and retrosigmoid (RS) approach, where the patient is left with bilateral profound hearing loss, but anatomical integrity of the cochlear nerve is suggested by intraoperative cochlear nerve monitoring measures. However, the decision for successful cochlear implantation in this setting is made if a functioning cochlear nerve after tumor removal is predicted[8-12] by intraoperative direct recording of CNAPs[13] or DNAP (as discussed in Chapter 3 "Nerve Monitoring for CPA Surgery) or after promontory stimulation following labyrinthectomy.[14] Cochlear implantation can be done both simultaneously and sequentially after tumor removal. If neither cochlear nerve is functional (cannot be stimulated), a multichannel ABI is considered.

Approach and Tumor Removal

The ABI insertion after resection of acoustic neuroma can be performed by both translabyrinthine (TL) and retrosigmoid (RS) approaches. The retrosigmoid approach and acoustic tumor removal have been discussed in Chapter 5 on acoustic neuroma. There have been proponents for translabyrinthine[8,15] and retrosigmoid approaches for insertion of ABI after removal of tumor. We feel that the size of the tumor, hearing status of both ears

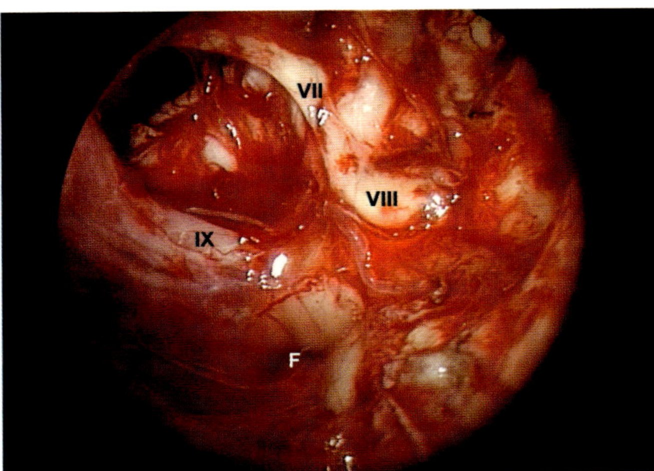

Fig. 8.10: Endoscopic view of foramen of Luschka (left side) with VIIth nerve anterosuperiorly and IXth nerve inferior to it. The cut stump of vestibulocochlear nerve after acoustic neuroma surgery can be appreciated superiorly

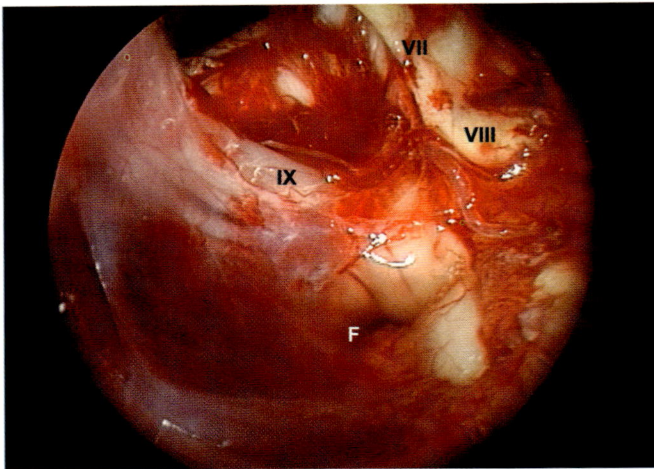

Fig. 8.11: Endoscopic view of foramen of Luschka (left side) with VIIth nerve anterosuperiorly and IXth nerve inferior to it. The cut stump of vestibulocochlear nerve after acoustic neuroma surgery can be appreciated superiorly

and presence of associated other CPA tumors are important factors in determining the decision for surgery, its time, the approach for tumor removal and consideration of nonsurgical options like radiotherapy. Proponents of the TL approach consider this to be the most direct access route to the foramen of Luschka and suggest the advantage of being able to perform simultaneous cochlear implantation from the same approach. The disadvantage with the TL approach compared to the retrosigmoid approach is to exclude the chance to perform hearing preservation surgery in NF2 patients. Residual hearing, even if it is severe on PTA, and poor discrimination on speech audiometry have importance in the patients of NF2. These patients can be implanted by cochlear implant later, if hearing aid is not useful. However, hearing preservation in NF2 subjects is more challenging than in single AN as here the tumoral process has a tendency to infiltrate the cochlear nerve. Therefore a surgical cleavage plane between tumor and nerves may be difficult to establish. The larger tumors distort the anatomy of the lateral pontomedullary junction and can occasionally make it difficult to identify the exact location of foramen of Luschka.

Although, RS approach provides more posterior view and less lateral access than TL approach, it gives excellent visualization of the lateral recess[16-18] of the fourth ventricle, especially when using a 30° endoscope with more direct appreciation of the implant site. The main advantage of the RS approach is the unique possibility of performing real-time intraoperative monitoring by direct recording of cochlear nerve or dorsal cochlear nucleus action potentials (CNAP and DNAP), which could prove useful in the attempt at hearing preservation. Unfortunately, if the intraoperative DNAP shows a poor cochlear nerve function, decision is made for simultaneous ABI.

Endoscopic Inspection of Foramen of Luschka/Terminal Recess

After tumor excision, dissection is necessary to reach the cochlear nucleus area. The cochlear nucleus complex is the site for electrical stimulation and is positioned on the surface of the lateral recess of the fourth ventricle. The ventral cochlear nucleus is the main target for stimulation by the electrode array. This nucleus lies superiorly along the anterior surface of the lateral part of the lateral recess. The lateral recess is defined by the VIIIth cranial nerve, the root of which forms its superior wall, and by the IXth cranial nerve, which exits the brain along its inferior edge. At the end of tumor removal, the surgeon must locate the foramen of Luschka as a guide to lateral recess. After tumor removal by TL approach, microscopic and endoscopic assessment of the lateral pontomedullary junction is carried out to confirm the position of foramen of Luschka based on anatomical landmarks (Figs 8.10 and 8.11). In an undistorted brainstem, this is usually not difficult; however, brainstem distortion from tumor, previous surgery, or previous stereotactic radiosurgery can present challenges. The foramen is in a cleft between the VIIIth cranial nerve above, and the rootlets of the IXth and Xth nerves below. Usually, the choroid plexus,

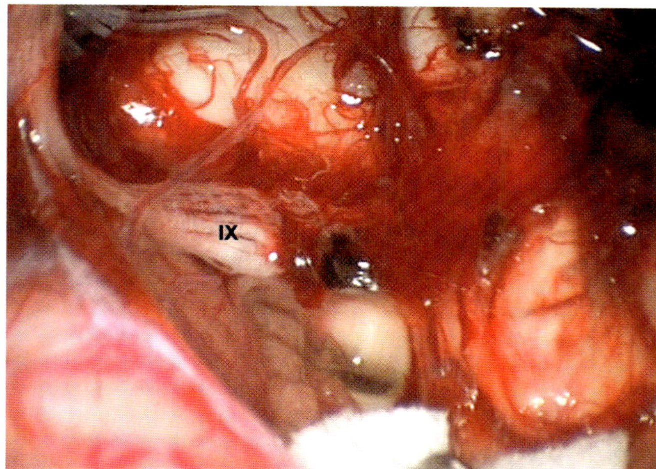

Fig. 8.12: Endoscopic view of foramen of Luschka through retrosigmoid approach with VIIth nerve anterosuperiorly and IXth nerve inferior to it. The choroid plexus can be seen on the posterior border of foramen of Luschka and entering into lateral recess

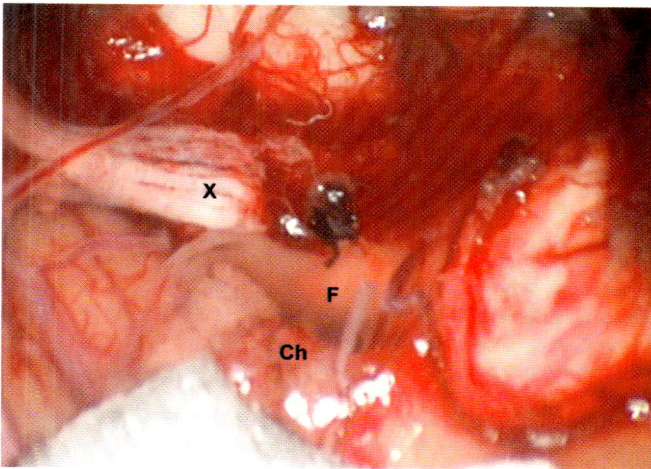

Fig. 8.13: Endoscopic view of foramen of Luschka through retrosigmoid approach with VIIth nerve anterosuperiorly (covered with blood in this picture) and IXth nerve inferior to it. The choroid plexus can be seen on the posterior border of foramen of Luschka and entering into lateral recess

which comes out of the foramen of Luschka, is the most important landmark for identifying the cochlear nucleus area. Any remaining cochlear nerve stump can be followed caudally to the glossopharyngeal nerve, which is followed cranially to where the choroid plexus usually will be found emerging from the foramen between the nerves.

When viewed from the RS approach, the entry of the cochlear nerve into the brainstem is usually obscured by the cerebellar flocculus and covered by the choroid plexus, which fills the lateral recess of the fourth ventricle and protrudes from the foramen of Luschka. However, when the VIIIth cranial nerve has been cut during AN removal, it may be difficult to identify the proximal stump. In this case, the flocculus must be retracted in a posterosuperior direction to reveal the proximal portion of the VIIIth nerve entering the lateral recess. Here, the nerve may be adherent with the surface of the pons and difficult to delineate. In this case, the choroid plexus protruding from the foramen of Luschka in the subarachnoid space constitutes an important landmark. The identification of the opening of Foramen of Luschka is often difficult in distorted tumor anatomy and the use of 30°-angled endoscope allows visualizing and confirming the position of lateral recess opening (Figs 8.12 and 8.13). Opening of the lateral recess may be confirmed by the outflow of cerebrospinal fluid. The anesthetist is asked sometimes to raise the intracranial pressure by performing modified Valsalva maneuver that can increase cerebrospinal fluid flow temporarily through the foramen of Luschka and can assist identification.

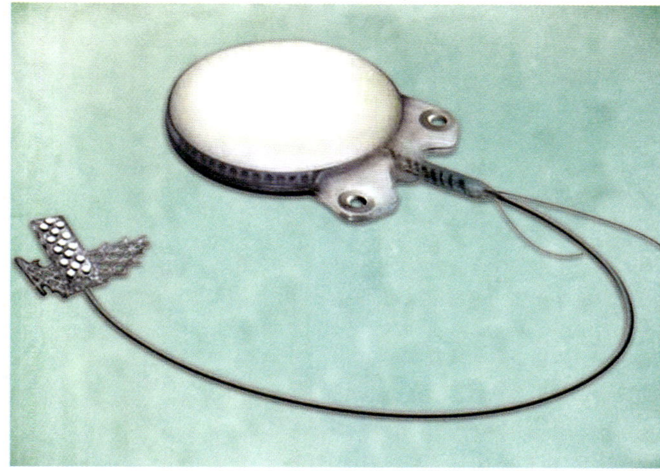

Fig. 8.14: Neurelec Digisonic SP auditory brainstem implant

Auditory Brainstem Implant

The Digisonic SP ABI (Fig. 8.14) is a transcutaneous implant that functions with an externally worn device and an implanted internal component. The external part of device consists of a behind the ear external processor (DIGI SP/SAPHYR SP) or microcontour remote battery (DIGI SPK) and a transmitter with a magnet. An internal device consists of receiver stimulator and the electrode array with ground electrode. The receiver stimulator unit is fixed by two self-tapping screws to the skull bone and is placed in a pocket created under the temporalis

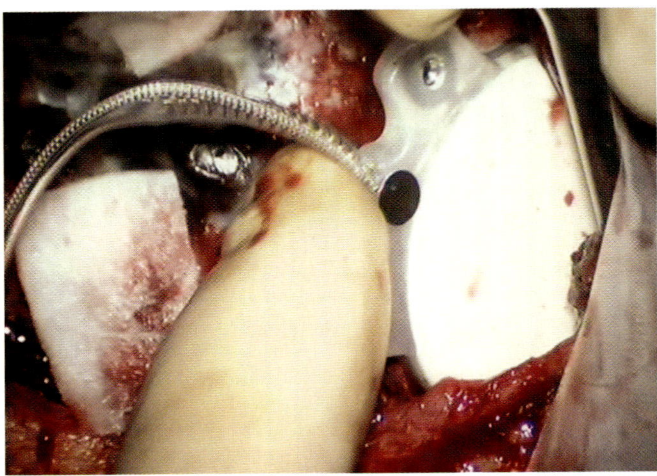

Fig. 8.15: Neurelec Digisonic SP ABI's ceramic body internal receiver slides under the pocket created under temporalis muscle in contact to the skull bone and needs to be fixed by two self-tapping screws

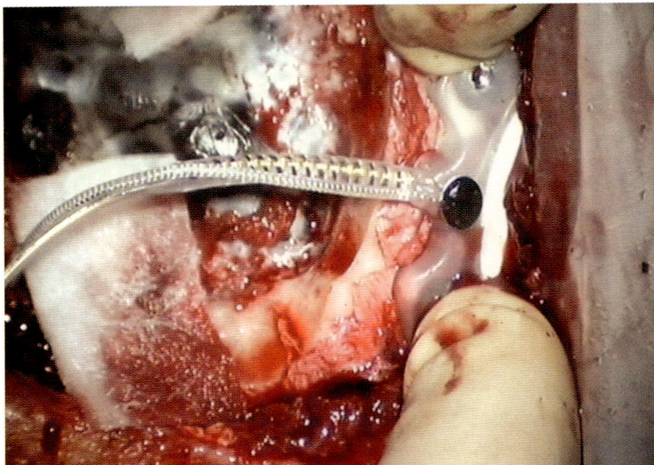

Fig. 8.16: Neurelec Digisonic SP ABI's internal receiver has been completely placed under the pocket created under temporalis muscle in contact to the skull bone

muscle. The external antenna and the receiver stimulator each contain a magnet and the external antenna is thus kept in place opposite the implanted device by magnetic attraction due to the permanent magnet within the implant. Sound received by the microphone is transduced into electrical signals that are further processed by the external speech processor and forwarded to the transmitting coil. The encoded signals are then delivered to the implanted receiver stimulator by radio-frequency electromagnetic induction. This signal is reconverted to an electrical signal, which is then delivered to the implanted electrode array to the cochlear nucleus complex. The electrode array (7.8 mm length, 3 mm wide) consists of a network of 15 electrodes and a polyester strip placed opposite the cochlear nuclei. Each electrode stimulates a different area of the cochlear nuclei, which corresponds to a frequency band of the sound signal processed by the external processor. Magnetic resonance imaging (MRI) examination in intense magnetic field is contraindicated. However, it is possible to perform an MRI at 1.5 T.

Preparation of Implant Bed for Receiver Unit

Once the position of the foramen is confirmed, the internal receiver of the ABI has to be secured by sliding in the pocket created under temporalis muscle in contact to the skull bone (Figs 8.15 and 8.16). Usually the skin and subcutaneous incision is extended in the superior part minimally and the periosteum under the temporalis muscle is elevated by the periosteal elevator. In nucleus or Medel ABI, one needs to drill the skull to make the receiver bed. Using Digisonic ABI (Neurelec Corporation), the ceramic body internal receiver device is very thin and can be fixed to the skull with two abutment screws (Fig. 8.17) to prevent it from displacement. This saves time and efforts within an already delicate surgical procedure. The implant is fixed to the skull bone and the ground electrode is placed under the temporalis muscle.

Auditory Brainstem Implant Array Insertion

The electrode of the Digisonic ABI has 15 channels (Fig. 8.18) and is secured till the location of lateral recess is confirmed. The implant array is then inserted by sliding the flat surface with electrode channels along the line of the cochlear nerve remnant along the anterior margin of foramen of Luschka facing toward the superior part of lateral recess of the fourth ventricle, with the electrodes pointing cranially to make contact with the cochlear nucleus (Figs 8.19 to 8.21). The Dacron mesh and a plug of soft tissue in the lateral recess provide stability to the electrode array and secure its positioning.

This insertion of the electrode array through the foramen of Luschka to the superior part of lateral recess of fourth ventricle is carried out under microscopic vision and is confirmed later with endoscope (Fig. 8.22) and nerve telemetry.

Confirmation of Position of Implant by Nerve Monitoring

Electrophysiological measures are then made intraoperatively to check that the electrode array is in the correct position. The electrically evoked auditory brainstem

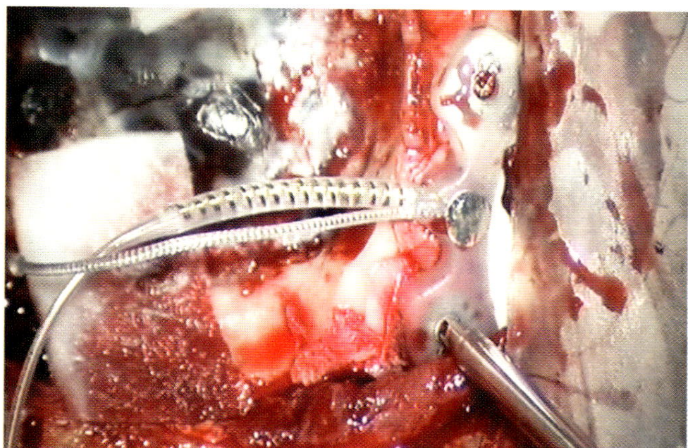

Fig. 8.17: Neurelec Digisonic SP ABI's ceramic body internal receiver is fixed by two abutment screws and there is no need to drill out the skull bone to create receiver bed

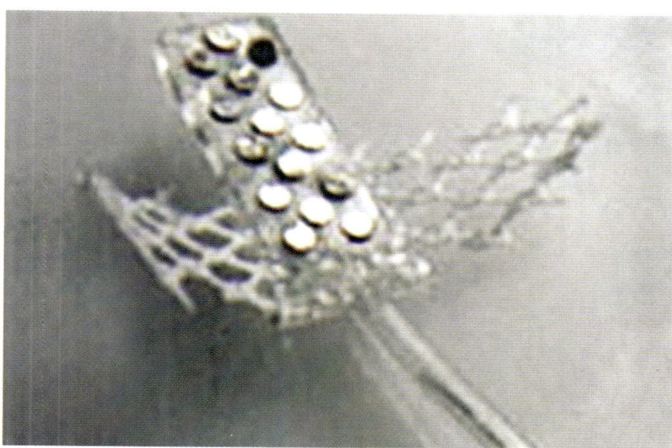

Fig. 8.18: The electrode array consists of a network of 15 electrodes and a polyester strip with dimensions of 7.8 mm by 3 mm to be placed opposite the cochlear nuclei

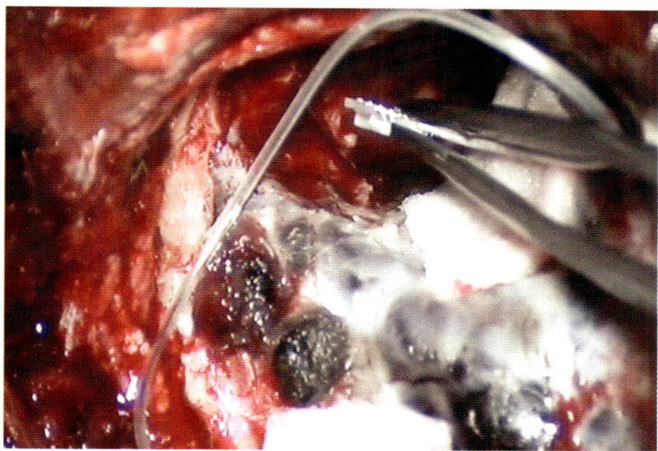

Fig. 8.19: After securing the internal receiver and ground electrode, the electrode array is ready to be inserted

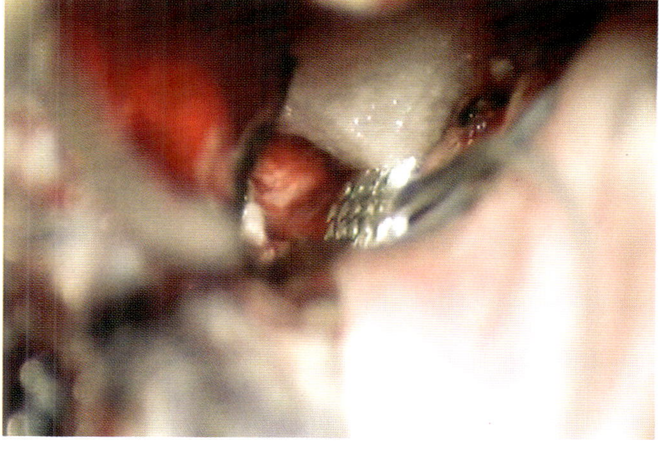

Fig. 8.20: The electrode array is placed close to foramen of Luschka before confirming the final position for insertion by endoscope

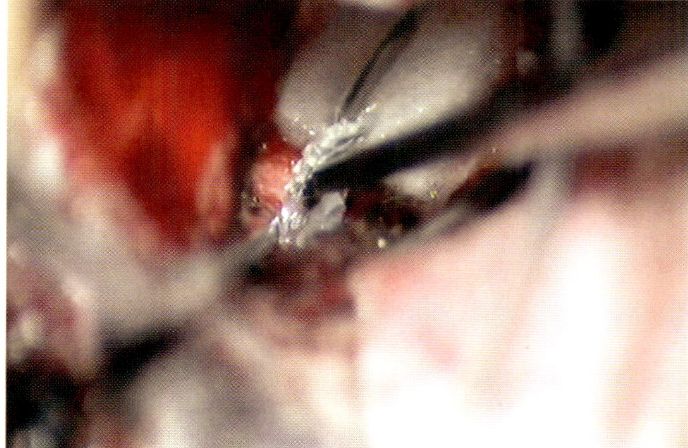

Fig. 8.21: After confirming the position of foramen of Luschka, the electrode array is inserted into lateral recess through foramen of Luschka under microscopic vision

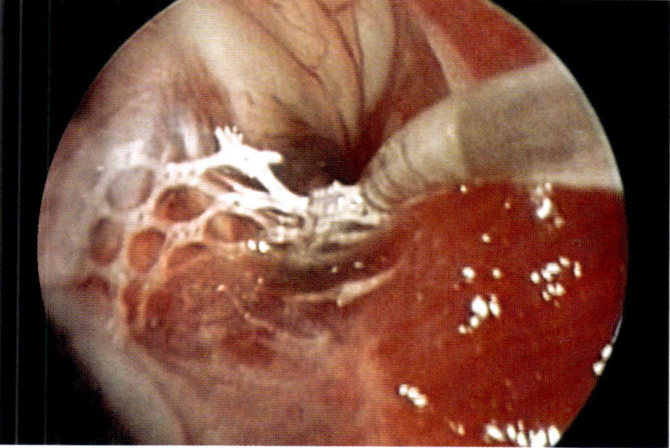

Fig. 8.22: The electrode array is inserted into lateral recess through foramen of Luschka and its position confirmed under endoscopic vision

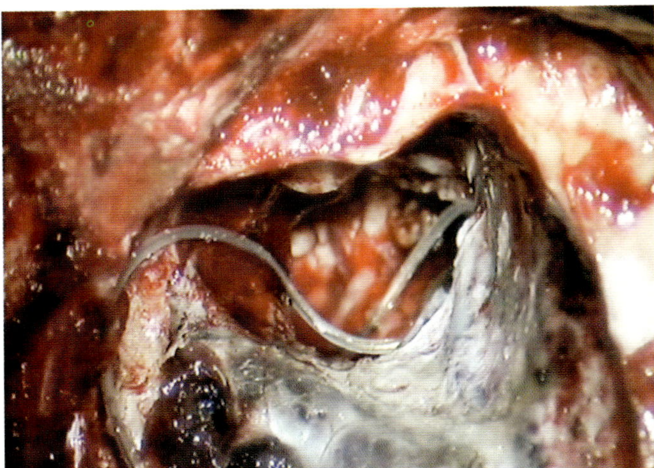

Fig. 8.23: Final picture after placement of ABI through translabyrinthine approach

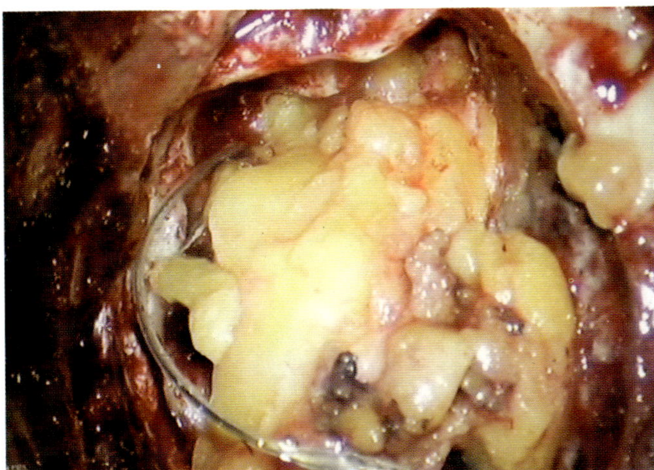

Fig. 8.24: Obliteration of the dural defect and the CPA after translabyrinthine approach with strips of abdominal fat

response (EABR) is recorded by stimulating the device through the external signal processor. Needle electrodes in the facial muscles, the soft palate and the sternomastoid muscle are connected to a multichannel cranial nerve electromyograph (EMG) monitor. A robust and reproducible EABR with no nonauditory responses from the EMG and no gross changes in vital signs on stimulation of electrodes indicates that the ABI is correctly positioned. Poor EABR quality or unwanted cranial nerve activity indicates that repositioning of the ABI may be necessary. Usually, some electrode combinations give a good EABR while others fail to give any response. The implant audiologist attempts to create a map of the responsive parts of the array, which may be useful for activating the implant postoperatively.

Final Evaluation

Once the electrode array is inserted and the position of implant confirmed by endoscopy and electrophysiological evaluation, hemostasis is reconfirmed in the CPA (Fig. 8.23) and the wound closed carefully with abdominal fat (Fig. 8.24) to prevent the high risk of meningocele or cerebrospinal fluid (CSF) leak.

AUDITORY BRAINSTEM IMPLANT FOR CONGENITALLY DEAF CHILDREN WITH BILATERAL COCHLEAR NERVE APLASIA

Though rare, bilateral cochlear nerve aplasia is being diagnosed more frequently due to thorough assessment of all the prelingually deaf patients with audiological and radiological assessment. Bilateral cochlear nerve aplasia is frequently associated with multiple other congenital anomalies (Fig. 8.25) and auditory deprivation significantly alters the rehabilitation of these children. The HRCT temporal bone along with MRI of inner ear and internal auditory meatus (IAM) can reliably predict the cochlear anomalies with presence/absence of cochlear nerve (Figs 8.26 to 8.28). The ABI is inserted through retrosigmoid approach as discussed in ABI for NF2 patients.

Device Activation and Programming

Initial stimulation using the ABI is performed 6–8 weeks after implantation. Owing to the possibility of eliciting changes in vital signs, initial stimulation is always performed with emergency medical assistance readily available. Initial stimulation tasks include setting of threshold and comfort levels, evaluation and management of nonauditory stimulation. Data are collected regarding the sound quality of auditory response, including level and pitch, and of nonauditory sensations. To minimize nonauditory responses while maintaining sound quality, stimulation parameters can be adjusted. Occasionally, it is necessary to deactivate individual electrodes because of annoying nonauditory responses.

Electrodes that elicit auditory responses are next pitch scaled. Variations in individual anatomy and electrode array positioning ensure that this process is generally not straightforward and requires significant time. The overall goal is to define a set of electrodes that represent a range of perceived pitches. At initial stimulation, patients are generally dissatisfied with the quality of their auditory sensation. However, they can be assured that with time and experience using the ABI, sound quality can be expected

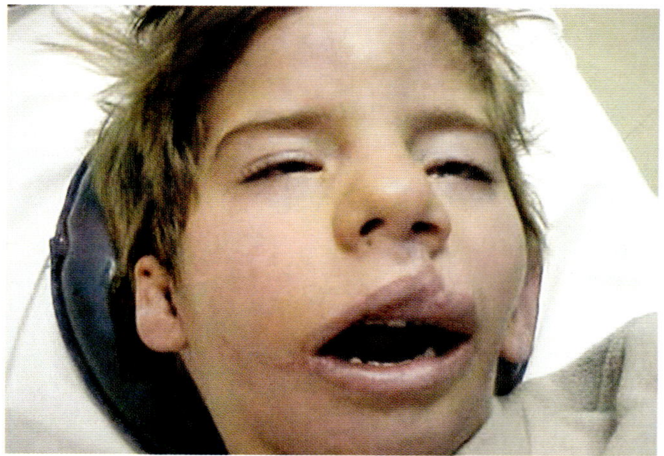

Fig. 8.25: A six-year child with CHARGE syndrome (coloboma of eye, heart defects, atresia of nasal choanae, retardation of growth, genital and/or urinary abnormalities, ear abnormalities and deafness) with bilateral cochlear nerve aplasia

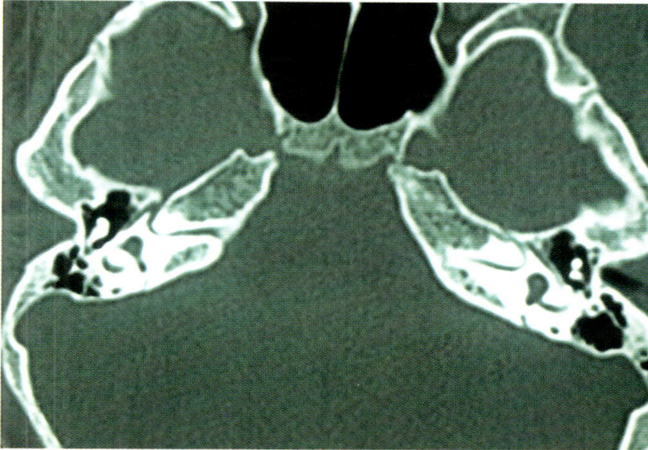

Fig. 8.26: Axial CT scan of temporal bone showing cochlea aplasia with only facial nerve in the IAM

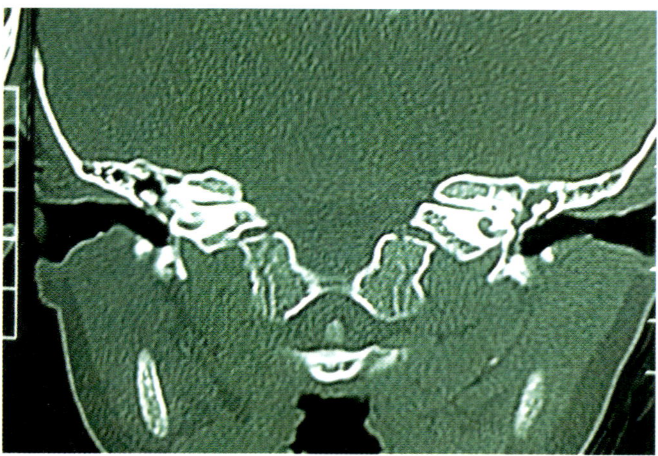

Fig. 8.27: Coronal CT scan of temporal bone showing cochlea aplasia with only facial nerve in the IAM

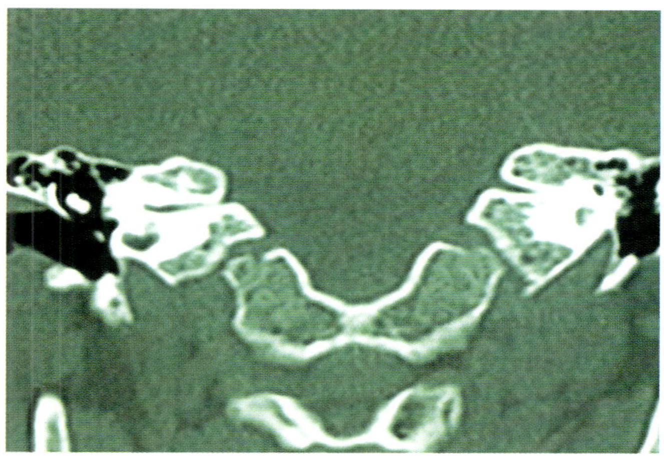

Fig. 8.28: Coronal CT scan of temporal bone showing cochlea aplasia with only facial nerve in the IAM

to improve, and any remaining nonauditory stimulation can be expected to ease generally.

Complications

The most common complications related to ABI surgery include CSF leak, electrode migration and nonauditory side effects. The CSF leak occurs usually along the electrode lead, from the subarachnoid space to the subcutaneous plane. These leaks are managed by pressure dressing, head elevation, bed rest and occasionally lumbar puncture and drainage. Rarely, revision surgery and exploration are necessary for control of the leak.

Migration of the electrode may occur as a result of unstable placement in lateral recess. Migration could be medial in the fourth ventricle secondary to the repositioning of the neural structures around the rigid electrode array or lateral in the cerebellopontine angle when the electrode was in fact only at the entrance of the foramen of Luschka and not well inserted in it. In both such situations, the implant will give no response. Electrode position may be confirmed on computed tomography (CT) scan (Fig. 8.30) and plain X-ray skull lateral view (Fig. 8.31).

Nonauditory side effects are relatively common after ABI activation. In patients with glossopharyngeal nerve stimulation owing to migration of the electrode in the lower part of the recess, symptoms of a sense of tingling or constriction in the throat appear. High electrode placement or migration causes facial twitching due to

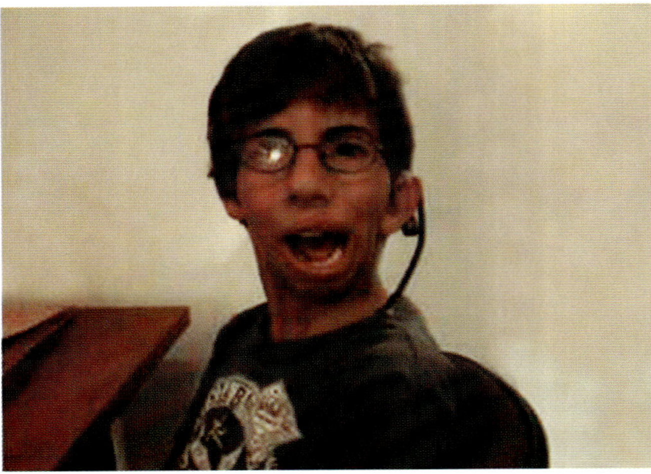

Fig. 8.29: Postoperative picture after 5 years of ABI

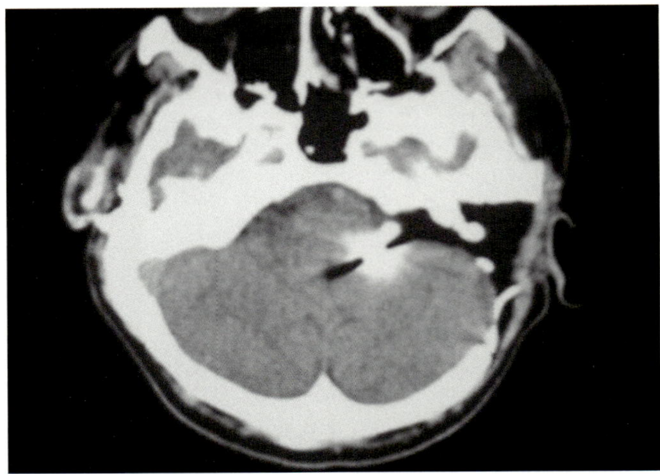

Fig. 8.30: Computed tomography scan picture showing ABI in lateral recess

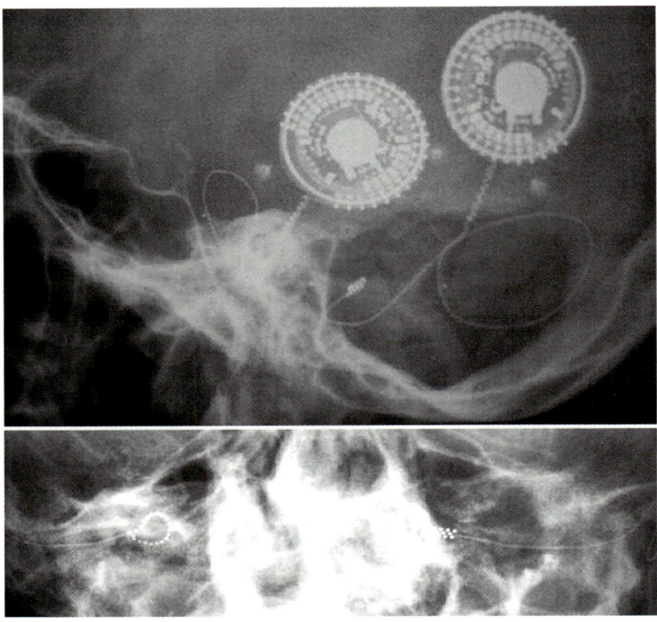

Fig. 8.31: X-ray skull lateral and anterior view in a patient with right cochlear and left brainstem implant

stimulation of the facial nerve or nucleus. Some patients complain of dizziness or tingling sensation in the arms or legs that may be due to stimulation of flocculus. Nonauditory side effects in the ABI generally occur with stimulation of the more medial or lateral electrodes. They can usually be reduced by switching reference electrodes or turning off the electrode. The severity of the nonauditory sensations often decreases over time, sometimes allowing for reactivation of electrodes previously turned off.

Results

The ABI was designed to restore hearing in patients with nonfunctional cochlear nerves in NF2 patients who were not candidates for cochlear implantation. Although ABI provides environmental sound and significant lip reading assistance, they have not reached consistent results in speech discrimination.[19-27] Notably, the group of patients implanted in the absence of acoustic neuromas has shown significantly greater auditory benefit than those with these tumors in the study by Colletti et al.[19] Although the reason for this difference between tumor and nontumor patients is unknown, hypotheses include subclinical brainstem injury related to tumor growth or resection and intrinsic maldevelopment of the cochlear nucleus related to the NF2 mutation. In the House Research Institute review on ABI, 85% of patients perceived auditory sensation.[20] Combined with lip reading cues, 93% of patients improved sentence understanding in 3–6 months. Most patients had environmental sound awareness and understanding of closed set words, consonants and vowels, while open set speech discrimination was difficult to achieve. In contrast, Lenarz et al.[21] reported better results with 2 out of 11 patients achieving some kind of telephone conversation. In general, open set speech recognition in the auditory mode alone is not common among patients implanted with ABI as reported by Sanna.[26,27]

Our experience on Digisonic ABI procedure is based on eight adults (seven NF2 patients and one nonNF2 patient) and four children with well-documented cochlear nerve aplasia (made in collaboration with Prof. Economides from Athens for three cases and with Dr Khashaba from Cairo for one case).

Table 8.1: Results of ABI in pediatric patients with cochlear nerve aplasia

S. No.	Age/Sex	Implantation Year	Associated Handicap	Perception	Discrimination	Language
1.	6 years/male	2005	Charge syndrome	Environment sounds, voices of family	Simple words	Short sentences
2.	5 years/male	2007	Cleft lip	Environment sounds, voices of family	All vowels, no consonants	A few words two syllables
3.	5 years/female	2007	Fallot tetralogy, esophageal and anal atresia	None	None	None
4.	6 years/female	2010	No handicap	Environment sound	Start a few words discrimination	None

Four children (two boys and two girls) with bilateral cochlear nerve aplasia were each 5 and 6 years old at the time of the surgery (Figs 8.26 to 8.29). After five years of follow-up, one child (Fig. 8.30) obtained sentence recognition, two children with less follow-up had only words recognition and one unfortunately never had no auditory response raising the question of perhaps cochlear nuclei aplasia (Table 8.1) Out of eight adults, two patients successfully utilize unilateral auditory brainstem implant with a contralateral cochlear implant revealing an improvement of their quality of life with activation of ABI.[25]

CONCLUSION

Early surgical intervention with preservation of the cochlear nerve function should be considered. Restoration of hearing using ABIs in NF2 patients is a safe and promising procedure for those who would otherwise be totally deaf. The ABI provides useful auditory sensations in most deaf NF2 patients and improves ability to communicate compared with "lip reading only." Auditory brainstem implant allows detection and recognition of many environmental sounds and can even offer significant ability to understand speech using only sound from the ABI. In rare cases excellent benefit with good speech discrimination and telephone use may be achieved. Surgical resection of NF2 tumor can be carried out through either TL or RS approach and does not affect speech test outcomes. Cochlear implantation in selected patients with NF2 and patients with vestibular schwannoma in the only hearing ear is a reasonable hearing rehabilitation option.

REFERENCES

1. Hitselberger WE, House WF, Edgerton BJ, et al. Cochlear nucleus implants. Otolaryngol Head Neck Surg.1984;92:52–4.
2. Colletti V, Carner M, Miorelli V, Colletti L, Guida M, Fiorino F. Auditory brainstem implant in posttraumatic cochlear nerve avulsion. Audiol Neurootol. 2004;9(4):247–55.
3. Colletti V, Carner M, Miorelli V, Guida M, Colletti L, Fiorino F. Auditory brainstem implant (ABI): new frontiers in adults and children. Otolaryngol Head Neck Surg. 2005;133(1):126–38.
4. Colletti V, Carner M, Fiorino F, Sacchetto L, Miorelli V, Orsi A, Cilurzo F, Pacini L. Hearing restoration with auditory brainstem implant in three children with cochlear nerve aplasia. Otol Neurotol. 2002;23(5):682–93.
5. Sennaroglu L, Colletti V, Manrique M, et al. Auditory brainstem implantation in children and non-neurofibromatosis type 2 patients - a consensus statement. Otol Neurotol. 2011;32(2):187–91.
6. Slattery W, Fisher L. Neurofibromatosis type 2. In: Jackler R, Brackman D (Eds.). Neurotology. USA: Elsevier; 2005:783–91.
7. Driscoll C, Jackler R, Pitts L, Brackmann D. Lesions of the internal auditory canal and cerebellopontine angle in an only hearing ear: is surgery ever advisable? Am J Otol. 2000;21(4):573–81.
8. Arriaga MA, Marks S. Simultaneous cochlear implantation and acoustic neuroma resection: imaging considerations, technique, and functional outcome. Otolaryngol Head Neck Surg. 1995;112:325–8.
9. Lustig LR, Yeagle J, Driscoll CL, et al. Cochlear implantation in patients with neurofibromatosis type 2 and bilateral vestibular schwannoma. Otol Neurotol. 2006;27:512–8.

10. Ahsan S, Telischi F, Hodges A, Balkany T. Cochlear implantation concurrent with translabyrinthine acoustic neuroma resection. Laryngoscope. 2003;113:472–4.
11. Neff BA, Wiet RM, Lasak JM, et al. Cochlear implantation in the neurofibromatosis type 2 patient: long-term follow-up. Laryngoscope. 2007;117:1069–72.
12. Vincenti V, Pasanisi E, Guida M, Di Trapani G, Sanna M. Hearing rehabilitation in neurofibromatosis type 2 patients: cochlear versus auditory brainstem implantation. Audiol Neurootol. 2008;13:273–80.
13. Piccirillo E, Guida M, Flanagan S, Lauda L, Fois P, Sanna M. CNAP to predict functional cochlear nerve preservation in NF2: cochlear implant or auditory brainstem implant. Case report. Skull Base. 2008;18(4):281–7.
14. Kartush JM, Linstrom CJ, Graham MD, Kulick KC, Bouchard KR. Promontory stimulation following labyrinthectomy: implications for cochlear implantation. Laryngoscope. 1990;100:5–9.
15. Schwartz M, Hitselberger W, Otto S, Brackmann D, Shannon R. Brainstem auditory implants. Oper Tech Otolaryngol Head Neck Surg. 2003;14(4):282–7.
16. Colletti V, Fiorino F, Carner M, Giarbini N, Sacchetto L, Cumer G. Advantages of the retrosigmoid approach in auditory brainstem implantation. Skull Base Surg. 2000;10(4):165–70.
17. Kuroki A, Moller AR. Microsurgical anatomy around the foramen of Luschka in relation to intraoperative recording of auditory evoked potentials from the cochlear nuclei. J Neurosurg. 1995;82:933–9.
18. Friedland DR, Wackym PA. Evaluation of surgical approaches to endoscopic auditory brainstem implantation. Laryngoscope. 1999;109:175–80.
19. Colletti V, Shannon R, Carner M, Veronese S, Colletti L. Outcomes in nontumor adults fitted with the auditory brainstem implant: 10 years' experience. Otol Neurotol. 2009;30(5):614–8.
20. Toh E, Luxford W. Cochlear and brainstem implantation. Neurosurg Clin North Am. 2008;19(2):317–29.
21. Lenarz M, Matthies C, Lesinski-Schiedat A, Frohne C, Rost U, Illg A, Battmer RD, Samii M, Lenarz T. Auditory brainstem implant part II: subjective assessment of functional outcome. Otol Neurotol. 2002;23:694–7.
22. Kanowitz SJ, Shapiro WH, Golfinos JG, Cohen NL, Roland JT Jr. Auditory brainstem implantation in patients with neurofibromatosis type 2. Laryngoscope. 2004;114(12):2135–46.
23. Nevison B, Laszig R, Sollmann WP, Lenarz T, Sterkers O, Ramsden R, Fraysse B, Manrique M, Rask-Andersen H, Garcia-Ibanez E, Colletti V, von Wallenberg E. Results from a European clinical investigation of the Nucleus multichannel auditory brainstem implant. Ear Hear. 2002;23:170–83.
24. Vincent C, Zini C, Gandolfi A, Triglia JM, Pellet W, Truy E, Fischer G, Maurizi M, Meglio M, Lejeune JP, Vaneecloo FM. Results of the MXM Digisonic auditory brainstem implant clinical trials in Europe. Otol Neurotol. 2002;23(1):56–60.
25. Ar S, Meller R, Cosso M, Magnan J. Cochlear implantation and contralateral auditory brainstem implantation. Otol Neurotol. 2012; 33(6):963-67.
26. Merkus P, Lella F, Trapani G, Pasanisi E, Beltrame M, Zanetti D, Negri M, Sanna M. Indications and contraindications of auditory brainstem implants: systematic review and illustrative cases. Eur Arch of OtoRhinoLaryngol. 2013;270(2).
27. Sanna M, Lella F, Guida M, Merkus P. Auditory Brainstem Implants in NF2 Patients: Results and Review of the Literature. Otol Neurotol. 2012; 33:154-64.

Index

Page numbers followed by *f* refer to figure and *t* refer to table

R

S

T

V

W

X

Z